PMHNP-BC™ Certification Practice Q&A

PMHNP-BC™ Certification Practice Q&A

SPRINGER PUBLISHING

Springer Publishing Company, LLC
11 West 42nd Street, New York, NY 10036
www.springerpub.com

Acquisitions Editor: Elizabeth Nieginski
Compositor: DiacriTech

ISBN: 9780826146168
ebook ISBN: 9780826146175
DOI: 10.1891/9780826146175

Printed by BnT

Medicine is an ever-changing science. Research and clinical experience are continually expanding our knowledge, in particular our understanding of proper treatment and drug therapy. The authors, editors, and publisher have made every effort to ensure that all information in this book is in accordance with the state of knowledge at the time of production of the book. Nevertheless, the authors, editors, and publisher are not responsible for any errors or omissions or for any consequence from application of the information in this book and make no warranty, expressed or implied, with respect to the content of this publication. Every reader should examine carefully the package inserts accompanying each drug and should carefully check whether the dosage schedules therein or the contraindications stated by the manufacturer differ from the statements made in this book. Such examination is particularly important with drugs that are either rarely used or have been newly released on the market.

Contact sales@springerpub.com to receive discount rates on bulk purchases.

Publisher's Note: **New and used products purchased from third-party sellers are not guaranteed for quality, authenticity, or access to any included digital components.**

Printed in the United States of America.

Contents

Preface

Welcome to *PMHNP-BC™ Certification Practice Q&A*! Congratulations on taking this important step on your journey to becoming a certified psychiatric-mental health nurse practitioner. This resource is based on the most recent American Nurses Credentialing Center (ANCC) exam blueprint and was developed by experienced psychiatric-mental health nurse practitioners. It is designed to help you sharpen your specialty knowledge with 350 practice questions organized by exam subject area, as well as strengthen your knowledge-application and test-taking skills with two 175-question practice tests. It also includes essential information about the Psychiatric-Mental Health Nurse Practitioner (Across the Lifespan) certification (PMHNP-BC™) exam, including eligibility requirements, exam subject areas and question distribution, and tips for successful exam preparation.

▶ PART I: PRACTICE QUESTIONS

Part I includes five chapters based on the exam blueprint: Scientific Foundation, Advanced Practice Skills, Diagnosis and Treatment, Psychotherapy and Related Theories, and Ethical and Legal Principles. Each chapter includes high-quality, exam-style questions and comprehensive answers with rationales that address both correct and incorrect answers. Part I is designed to strengthen your specialty knowledge and is formatted for ultimate studying convenience—answer the questions on each page and simply turn the page for the corresponding answers and rationales. No need to refer to the back of the book for the answers.

▶ PART II: PRACTICE TESTS

Part II includes two 175-question practice tests that align with the content domains and question distribution on the most recent PMHNP-BC™ exam blueprint. These chapters are designed to help you strengthen your knowledge-application and test-taking skills. Maximize your preparation and simulate the exam experience by setting aside 3.5 hours to complete each practice test. Comprehensive answers and rationales that address both correct and incorrect answers are located in the chapters immediately following each practice test.

We know life is busy, and being able to prepare for your exam efficiently and effectively is paramount. This resource will give you the tools and confidence you need to succeed. For additional exam preparation resources, including self-paced online courses, online QBanks, comprehensive review texts, and high-yield study guides, visit www.springerpub.com/exam prep. Best of luck to you on your certification journey!

Introduction: Certification Examination and Tips for Preparation

▶ ELIGIBILITY REQUIREMENTS

The Psychiatric-Mental Health Nurse Practitioner (Across the Lifespan) certification (PMHNP-BC™) exam is developed and administered by the American Nurses Credentialing Center (ANCC). To qualify to take the exam, you must meet the following requirements:

- A master's, post-graduate certificate, or DNP from a psychiatric-mental health nurse practitioner (PMHNP) program accredited by the Commission on Collegiate Nursing Education (CCNE), the Accreditation Commission for Education in Nursing (ACEN), or the National League for Nursing (NLN) Commission for Nursing Education Accreditation (CNEA).
- At least 500 faculty-supervised clinical hours included in the PMHNP program.
- Completion of graduate-level courses in advanced physiology/pathophysiology, advanced health assessment, and advanced pharmacology. Courses must cover health promotion, differential diagnosis, and management and treatment.
- Clinical training in at least two psychotherapeutic modalities.

Qualified applicants may submit an online application. Successful candidates will receive instructions on how to schedule their exam at a Prometric Test Center or via live remote proctoring. The exam fee is $395; however, ANCC offers discounted rates for members of select associations. Refer to the ANCC website for complete eligibility requirements, pricing and discounts, and certification information: https://www.nursingworld.org/our-certifications/psychiatric-mental-health-nurse-practitioner/.

▶ ABOUT THE EXAMINATION

The PMHNP-BC™ exam is 3.5 hours and consists of 175 multiple-choice questions with four answer options. You must select the single best answer. Only 150 questions are scored, and the remaining 25 questions are used as pretest questions. It is impossible to know which questions are scored, so be sure to answer all questions to the best of your ability.

See Table 1 for exam content domains and question distribution. For the list of skill and knowledge statements, refer to the test content outline on the ANCC website.

Table 1 PMHNP-BC™ Exam Content Domains and Question Distribution

Content Domain	% of Questions
Scientific Foundation	20%
Advanced Practice Skills	25%
Diagnosis and Treatment	25%
Psychotherapy and Related Theories	15%
Ethical and Legal Principles	15%

Source: Data from American Nurses Credentialing Center. PMHNP-BC™ Board Certification Examination Test Content Outline. 2019. https://www.nursingworld.org/~49eb43/globalassets/certification/certification-specialty-pages/resources/test-content-outlines/exam-35-pmhnp-tco-10-15-2018_for-webposting.pdf

▶ TIPS FOR EXAM PREPARATION

You know the old joke about how to get to Carnegie Hall—practice, practice, practice! The same is true when seeking certification. Practice and preparation are key to your success on exam day. Here are ten tips to help you prepare:

1. Allow at least 6 months to fully prepare for the exam. Do not rely on last-minute cramming sessions.
2. Thoroughly review the ANCC General Testing and Renewal Handbook and the Test Content Outline so that you know exactly what to expect. Pay close attention to the content domains and list of skill and knowledge statements. Identify your strengths, weaknesses, and knowledge gaps, so you know where to focus your studies. Review all of the supplementary resources available on the ANCC website, including exam references and sample questions.
3. Create a study timeline with weekly or monthly study tasks. Be as specific as possible—identify *what* you will study, *how* you will study, and *when* you will study.
4. Use several exam prep resources that provide different benefits. For example, use a comprehensive review to build your specialty knowledge, use this resource and other question banks to strengthen your knowledge-application and test-taking skills, and use a high-yield review to brush up on key concepts in the days leading up to the exam. Springer Publishing offers a wide range of print and online exam prep products to suit all of your study needs; visit https://www.springerpub.com/examprep.
5. Assess your level of knowledge and performance on practice questions and tests. Carefully consider why you may be missing certain questions. Continually analyze your strengths, weaknesses, and knowledge gaps, and adjust your study plan accordingly.
6. Minimize distraction as much as possible while you are studying. You will feel more calm, centered, and focused, which will lead to increased knowledge retention.
7. Engage in stress-reducing activities, particularly in the month leading up to the exam. Yoga, stretching, and deep-breathing exercises can be beneficial. If you are feeling frustrated or anxious while studying, take a break. Go for a walk, play with your child or pet, or finish a chore that has been weighing on you. Wait until you feel more refreshed before returning to study.

8. Focus on your health in the weeks and days before the exam. Eat balanced meals, stay hydrated, and minimize alcohol consumption. Get as much sleep as possible, particularly the night before the exam.
9. Eat a light meal before the exam but limit your liquid consumption. The clock does not stop for restroom breaks! Ensure that you know exactly where you are going and how long it will take to get there. Leave with plenty of time to spare to reduce travel-related stress and ensure that you arrive on time.
10. Remind yourself to relax and stay calm. You have prepared, and you know your stuff. Visualize the success that is just ahead of you and make it happen. When you pass, celebrate!

Pass Guarantee

If you use this resource to prepare for your exam and do not pass, you may return it for a refund of your full purchase price, excluding tax, shipping, and handling. To receive a refund, return your product along with a copy of your exam score report and original receipt showing purchase of new product (not used). Product must be returned and received within 180 days of the original purchase date. Refunds will be issued within 8 weeks from acceptance and approval. One offer per person and address. This offer is valid for U.S. residents only. Void where prohibited. To initiate a refund, please contact Customer Service at csexamprep@springerpub.com.

Part I
Practice Questions and Answers With Rationales

Scientific Foundation

1. The suprachiasmatic nucleus is located in the:

   A. Amygdala
   B. Pineal gland
   C. Hypothalamus
   D. Hippocampus

2. An 11-year-old patient with autism is brought to the clinic to be seen by the psychiatric-mental health nurse practitioner for extreme agitation and possible Tourette's syndrome. The patient has previously tried several medications. The patient's parent asks about aripiprazole (Abilify). The nurse practitioner explains that:

   A. Aripiprazole can be used for patients age 10 years and older with autism and Tourette's
   B. Aripiprazole is not an option because it is not an effective treatment for autism
   C. Aripiprazole is effective for Tourette's but not for autistic behaviors
   D. Aripiprazole can only be used for patients age 20 years and older for treatment of autism

3. In general, first-generation antipsychotic medicines block the:

   A. 5 hydroxytryptamine-2 receptor
   B. Muscarinic-2 receptor
   C. Alpha1 adrenergic receptor
   D. Dopamine D2 receptor

4. The part of a neuron that forms the command center of the nerve is the:

   A. Dendrite
   B. Axon
   C. Cell body
   D. Axonal terminal

5. An important tool for assessing patient or family history is:

   A. A genogram
   B. An EKG
   C. CT
   D. An EEG

1. C) Hypothalamus

The suprachiasmatic nucleus is located at the hypothalamus of the brain. Its function is to maintain the regulation of the sleep—wake cycle. It is present in the hypothalamus as a cluster of many cells. This nucleus is not a part of the amygdala or the hippocampus. It is not present in the pineal gland; rather, it controls the secretion of the hormone known as melatonin from this gland.

2. A) Aripiprazole can be used for patients age 10 years and older with autism and Tourette's

Aripiprazole can be used for patients age 10 years and older for behaviors associated with autism; it is also approved for Tourette's syndrome. Aripiprazole is effective and approved for both autism and Tourette's syndrome in both children and adults.

3. D) Dopamine D2 receptor

First-generation antipsychotic medicines perform their activities by blocking the dopamine D2 receptors. 5 hydroxytryptamine-2 receptors are serotonin receptors, which can be blocked by second-generation antipsychotic medicines, not by first-generation ones. Muscarinic-2 receptors are acetylcholine receptors, which are not blocked by first-generation antipsychotic medicines. First-generation antipsychotic medications also do not block the alpha1 adrenergic receptors of epinephrine or norepinephrine.

4. C) Cell body

The cell body, also called the soma, forms the command center of a nerve. Dendrites transfer information from other neurons to the cell body. Axons transfer information from the cell body to other neurons. Axonal terminals are bulb-like structures at the ends of axons, and they store neurotransmitters.

5. A) A genogram

A genogram is a representation of a person's family history in a diagram. It provides a picture of how the hereditary patterns of behavioral, medical, and psychological factors run through the family. An electrocardiogram is the transmitted waveform that provides a reading on the functioning of the heart muscles. CT is an imaging technique that provides an image of the internal organs. An electroencephalogram is a test used to detect brain waves. It is used to diagnose conditions like sleep disorders, epilepsy, and brain tumors.

6. A decrease in the neurotransmitter dopamine as a result of the death of brain cells in a mental health condition is known as:

   A. Parkinson's disease
   B. Depression
   C. Anxiety
   D. Attention deficit/hyperactivity disorder

7. The pathway involved in reward motivation is called:

   A. Nigrostriatal
   B. Mesocortical
   C. Mesolimbic
   D. Tuberoinfundibular

8. A group of neuron cell bodies located mostly in the peripheral nervous system is known as the:

   A. Cerebellum
   B. Medulla oblongata
   C. Pons
   D. Ganglion

9. The psychiatric-mental health nurse practitioner is asked to evaluate an older patient with Alzheimer's disease who is scheduled for a hip replacement after a fall. The patient has a history of migraines, hyperlipidemia, and dementia-related psychosis. The medication consistent with the patient's psychiatric diagnosis of Alzheimer's disease is:

   A. Topiramate (Topamax)
   B. Quetiapine (Seroquel)
   C. Rivastigmine (Exelon)
   D. Atorvastatin (Lipitor)

10. The psychiatric-mental health nurse practitioner is reviewing the medical record of a 5-year-old and notes that the gene study detects inactivation of the *FMR-1* gene. Based on this information, the nurse practitioner refers the patient to a genetic specialist to test for:

   A. Rett syndrome
   B. Down syndrome
   C. Prader-Willi syndrome
   D. Fragile X syndrome

(See answers next page.)

6. A) Parkinson's disease
Death of brain cells occurs in parkinsonism due to neurodegeneration. The affected area is the substantia nigra, and these cells are critical to producing dopamine. Depression is a mood disorder that may be associated with family history, illness, health issues, medications, and personality disorders. Anxiety can run in families and may be related to serotonin, norepinephrine, and gamma-aminobutyric acid levels, as well as environmental factors including medical conditions. Attention deficit/hyperactivity disorder may be caused by family history, exposure to environmental toxins, or maternal smoking or drug use during pregnancy.

7. C) Mesolimbic
The mesolimbic pathway is involved in reward motivation. It is stimulated by rewarding actions or behavior, and the main neurotransmitter involved in this is dopamine. The nigrostriatal pathway is involved in purposeful movement. The mesocortical pathway is involved in cognitive functions. The tuberoinfundibular pathway is involved in the regulation of prolactin secretion.

8. D) Ganglion
A ganglion is a group of neuron cell bodies in the peripheral nervous system. A ganglion provides intermediary connection between neurological structures in the body. The cerebellum, as the name suggests, is the "little brain." The cerebellum helps in maintaining the balance of the body. The medulla oblongata is between the brain and the spinal cord. It transmits signals between them and also plays a role in the regulation of autonomic functions like respiration and breathing. The pons is a part of the brain stem. The pons, along with the medulla oblongata, relays information between the brain and spinal cord. It also helps in functions like respiration and breathing along with the medulla oblongata.

9. C) Rivastigmine (Exelon)
Rivastigmine (Exelon) is an FDA-approved drug to treat Alzheimer's disease. Topiramate is an anticonvulsant (antiepileptic drug) used to treat seizure disorders and occasionally mood disorders. Quetiapine is an atypical antipsychotic used for schizophrenia and mood disorders. It is used off label for dementia patients who become aggressive. However, it is not approved by the FDA for treatment of dementia-related psychosis. Atorvastatin (Lipitor) is statin medicine that lowers cholesterol in the blood. It may reduce the risk of myocardial infarction or stroke.

10. D) Fragile X syndrome
Inactivation of the FMR-1 gene is seen in fragile X syndrome and results from a mutation on the X chromosome in an area known as the fragile site, which is expressed in only some cells; that is why it is seen in both males and females. Some may be carriers without the phenotype expression of the disease. Rett syndrome is caused by a dominant X-linked gene mutation. Down syndrome, or Trisomy 21, indicates an extra copy of chromosome 21. Prader—Willi syndrome is a deletion in chromosome 15q12.

11. Cannabis disrupts short-term memory due to:

    A. Cannabinoid (CB2) receptor effects
    B. Abundance of cannabinoid (CB1) receptors in the hippocampus
    C. Cannabidiol (CBD) antioxidative activity and neurodegeneration
    D. Increases in potency of cannabis over the past decade

12. After completing an initial psychiatric evaluation of a patient, the psychiatric-mental health nurse practitioner differentiates bipolar I disorder from bipolar II disorder because:

    A. At least one major depressive episode has been documented
    B. One past hospitalization for mania has occurred
    C. There has been a history of suicide attempt
    D. There has been one identifiable episode of mania

13. Concerned parents brings their infant in for evaluation by the psychiatric-mental health nurse practitioner and report that their daughter, who is 1 year old, appears to be declining, as she has lost her ability to communicate and is no longer attempting to walk. She is noted to have stereotypic hand movements and does not maintain eye contact, and her head circumference reveals microcephaly. Understanding the genetics of this disease, the nurse explains that it is caused by:

    A. Recessive X-linked gene
    B. Dominant X-linked gene
    C. An extra chromosome 21
    D. Inactivation of the *FMR-1* gene

14. The risk of an infant being born with a neurological disorder can be reduced if, before and during pregnancy, the pregnant patient takes:

    A. Thiamine (vitamin B1)
    B. Folic acid (vitamin B9)
    C. Cyanocobalamin (vitamin B12)
    D. Niacin (vitamin B6)

15. To assess for normal behavioral development of a 3 year old, the psychiatric-mental health nurse practitioner asks the toddler to perform a task such as:

    A. Build a tower of nine cubes
    B. Skip using feet alternately
    C. Stand on one foot for 5 seconds
    D. Tie their shoelaces

16. Spina bifida is a common defect found in neonates exposed during the first trimester to:

    A. Carbamazepine (Tegretol)
    B. Folic acid (Folacin)
    C. Paroxetine (Paxil)
    D. Lamotrigine (Lamictal)

(See answers next page.)

11. B) Abundance of cannabinoid (CB1) receptors in the hippocampus

Cannabinoid receptors (CB1) found in brain regions with an abundance found in the hippocampus are involved in mood, motor control, pain modulation, and memory formation, among other effects. Cannabinoid receptors (CB2) receptors are associated with the immune system to modulate inflammatory responses. Cannabidiol (CBD) compounds are neuroprotective through their antioxidative activity. Increased potency has not been proven and, therefore, is not a viable option.

12. D) There has been one identifiable episode of mania

Bipolar I disorder requires that the DSM-5 criterion for at least one manic episode must be met. A depressive episode is not required for a diagnosis of bipolar I disorder. Hospitalization is not required for all manic episodes and is therefore not a criterion for bipolar I disorder. Although the lifetime suicide risk for individuals with bipolar disorder is 15 times higher than for the general population, history of suicide attempt is not a criterion for either bipolar I or bipolar II disorder.

13. B) Dominant X-linked gene

Rett syndrome is caused by a dominant, not recessive, X-linked gene mutation, and is therefore seen only in girls. Patients have clinical features including normal development for the first 5 months followed at 6 months to 2 years of age by a progressive encephalopathy leading to stereotypic hand movements, such as wringing of the hands or spastic hand movements. They also lose gait coordination and the ability to communicate both expressively and receptively (poor eye contact). They have growth deceleration of the head, producing microcephaly, which is a defining symptom of this disorder. Trisomy 21 or having an extra 21st chromosome indicates Down syndrome. Inactivation of the FMR-1 gene is seen in fragile X syndrome.

14. B) Folic acid (vitamin B9)

Folic acid is a B vitamin that is known for neuroprotection of the fetus. Although all B vitamins are vital to fetal development, folic acid is needed for the process of neurulation, which is when the neural tube is developed in utero at 3 to 4 weeks' gestation. A diet deficient in folic acid will produce neurulation defects; therefore, it is important to advise all pregnant patients to take an adequate supply of folic acid.

15. A) Build a tower of nine cubes

A 3-year-old is able to build a tower of 9 to 10 cubes, copy a circle and a cross, ride a tricycle, jump from the bottom step, alternate feet going upstairs, put on their shoes, unbutton buttons, and feed self. A 5-year-old can skip using feet alternately, a 4-year-old can stand on one foot for 5 to 8 seconds, and a 6-year-old can tie their shoelaces.

16. A) Carbamazepine (Tegretol)

Carbamazepine is associated with neural tube defects, such as spina bifida. Folic acid is used to protect the neural development of a fetus, and all pregnant patients should be instructed to take folic acid. Though paroxetine is a teratogen, it does not cause neural tube defects, but is associated with cardiac malformations. Lamotrigine is associated with cleft palate.

17. The psychiatric-mental health nurse practitioner is assessing a 6-year-old patient who is cognitively impaired, makes poor eye contact, and does not interact socially with peers. His mother took medications for a seizure disorder and depression while pregnant. To determine exposure to a neurological teratogen, the nurse practitioner will assess for:

    A. Spina bifida at birth
    B. History of cleft palate
    C. Congenital Ebstein's anomaly
    D. Neonatal withdrawal syndrome

18. The psychiatric-mental health nurse practitioner is reviewing the chart of a 7-year-old patient and notes that genetic testing reveals an extra chromosome 21, which indicates:

    A. Down syndrome
    B. Rett syndrome
    C. Fragile X syndrome
    D. Prader-Willi syndrome

19. The psychiatric-mental health nurse practitioner is performing a physical assessment on a child who is able to print their name, tie their shoelaces, and count 10 objects accurately. These developmental milestones would indicate the child is age:

    A. 3 years
    B. 4 years
    C. 5 years
    D. 6 years

20. In guanine nucleotide-binding proteins (G proteins), reduction of response in the continued presence of an agonist is known as:

    A. An affinity
    B. A mutation
    C. Receptor desensitization
    D. Inverse agonism

21. The term *pharmacodynamics* describes the:

    A. Effects of drugs on plasma concentrations
    B. Time, course, and intensity of a drug's effects
    C. Individual way drugs are metabolized
    D. Propensity for drug–drug interactions

22. Antipsychotic-induced movement disorders result primarily from:

    A. Blockade of muscarinic acetylcholine receptors
    B. Skeletal muscle relaxation and neurogenic pain
    C. Antagonism of histamine (H1) receptors
    D. Dopamine (D1) receptor blockage in the extrapyramidal tract

(See answers next page.)

17. A) Spina bifida at birth

Spina bifida is a common neuronal defect seen in neonates who have been exposed in utero to valproate (Depakote) or carbamazepine (Tegretol), both of which are well known neuronal teratogens used to treat seizure disorders. Cleft palate is not a neurological disorder and may be seen with various medications when given in utero, including lamotrigine, a neuroleptic medication that can be used to treat seizures. Ebstein's anomaly is a cardiac abnormality seen in patients exposed to lithium in utero; lithium is used to treat mood disorders and may be used adjunctly in the treatment of depression. Neonatal withdrawal syndrome may occur with controlled substances or other drugs such as selective serotonin reuptake inhibitors (SSRIs), which are used to treat depression. However, SSRIs are not considered neurological teratogens.

18. A) Down syndrome

Down syndrome or Trisomy 21 is caused by an extra copy of chromosome 21. Rett syndrome is caused by a dominant X-linked gene mutation. Inactivation of the FMR-1 gene is seen in fragile X syndrome, and Prader-Willi syndrome is a deletion in chromosome 15q12.

19. D) 6 years

By 6 years old, a child should be able to ride a two-wheel bicycle, count 10 objects correctly, print their name, copy a triangle, and tie shoelaces. A 3-year-old is able to build a tower of 9 to 10 cubes, copy a circle and a cross, ride a tricycle, jump from the bottom step, alternate feet going upstairs, put on their shoes, unbutton buttons, and feed self. A 4-year-old can walk downstairs one step at a time, stand on one foot for 5 to 8 seconds, copy a cross, repeat four digits, count three objects correctly, brush their own teeth, and wash and dry their face. A 5-year-old will skip using feet alternately, have complete sphincter control, copy a square, dress and undress self, and print a few letters.

20. C) Receptor desensitization

Attenuation of receptor response for G proteins in the continued presence of an agonist is known as receptor desensitization. Affinity is the extent to which a drug binds to receptors at a given concentration. A mutation is a structural alteration. Inverse agonism induces a pharmacological response opposite to that of an agonist.

21. B) Time, course, and intensity of a drug's effects

The time, course, and intensity of a drug's effects compose pharmacodynamics. Effects of drugs on plasma concentrations and the propensity for drug–drug interactions are aspects of pharmacokinetics. Pharmacogenetics is concerned with why drugs are metabolized differently among individuals.

22. D) Dopamine (D1) receptor blockage in the extrapyramidal tract

D1 blockage in the extrapyramidal tract can cause antipsychotic-induced movement disorders. Anticholinergic agents act to block muscarinic acetylcholine receptors that can lead to mydriasis and bronchodilation. H1 antagonism results in inhibition of the effects of histamine. Skeletal muscle relaxation and neurogenic pain are not typical manifestations because antipsychotic induced movements are typically tics and tremors.

23. In the study of drugs, response, therapeutic index, and development of the dependence, tolerance, and withdrawal phenomena are all recognized as aspects of:

    A. Pharmacokinetics
    B. Therapeutics
    C. Efficacy
    D. Pharmacodynamics

24. Inattention, restlessness, and impulsivity associated with attention deficit/hyperactivity disorder (ADHD):

    A. Diminish as the individual ages
    B. Are not usually seen in younger children
    C. Usually resolve in adolescence
    D. Can remain problematic into adulthood

25. Pharmacokinetics is the study of:

    A. The time, course, and intensity of a drug's effects
    B. How drugs are metabolized differently among patients
    C. The effects of drugs on plasma concentrations of other drugs
    D. Response and sensitivity to side effects

26. The major inhibitory neurotransmitter in the central nervous system is:

    A. Dopamine
    B. G-aminobutyric acid (GABA)
    C. 5-hydroxytryptamine (5-HT)
    D. Norepinephrine

27. Sexual side effects resulting from use of a selective serotonin reuptake inhibitor (SSRI) can be treated with the adjunctive medication:

    A. Buspirone (Buspar)
    B. Verapamil (Isoptin)
    C. Bupropion (Wellbutrin)
    D. Carbamazepine (Tegretol)

28. A first-line treatment of Alzheimer's disease is:

    A. Methylphenidate
    B. Donepezil
    C. Carbidopa-levodopa
    D. Lithium

(See answers next page.)

23. D) Pharmacodynamics

Pharmacodynamics of a drug include receptor mechanisms, response, therapeutic index, and development of the dependence, tolerance, and withdrawal phenomena. Effects of a drug on plasma concentrations and the propensity for drug–drug interactions are aspects of pharmacokinetics. Therapeutics refers to a treatment, therapy, or drug. Efficacy is the ability to produce a desired effect.

24. D) Can remain problematic into adulthood

Along with inattention and restlessness, symptoms of impulsivity may continue to be challenging for patients with ADHD into adulthood. These symptoms are usually seen in even young patients.

25. C) The effects of drugs on plasma concentrations of other drugs

The effect of a drug on plasma concentrations of other drugs is referred to as pharmacokinetics. Time, course, and intensity of a drug's effects are aspects of pharmacodynamics. Pharmacogenetics refers to how drugs are metabolized differently among patients. Response and sensitivity to side effects are patient-related factors of pharmacological actions.

26. B) G-aminobutyric acid (GABA)

GABA is the primary neurotransmitter that reduces the neuronal excitability throughout the nervous system. Dopamine, serotonin (5-HT), and norepinephrine strongly influence mental behavior and are fundamental to normal brain function.

27. C) Bupropion (Wellbutrin)

Bupropion (Wellbutrin) is commonly used in the treatment of SSRI-induced sexual side effects. Buspirone (Buspar) is used in the treatment of generalized anxiety disorder and anxiety related to depression. Verapamil (Isoptin) is a calcium channel blocker that, while not officially recognized as psychotropic, is commonly used to treat some psychiatric disorders. Carbamazepine (Tegretol) is an anticonvulsant.

28. B) Donepezil

Being a cholinesterase inhibitor, donepezil becomes a part of the first-line treatment of Alzheimer's disease. Methylphenidate is a psychostimulant used in the first-line treatment of attention deficit/hyperactivity disorder. Carbidopa-levodopa is a combination of medicines that belongs to the first-line treatment of Parkinson's disease. The mood stabilizer lithium is the first-line treatment of bipolar disorder.

29. A biological risk factor contributing to the development of disruptive behavior disorders is:

   A. Stress experiences at home and school
   B. Living with an alcoholic parent
   C. Family systems discord
   D. Abnormalities in the prefrontal cortex

30. In general, the neurotransmitter dopamine is increased in patients with:

   A. Parkinson's disease
   B. Depression
   C. Schizophrenia
   D. Attention deficit/hyperactivity disorder

31. Complications occurring within days of beginning antipsychotic treatment can include moderate to severe elevation of temperature, muscle rigidity, altered consciousness, and autonomic instability that are most likely related to:

   A. Serotonin syndrome
   B. Neuroleptic malignant syndrome
   C. Anticholinergic syndrome
   D. Malignant hyperthermia

32. On an inpatient psychiatric unit, a recently admitted patient is elated, sarcastic, using abusive language, and verbally harassing other patients The previous day's lithium and carbamazepine levels are determined to be within therapeutic range. In managing the patient's acute mania, the psychiatric-mental health nurse practitioner would:

   A. Increase the patient's current dose of lithium
   B. Start the patient on a benzodiazepine
   C. Discontinue current medications and begin an antipsychotic
   D. Consult with a collaborating psychiatrist

33. Based on its mechanism of action, sertraline is a:

   A. Norepinephrine and dopamine uptake inhibitor
   B. Norepinephrine and serotonin specific antidepressant
   C. Serotonin-norepinephrine reuptake inhibitor
   D. Selective serotonin reuptake inhibitor

34. Amphetamine (d,l) (Adderall XR) works by blocking reuptake and increasing the release of:

   A. Epinephrine and serotonin
   B. Epinephrine and dopamine
   C. Dopamine and serotonin
   D. Dopamine and glutamate

(See answers next page.)

29. D) Abnormalities in the prefrontal cortex

Abnormality in the prefrontal cortex is one biological factor that may contribute to the development of disruptive behavior disorders. Stress experiences, an alcoholic parent, and family discord are psychodynamic contributing factors.

30. C) Schizophrenia

In patients with schizophrenia, the enhanced subcortical release of the neurotransmitter dopamine brings the symptoms of delusions and hallucinations. Parkinson's disease occurs as the cells giving birth to dopamine die. Feeling hopeless and losing motivation are some symptoms of depression, and a decrease in dopamine level enhances these issues. A lower level of dopamine is a sign of attention deficit/hyperactivity disorder as well.

31. B) Neuroleptic malignant syndrome

Neuroleptic malignant syndrome typically occurs within days after exposure to an antipsychotic, with core symptoms including severe muscle rigidity, altered consciousness, elevated temperature, and autonomic dysregulation. Although muscle rigidity is a possible indication of serotonin syndrome, symptoms of this condition usually occur within several hours of taking a new drug or increasing dosage. Antipsychotics may cause anticholinergic syndrome; however, symptoms of this condition include flushing, dry mucous membranes, hypertension, tachycardia, and urinary retention. Malignant hyperthermia can occur when exposed to drugs usually used for anesthesia, and symptoms include severe muscle rigidity, shallow and rapid breathing, tachycardia, arrhythmia, dangerously high body temperature, and excessive sweating.

32. B) Start the patient on a benzodiazepine

Benzodiazepines are frequently used in an inpatient setting for rapid control of certain symptoms related to mania, such as agitation, restlessness, and insomnia. An increase in lithium would not have an immediate impact on the patient's disruptive and manic behaviors. Adjunct treatment to the current regimen may be necessary before discontinuing any medications. Managing a manic patient is within the scope of practice of the psychiatric-mental health nurse practitioner, and consultation or referral should be done when evidence-based approaches are unsuccessful.

33. D) Selective serotonin reuptake inhibitor

Because sertraline possesses the capability of blocking serotonin reuptake, more of this neurotransmitter becomes available at the synapse; thus, it is a selective serotonin reuptake inhibitor. It does not inhibit the reuptake of norepinephrine and dopamine. Although it increases the neurotransmission of serotonin, it does not do the same in the case of norepinephrine; hence, it is not a norepinephrine and serotonin-specific antidepressant. It can only inhibit the reuptake of serotonin, not of norepinephrine.

34. B) Epinephrine and dopamine

Amphetamine (d,l), or Adderall XR, works by increasing both epinephrine and dopamine. This is accomplished by blocking the reuptake and aiding the presynapse in releasing more of these neurotransmitters. Serotonin and glutamate, although possibly implicated in attention deficit hyperactivity disorder, are not impacted by amphetamine (d,l).

35. The medication that increases the inhibitory effect of g-aminobutyric acid (GABA) is:

    A. Alprazolam (Xanax)
    B. Buspirone (Buspar)
    C. Sertraline (Zoloft)
    D. Vilazodone (Viibryd)

36. Antipsychotics, tricyclic antidepressants (TCAs), monoamine oxidase inhibitors (MAOIs), and the atypical antidepressant trazodone share a common side effect that is especially dangerous in older patients. This side effect is:

    A. Elevated temperature
    B. Orthostatic hypotension
    C. Increased respiratory rate
    D. Decreased oxygen saturation

37. Korsakoff's syndrome is caused by a deficiency of:

    A. Vitamin A
    B. Vitamin B1
    C. Vitamin C
    D. Vitamin D

38. The regulated process that results in a single gene coding for multiple proteins is known as gene:

    A. Expression
    B. Transcription
    C. Splicing
    D. Translation

39. Effective treatment in front temporal dementia includes:

    A. Antisense oligonucleotide therapy
    B. Cholinesterase
    C. Chemotherapy
    D. Carbidopa

40. The drug fluoxetine (Prozac) belongs to the class of:

    A. Selective serotonin reuptake inhibitors (SSRIs)
    B. Serotonin and norepinephrine reuptake inhibitors (SNRIs)
    C. Tricyclic antidepressants (TCAs)
    D. Monoamine oxidase inhibitors (MAOIs)

(See answers next page.)

35. A) Alprazolam (Xanax)

Alprazolam (Xanax) is the medication that impacts the inhibitory effect of GABA by binding to the benzodiazepine receptor at the GABA-A ligand gate. Buspirone, vilazodone, and sertraline all affect serotonin.

36. B) Orthostatic hypotension

Orthostatic hypotension in older patients requires careful attention because of potential underlying gait disturbances, poor reflexes, and increased risk of falls. Elevated temperature, increased respiratory rate, and decreased oxygen saturation are not effects that are associated with antipsychotics, TCAs, MAOIs, or trazodone.

37. B) Vitamin B1

Korsakoff's syndrome usually results from a deficiency of thiamine (vitamin B1) and may be caused by alcohol abuse, dietary deficiencies, prolonged vomiting, eating disorders, or effects of chemotherapy. Alcohol intake causes inflammation of the stomach lining and reduces the body's ability to absorb vitamin B1. The symptoms include mental confusion, vision problems, hypothermia, low blood pressure, and a lack of muscle coordination. Other vitamin deficiencies do not contribute to Korsakoff's syndrome. Vitamin A deficiency is related to night blindness and poor immunity. Vitamin C deficiency contributes to scurvy, lethargy, myalgia, easy bruising, fatigue, and poor mood. Vitamin D deficiency contributes to rickets and osteomalacia.

38. C) Splicing

During gene splicing, some of the genes are included or excluded from the final messenger RNA produced in the nucleotide sequence. Because proteins translated from alternatively spliced RNA contain different amino acid sequences, splicing allows the synthesis of many more proteins than would be expected from the human genomics. Turning on a gene to produce is called gene expression. Transcription is when the information in a strand of DNA is copied into a new molecule of messenger RNA. Translation relates to the process in which the RNA decoding takes place and is used for building a polypeptide or chain of amino acid.

39. A) Antisense oligonucleotide therapy

Antisense oligonucleotide therapy (ASO) may treat gain of function disorders by silencing the causative gene, either by acting on both of the alleles for nonessential genes or by selectively acting on the mutant allele in the case of essential genes. For certain loss of function of disease, there is the possibility of using ASO splice modulation, which can in certain cases restore the gene function or otherwise compensate for its loss. Cholinesterases are a group of medications that block the normal breakdown of acetylcholine, a neurotransmitter that has action on both central and peripheral nervous systems. Chemotherapy is a cancer treatment. Carbidopa is a dopa decarboxylase inhibitor used to treat symptoms of Parkinson's disease.

40. A) Selective serotonin reuptake inhibitors (SSRIs)

Fluoxetine is an example of an SSRI, an important class of antidepressants. Serotonin and norepinephrine reuptake inhibitors are another class of antidepressant that includes medications such as duloxetine. Tricyclics are a third class of antidepressant, which includes drugs such as amoxapine and clomipramine. Monoamine oxidase inhibitors are also a class of antidepressant and include drugs like phenelzine (Nardil) and selegiline.

41. Trisomy, mosaicism, and translocation are types of:

    A. Parkinsonism
    B. Metabolic disorder
    C. Intellectual and cognitive disability
    D. Down syndrome

42. A majority of antipsychotics block:

    A. D1 receptors
    B. D2 receptors
    C. D3 receptors
    D. D4 receptors

43. The class of antidepressants that reduces the breakdown of presynaptic amines is:

    A. Selective serotonin reuptake inhibitors (SSRIs)
    B. Serotonin and norepinephrine reuptake inhibitors (SNRIs)
    C. Tricyclic antidepressants (TCAs)
    D. Monoamine oxidase inhibitors (MAOIs)

44. The lobe that is associated with the sensation of touch is the:

    A. Frontal
    B. Temporal
    C. Parietal
    D. Occipital

45. Benzodiazepines produce their effect by increasing levels in the brain of:

    A. Gamma-aminobutyric acid
    B. Serotonin
    C. Dopamine
    D. Norepinephrine

46. The drug that causes gingival hyperplasia as a side effect in almost 50% of patients is:

    A. Lithium citrate
    B. Phenytoin sodium
    C. Phenelzine
    D. Diazepam

(See answers next page.)

41. D) Down syndrome

Trisomy includes one extra chromosome 21 and is a common type of Down syndrome. The total number of chromosomes present is 47 instead of 46 chromosomes. In mosaicism, some cells have 46 chromosomes and some cells have 47 chromosomes. In translocation, an extra part of the chromosome 21 attaches to a different chromosome. A total of 46 chromosomes are present, of which one is abnormal. Familial Parkinson's disease is associated with two genes: one is the alpha-synuclein gene located in the long arm of chromosome 4, and the other is the parkin gene located in the long arm of chromosome 6. There are many metabolic disorders; for example, Albinism deafness disorder characterized by congenital nerve deafness is transmitted though the X-linked chromosome. Intellectual and cognitive disability is a symptom resultant of many different neurological conditions.

42. B) D2 receptors

Dopamine receptors are widely studied because of their impact on psychosis. Psychotic behavior is usually attributed to the D2 dopamine receptor. Antipsychotic drugs block this receptor in order to be effective. However, with advancements in research, other dopamine receptors are also targeted by antipsychotics. How these receptors contribute to the effectiveness of the antipsychotics is not well studied, but D1, D3, and D4 are also blocked by some, but not a majority of, antipsychotics.

43. D) Monoamine oxidase inhibitors (MAOIs)

MAOIs work by reducing the activity of monoamine oxidase in breaking the presynaptic amine. SSRIs work by blocking the uptake of serotonin. SNRIs work by preventing the presynaptic reuptake of amines noradrenaline and serotonin. TCAs work by increasing serotonin and norepinephrine in the brain.

44. C) Parietal

The cerebral cortex has four lobes, each performing specific sensory and motor functions. The parietal lobe is associated with the sensation of touch. The frontal lobe is associated with conscious or voluntary sensations and movement. The temporal lobe is associated with the sensation of sound. The occipital lobe is associated with vision sensation.

45. A) Gamma-aminobutyric acid

Antianxiety drugs (benzodiazepines) work by increasing the level of gamma-aminobutyric acid levels in the brain. This increased level causes calmness and relaxes the patient. Selective serotonin reuptake inhibitors (SSRIs) work by increasing the amount of serotonin. Monoamine oxidase inhibitors (MAOIs) work by increasing dopamine as well as serotonin. Tricyclic antidepressants (TCAs) increase the amount of serotonin and norepinephrine in the brain to improve mood. SSRIs, MAOIs, and TCAs are different classes of antidepressants.

46. B) Phenytoin sodium

Phenytoin sodium is an antiepileptic drug that causes gingival hyperplasia as a side effect in almost 50% of patients. Lithium citrate is a mood stabilizer that has side effects like goiter and hyperthyroidism. Phenelzine is an antidepressant that causes constipation and arrhythmia as side effects. Diazepam is a benzodiazepine that is used to treat anxiety and seizures. It can cause nausea and vomiting as side effects.

47. Schizophrenia is usually treated with the help of:

   A. Antipsychotics
   B. Antidepressants
   C. Anxiolytics
   D. Mood stabilizers

48. The first-line treatment for obsessive-compulsive disorder (OCD) includes:

   A. Tricyclic antidepressants (TCAs)
   B. Selective serotonin reuptake inhibitors (SSRIs)
   C. Monoamine oxidase inhibitors (MAOIs)
   D. Selective serotonin reuptake inhibitors (SSRIs) with lithium

49. The brain structure that plays a role in executive function is the:

   A. Hippocampus
   B. Amygdala
   C. Prefrontal cortex
   D. Pons

50. The structure of the brain located on top of and surrounding the brainstem is the:

   A. Pons
   B. Medulla oblongata
   C. Cerebrum
   D. Cerebellum

51. The lobe where auditory sensation is based is the:

   A. Frontal
   B. Parietal
   C. Temporal
   D. Occipital

52. The part of the brain that is involved in long-term memory formation and emotional responses is the:

   A. Hypothalamus
   B. Hippocampus
   C. Thalamus
   D. Medulla oblongata

53. The cranial nerve that is responsible for the homeostatic control of the organs of the thoracic and upper abdominal cavities is the nerve known as:

   A. Vagus
   B. Spinal accessory
   C. Hypoglossal
   D. Glossopharyngeal

(See answers next page.)

47. A) Antipsychotics
Schizophrenia is a mental disorder in which the thinking ability of a person is affected. Thought process, behavior, and speech are highly affected. Antipsychotics are the best medicine to treat such disorders, which mainly affect the central nervous system. Antidepressants are used to treat depression. Anxiolytics are used to treat anxiety disorders. Mood stabilizers like lithium are used to prevent major mood episodes.

48. B) Selective serotonin reuptake inhibitors (SSRIs)
OCD is treated with SSRIs as a first-line treatment. Tricyclic antidepressants are used in second-line treatment. MAOIs are preferred for later stages. These can be augmented by higher doses of SSRIs when the first line of treatment has failed. SSRIs with benzodiazepine or lithium are also considered when the patient does not respond well to SSRIs.

49. C) Prefrontal cortex
The prefrontal cortex is involved in executive function. The hippocampus is associated with memory processes. The amygdala is associated with emotional processes such as fear. The pons connects the spinal cord and brain, and it plays a role in autonomic functions like respiration.

50. C) Cerebrum
The cerebrum is located on top of and surrounding the brainstem. The pons is a part of the brainstem located below the midbrain. The medulla oblongata is a part of the brainstem located below the pons. The cerebellum is located behind the brainstem at the junction of the spinal cord and brain.

51. C) Temporal
The temporal lobe is associated with auditory memories or sensations. The cerebral cortex has four major lobes, which are interconnected: frontal, parietal, temporal, and occipital. The frontal lobe controls behavior and voluntary movements. The parietal lobe controls sensations in the body. The occipital lobe is responsible for vision-related responses in the body.

52. B) Hippocampus
The hippocampus is involved in long-term memory formation and emotional responses. The hypothalamus is a collection of nuclei that are largely involved in regulating homeostasis. The thalamus is important for relaying signals to and from the cerebral cortex. All sensory information, except for the sense of smell, passes through the thalamus before processing by the cortex. The main function of the medulla oblongata is to transmit signals between the spinal cord and the brain. It is a part of the brain stem.

53. A) Vagus
The vagus nerve is responsible for contributing to homeostatic control of the organs of the thoracic and upper abdominal cavities. The spinal accessory nerve is responsible for controlling the muscles of the neck, along with cervical spinal nerves. The hypoglossal nerve is responsible for controlling the muscles of the lower throat and tongue. The glossopharyngeal nerve is responsible for controlling muscles in the oral cavity and upper throat, as well as for part of the sense of taste and the production of saliva.

54. Electrodes are attached to the scalp in:

A. CT

B. MRI

C. EEG

D. PET

55. A neurodevelopmental disorder characterized by aneuploidy is:

A. Williams–Beuren syndrome

B. Down syndrome

C. Fragile X syndrome

D. Autism

56. Flurazepam is prescribed for sleep-related problems like insomnia or inability to sleep due to an acute medical condition. The psychiatric-mental health nurse practitioner prescribes flurazepam to a patient, but after a week the patient's condition has not improved. The nurse practitioner should now:

A. Prescribe a central nervous system depressant as well

B. Increase the dose of flurazepam

C. Replace the flurazepam with another drug since it is a Schedule IV drug

D. Prescribe trazodone

57. The psychiatric-mental health nurse practitioner is counseling a 20-year-old pregnant patient. It is the patient's first pregnancy. The patient asks if she can drink wine during the pregnancy. The nurse practitioner explains that:

A. Alcohol can harm the fetus at any stage of pregnancy, including the earliest stages before the pregnancy is known

B. The patient can reduce her risk of harming the fetus by drinking no more than 10 drinks a week, with no more than 2 drinks per day

C. The patient should not drink until the last trimester, when the risk of harming the fetus has passed

D. Having an occasional drink of wine or other alcohol will not harm the fetus

58. The most frequently diagnosed neurodevelopmental disability (NDD) is:

A. Developmental language disorders

B. Autism spectrum disorders (ASD)

C. Attention deficit/hyperactivity disorder (ADHD)

D. Learning disorders

(*See answers next page.*)

54. C) EEG

EEG is a procedure that involves attaching electrodes to the patient's scalp and recording electrical impulses from the brain. The distinctive patterns of current differ based on the state the patient is in: sleeping, awake, or anesthetized. CT is a type of imaging that uses a series of x-ray scans of the brain, from which a computer analysis generates "slices" that allow for an accurate 3D-like reconstruction of each part. CT is capable of detecting lesions, abrasions, areas of infarct, and aneurysm. MRI uses a magnetic field to be applied to the brain. The nuclei of hydrogen atoms absorb and emit radio waves that are analyzed by the computer, which provides 3D visualization of brain structure in sectional images. MRI is used to detect brain edema, ischemia, infection, neoplasm, and trauma. PET is used to detect oxygen utilization, glucose metabolism, blood flow, and neurotransmitter-receptor interaction.

55. B) Down syndrome

Neurodevelopmental disorders are classified by (theoretical) cellular causes. The first group is caused aneuploidy, which is an abnormal number of chromosomes. The most well-known neurodevelopmental aneuploidy is Down syndrome, with a trisomy of chromosome 21. Disorders of the second subgroup involve deletion of a chromosome region, such as the deletion of chromosomal region 7q11.2 in Williams-Beuren syndrome. The third group is hypothesized to be due to a single affected gene. An example is the fragile X syndrome mental retardation. The last group is theorized to be caused by complex etiology genetic, environmental, and epigenetic factors such as autism and schizophrenia.

56. B) Increase the dose of flurazepam

Flurazepam is a Schedule IV drug and is not prescribed for more than a month. Long-term use can affect the cognitive abilities of the patient and cause dependence. However, the drug is initially prescribed for 7 to 10 days to see its effects at the lowest dose. If the patient's condition is not improved, the dose is increased but is always prescribed at the lowest effective dose. A central nervous system (CNS) depressant and flurazepam combination can cause respiratory sedation, so flurazepam is avoided when the patient is using a CNS depressant. Trazodone is prescribed only when the flurazepam has failed to have any thera-peutic effect. First, the dose of the flurazepam is increased to see its effects, and if the dose increase is not effective, replacement with trazodone may be implemented.

57. A) Alcohol can harm the fetus at any stage of pregnancy, including the earli-est stages before the pregnancy is known

Alcohol causes neuronal damage and cell loss in the fetal brain through direct action as a toxin. No prenatal period has been shown to be safe from the deleterious effects of alcohol. Central nervous system damage to the fetus may result from alcohol exposure in any trimes-ter, even before the time of a pregnancy test. Pregnant patients should be advised not to drink from the time of conception to birth. Because this is the patient's first pregnancy, it is a timely opportunity to investigate the patient's history of alcohol and/or other recreational drug use.

58. D) Learning disorders

Collectively, NDDs make up the largest category of disorders seen in the pediatric pop-ulation. The most frequently diagnosed NDD is learning disorders, with an estimated prevalence of 8%. Developmental language disorders are a close second, with incidence of approximately 7% of the population. ASDs constitute 1% to 2% of the population, followed by ADHD with an incidence of approximately 2% worldwide.

59. Cell synaptogenesis:

    A. Begins in utero and continues during the first 2 postnatal years
    B. Forms the neural tube at 3 to 4 weeks' gestation
    C. Is the birth of new neuronal cells occurring throughout the life span
    D. Occurs when the brain eliminates extra synapses during early childhood and early adulthood

60. A fatal neural tube discord (NTD) that results from a failure of the anterior (rostral) portion of the embryonic neural tube (anterior neuropore) to close properly is:

    A. Spina bifida
    B. Myelomeningocele
    C. Talipes equinovarus
    D. Anencephaly

61. Primary prevention of central nervous system (CNS) anomalies involving neural tube defects requires:

    A. Prenatal ultrasound screening
    B. Prenatal care
    C. Prevention of maternal diabetes mellitus
    D. Folic acid supplementation

(See answers next page.)

59. A) Begins in utero and continues during the first 2 postnatal years

Synaptogenesis is the formation of synaptic connections in the human cortex. It begins in utero and continues during the first 2 postnatal years. Neurulation causes changes in intracellular cytoskeleton and cell-extracellular matrix attachment. This process causes the formation of the neural tube from the ectoderm of the embryo. Neurogenesis is the birth of new neurons, which occurs in the brain throughout our life span. Synaptic pruning is another natural process that occurs in the brain between early childhood and early adulthood. During this time period, the brain eliminates extra synapses.

60. D) Anencephaly

Anencephaly is a condition characterized by a total or partial absence of the brain with absence of the cranial vault and covering skin. Anencephaly is an NTD that results from a failure of the anterior portion of the embryonic neural tube to close properly. Many affected fetuses are either stillborn or die shortly after birth. Spina bifida is a general term used to describe an NTD of the spine, in which part of the meninges or spinal cord or both protrudes through an opening in the vertebral column. Myelomeningocele is the most common type of spina bifida, constituting about 90% of all cases. Myelomeningoceles, which are usually open, can be clinically severe and disabling, and can cause a sequence of related findings (e.g., Chiari II malformation, hydrocephalus, hip dislocation, talipes, lower limb paralysis, loss of sphincter control including neurogenic bladder). For infants with myelomeningocele, nerve function is intact above the lesion; therefore, lower lesions have greater preservation of neurologic function. Talipes equinovarus is the most common congenital deformity of the feet.

61. D) Folic acid supplementation

Periconceptional folic acid supplementation and/or food fortification with folic acid has significantly reduced neural tube defects. Prenatal ultrasound screening is a secondary prevention. Prenatal care is important with all pregnancies; early identification and guidance is not primary prevention. CNS malformations may be associated with metabolic diseases, like agenesis of corpus callosum. Maternal diabetes mellitus is an important risk factor for the development of CNS malformations, but it is present prior to pregnancy. Other risk factors are fetal alcoholism, maternal age over 35 years, multiple pregnancy, oligohydramnios, hydramnios, maternal hyperthermia, and use of valproate by patients with epilepsy during pregnancy. Nongenetic risk factors include pregestational diabetes, folate insufficiency/deficiency, and hyperthermia (fever) in early pregnancy.

62. Most congenital anomalies of the central nervous system (CNS) are due to:

   A. Oligohydramnios
   B. Maternal diabetes mellitus
   C. Noxious exposure
   D. Neural tube defects

63. A factor with potential impact on the child's ability to visually follow an object is:

   A. Shared gaze between infant and primary caregiver at age 1 to 2 months
   B. Environmental stimulation from birth to 6 months
   C. Shared gaze between infant and primary caregiver from birth to 2 months
   D. Environmental stimulation at age 2 to 3 months

64. A patient presents with numbness, weakness, ataxia, and visual changes that are resolved within hours. The psychiatric-mental health nurse practitioner suspects a diagnosis of:

   A. Ischemic stroke
   B. Transient ischemic attack
   C. Embolic stroke
   D. Thrombotic stroke

(See answers next page.)

62. D) Neural tube defects

CNS congenital anomalies are birth defects of the physical structure of the brain or spinal cord that develop in utero. The different categories of congenital malformations of the CNS reflect the time at which a noxious event disrupted the normal sequence of CNS development rather than the nature of the noxious event itself. Neural tube defects account for the most congenital anomalies of the CNS and result from failure of the neural tube to close spontaneously between the 3rd and 4th week of embryonic development. Examples include spina bifida occulta, meningocele, myelomeningocele, and encephalocele. Less frequently occurring CNS malformations may be associated with metabolic diseases, like agenesis of corpus callosum. Maternal diabetes mellitus is an important risk factor for the development of CNS malformations. Oligohydramnios or low amniotic fluid is a less predominant risk factor. Secondary microcephaly results from a large number of noxious agents that may affect the fetus in utero, such as the use of valproate by patients with epilepsy during pregnancy, and are less frequent risk factors for the development of CNS malformations.

63. D) Environmental stimulation at age 2 to 3 months

Brain plasticity is maximal at specific time windows during early development, known as critical periods, during which sensory experience though environmental input is necessary to establish normal and optimal cortical representations of the surrounding environment. From the age of 2 to 3 months, metabolic activity in the visual and parietal cortex requires stimulation for normal development of the ability to visually follow an object. Without stimulation, circuitry will not be established. A shared gaze between infant and primary caregiver begins the process of attachment. It should continue past 1 to 2 months of age. Infants cannot see at birth; environmental stimulation related to visual fields is a critical period from age 2 to 3 months.

64. B) Transient ischemic attack

A transient ischemic attack has the same origins as an ischemic stroke, which is the most common type of stroke. In an ischemic stroke, a clot blocks the blood supply to part of the brain. In a transient ischemic attack, unlike a stroke, the blockage is brief, and there is no permanent damage. Embolic stroke is caused by a clot that develops in another part of the body and travels to and becomes lodged in a blood vessel in the brain; a clot that forms in the brain itself is known as a thrombosis and causes a thrombotic stroke. The physical and neurological damage caused by these strokes does not resolve.

65. A 27-year-old patient is the owner of several gas stations. She worked until she delivered her child 4 months ago. The patient received prenatal care and had no complications prior to delivery 4 weeks early. The patient denies any alcohol use, trauma, or infections during pregnancy and has no history of substance abuse. The infant was born with microcephaly, flat nasal bridge, deep-set eyes, small palpebral fissures, facial anomalies, and hypoplastic nails. The psychiatric-mental health nurse practitioner suspects:

A. Fetal alcohol spectrum disorders
B. Di Sala syndrome
C. Holoprosencephaly
D. Toluene embryopathy

66. An adverse effect frequently seen following prenatal exposure to neurotoxic drugs and teratogenic conditions is:

A. Abnormalities of finger ridges
B. High-steepled palate
C. Curved little finger
D. Microcephaly

67. Physical examination of a patient with bulimia nervosa purging subtype often includes findings of:

A. Lanugo
B. Acrocyanosis
C. Short stature
D. Russell's sign

(See answers next page.)

65. D) Toluene embryopathy

Toluene (toluol; methylbenzene; phenylmethane) is an aromatic hydrocarbon that is a component of gasoline. Inhalation of airborne toluene is the main source of human exposures, which may occur during the production, transport, and use of gasoline or toluene or by deliberate inhalation. The greatest risk of accidental exposure to toluene is likely to occur among those in the petroleum industry, such as gas station workers. Environmental prenatal exposure has evidenced premature delivery and congenital cranio-facial, limb, cardiac, renal, and central nervous system malformations. The characteristics reported are similar to fetal alcohol syndrome (microcephaly, flat nasal bridge, deep-set eyes, small palpebral fissures, facial anomalies, micrognathia, and hypoplastic nails); however, the patient denies alcohol use. Warfarin embryopathy, also known as fetal warfarin syndrome or Di Sala syndrome, is primarily characterized by nasal hypoplasia and skeletal abnormalities, including short limbs and digits (brachydactyly) and stippled epiphyses. Holoprosencephaly is the failure of the prosencephalon, or forebrain, to develop normally. It affects facial features, causing closely spaced eyes, small head size, and sometimes clefts of the lip and roof of the mouth. This malformation is thought to be genetic but can occur in fetal alcohol syndrome or with high doses of vitamin A during early embryonic development.

66. D) Microcephaly

Microcephaly is caused by prenatal exposure to neurotoxic drugs and by teratogenic conditions such as congenital rubella, congenital cytomegalovirus, congenital Zika, and congenital toxoplasmosis infections. Congenitally imperfect ridge formation is a result of disturbances in embryologic development during the period of ridge differentiation. This trait is suspected in future development of schizophrenia. There are no linked neurotoxic drugs or teratogenic conditions. A high-steepled palate occasionally occurs in association with congenital syndromes such as Marfan syndrome. Marfan syndrome is a disorder of the body's connective tissues, a group of tissues that maintain the structure of the body and support internal organs and other tissues. Children usually inherit the disorder from one of their parents. A curved little finger (clinodactyly) may be genetic or a syndrome. About 35% to 70% of children with Down syndrome have clinodactyly. Clinodactyly is linked with multiple congenital chromosomal disorders and prenatal exposure to neurotoxic drugs, but teratogenic conditions are not a factor.

67. D) Russell's sign

Bulimia nervosa is characterized by frequent binge eating followed by inappropriate compensatory behaviors to prevent weight gain, such as vomiting, use of laxatives or diuretics, fasting, or excessive exercise. The purging subtype is characterized by the use of self-induced vomiting, laxatives, enemas, or diuretics. The most characteristic cutaneous sign of vomiting is Russell's sign (knuckle calluses). Acrocyanosis is a bluish discoloration of the extremities due to decreased amounts of oxygen delivered to the peripheral part. It is seen in patients with anorexia nervosa. Lanugo, a symptom of deep starvation, is characterized by a soft, downy, fine, white/light hair that grows mainly on the arms, chest, back, and face of a patient with an eating disorder. The body grows lanugo as a means of insulating itself to maintain body temperature as fat stores are depleted. It is most commonly seen in patients with anorexia nervosa. Prader-Willi syndrome is a leading genetic cause of food craving and weight gain and is associated with short stature.

68. A patient is brought to the emergency department after the family calls 911. The patient is unable to provide history. The nurse practitioner notes pupillary dilation, sensitivity to light, persistent yawning, and rhinorrhea. The patient is sweating. Vital signs are abnormal (tachycardia, hypertension, hyperthermia). The nurse practitioner will diagnose:

    A. Cocaine intoxication
    B. Cannabis toxicity
    C. Anticholinergic overdose
    D. Opioid withdrawal

69. A patient has been treated with haloperidol (Haldol) for several years. During the physical examination, the patient exhibits drooling, nonresting hand tremor, upper extremity stiffness, and pill rolling movements of the fingers. These are extrapyramidal symptoms known as:

    A. Anticholinergic effects
    B. Parkinson's disease
    C. Dystonic reaction
    D. Pseudoparkinsonism

70. A patient diagnosed with schizophrenia has been on fluphenazine (Prolixin) for decades. The patient denies any physical problems. Physical examination reveals abnormal finger movements (as if playing the guitar), tooth decay, and chapped lips. The patient is unable to bear weight on the right ankle, and the ankle appears twisted. The psychiatric-mental health nurse practitioner suspects:

    A. Dyskinesias
    B. Parkinson's disease
    C. Tardive dyskinesia
    D. Dysdiadochokinesia

(See answers next page.)

68. D) Opioid withdrawal

When a patient who is dependent on opioids suddenly stops taking them, the patient will experience lacrimation or rhinorrhea, piloerection "goose flesh," myalgia, diarrhea, nausea/vomiting, photophobia, insomnia, and autonomic hyperactivity (tachypnea, hyperreflexia, sweating, and yawning). Cocaine intoxication presents with great dilation of pupils, elevated blood pressure, increased pulse, raised temperature, sweating, and tremor. Cannabis toxicity presents with shallow breathing, drooling, dizziness, itching/scratching, slow pulse, and lowered temperature. Anticholinergic overdose presents with dry skin, hyperthermia, mydriasis, tachycardia, delirium, thirst, and urinary retention.

69. D) Pseudoparkinsonism

Pseudoparkinsonism is caused by reaction to a drug such as haloperidol. Anticholinergic effects are also a drug reaction whose classic physical presentation includes pupillary dilation and visual defects, flushing, hyperthermia, dry mucosa/skin, and tachycardia. Parkinson's disease symptoms may be difficult to distinguish from pseudoparkinsonism. While resting tremors are common in patients with Parkinson's disease, they are not as common in pseudoparkinsonism. This is one way to tell the two conditions apart during the diagnostic process. Dystonic movements are defined as sustained muscle contractions, frequently causing twisting and repetitive movements or abnormal postures.

70. C) Tardive dyskinesia

Fluphenazine is in the class of drugs called antipsychotic, first-generation agents. The most frequent problems associated with the older generation of antipsychotic agents are extrapyramidal side effects and tardive dyskinesia. Patients taking these medications often have chronic, severe, persistent mental illness, such as schizophrenia. They may be poor historians or unable to describe symptoms that are abnormal; the physical exam is critical in these cases. This patient has classic symptoms of movement disorder (dystonia) as evidenced by abnormal finger movements and the twisted right ankle. One of the most common manifestations is an ankle that twists and won't bear weight. Patients with localized movement disorders affecting the oral-facial area, such as lip smacking, can have chapped lips. The patient is likely grinding his teeth (bruxism), causing erosion and tooth decay. Dyskinesias are involuntary, often hyperkinetic movements of various types that have no purpose and are not fully controllable by the patient. While this may describe some of the patient's symptoms, it does not describe the multiple symptoms of this patient. Patients with Parkinson's disease may have dyskinesia with uncontrolled movement; however, the patient's additional symptoms are not classic signs of Parkinson's disease. Dysdiadochokinesia is the inability to perform rapidly alternating hand movements.

Advanced Practice Skills

1. The patient will be starting a second-generation antipsychotic/mood stabilizer. The psychiatric-mental health nurse practitioner that explains ongoing monitoring will include weight and height, waist circumference, blood pressure, fasting plasma glucose, and fasting lipid profile. The nurse is explaining the risk of:

   A. Metabolic syndrome
   B. Tardive dyskinesia (TD)
   C. Extrapyramidal symptoms (EPS)
   D. Stevens-Johnson syndrome

2. The psychiatric-mental health nurse practitioner reviews the health record of a new patient diagnosed with major depressive disorder and documented psychomotor agitation. The nurse practitioner should expect to observe:

   A. Hypersomnia, leaden paralysis, or significant weight gain/increased appetite
   B. Rubbing or pulling of skin, difficulty sitting still, or wringing of hands
   C. Difficulty controlling worry, muscle tension, and irritability
   D. Repetitive hand washing, counting, or repeating words silently

3. An older adult presents with rapid-onset psychosis, ataxia, myoclonus, and dementia. The patient's condition, which is known to be rapidly progressive and fatal within a year, is:

   A. Thiamine deficiency
   B. Lyme disease
   C. Creutzfeldt-Jakob disease
   D. Urinary tract infection

4. The psychiatric-mental health nurse practitioner discontinues venlafaxine (Effexor) due to lack of positive response from the patient. The nurse practitioner advises the patient to expect the possibility of symptoms such as nausea, dizziness, "shock-like feeling," irritability, tremor, confusion, headache, or sweating. The nurse practitioner is reviewing symptoms of:

   A. Discontinuation syndrome
   B. Influenza
   C. Panic attack
   D. Sleep deprivation

1. A) Metabolic syndrome

Metabolic syndrome can occur with all second-generation antipsychotics and includes conditions such as high blood pressure, high blood sugar, and high cholesterol. TD, EPS, and Stevens-Johnson syndrome are not monitored by height and weight, waist circumference, blood pressure, fasting plasma glucose, or fasting lipid profile.

2. B) Rubbing or pulling of skin, difficulty sitting still, or wringing of hands

Rubbing or pulling of skin, difficulty sitting still, and wringing hands are all examples of psychomotor agitation. Hypersomnia, leaden paralysis, and significant weight gain/increased appetite are examples of atypical features of depression. Difficulty controlling worry, muscle tension, and irritability together are features of generalized anxiety disorder. Repetitive hand washing, counting, or repeating words silently are compulsions that can occur in patients with obsessive-compulsive disorder.

3. C) Creutzfeldt-Jakob disease

Patients with Creutzfeldt-Jakob disease feature rapidly progressive dementia with progressive neurological deficits. Ataxia and myoclonic jerks are present only in Creutzfeldt-Jakob disease. Thiamine deficiency is a clinical manifestation of Wernicke—Korsakoff syndrome. The hallmark of Lyme disease is an erythema migrans rash after a tick bite. Urinary infections are frequent and problematic in older adults. Confusion is commonly reported; however, ataxia, myoclonus, dementia, and evidential lethality are not symptoms of urinary tract infection.

4. A) Discontinuation syndrome

Discontinuation syndrome is frequently reported with venlafaxine (Effexor). Antidepressant discontinuation syndrome can include flu-like symptoms or symptoms similar to those of panic attacks, but the most likely cause of these symptoms in this patient would be discontinuation syndrome. Sleep deprivation can cause mood changes; however, only discontinuation syndrome includes shock-like symptoms.

5. When prescribing a stimulant, the psychiatric-mental health nurse practitioner explains that the patient may experience mydriasis if they take more than the dosage prescribed. Mydriasis is:

    A. Abnormally large and dilated pupils
    B. Excessive constriction of pupils
    C. Amblyopia
    D. Strabismus

6. The psychiatric-mental health nurse practitioner discusses with a patient the possible side effects of a prescribed medication, which include polyuria, polydipsia, weight gain, cognitive problems, tremor, sedation or lethargy, impaired coordination, gastrointestinal distress, hair loss, benign leukocytosis, acne, and edema. The medication most likely prescribed is:

    A. Valproate (Depakote)
    B. Lamotrigine (Lamictal)
    C. Lithium (Eskalith)
    D. Carbamazepine (Tegretol)

7. A middle-aged patient presents to the emergency department following an overdose of benztropine (Cogentin) and is diagnosed with atropine psychosis. The cluster of symptoms the psychiatric-mental health nurse practitioner documents are:

    A. Oculogyric crisis, torticollis, restlessness, and opisthotonus
    B. Rigidity, myoclonus, and restlessness
    C. Confusion, diplopia, flush, and delirium
    D. Lead-pipe rigidity, hyperthermia, elevated creatine phosphokinase, and elevated white blood cell count (WBC)

8. The psychiatric-mental health nurse practitioner is completing a mental status examination in an initial evaluation. The patient complains of being "down in the dumps" and is pulling and rubbing her skin, has difficulty sitting still, and is wringing her hands. The patient is exhibiting signs of:

    A. Comorbid generalized anxiety disorder
    B. Compulsions related to obsessive–compulsive disorder (OCD)
    C. Psychomotor agitation
    D. Atypical features of major depressive disorder

9. The nurse practitioner receives a call from a patient with schizophrenia who has taken clozapine (Clozaril) 400 mg daily for over a year. The patient reports feeling physically ill, including malaise, sore throat, and fever. The nurse practitioner orders a complete blood count stat to rule out agranulocytosis. The result is an absolute neutrophil count (ANC) <500. The nurse practitioner explains that the patient:

    A. Needs to be evaluated for possible myocarditis
    B. Must discontinue the clozapine and be referred to hematology
    C. Must decrease the dosage of clozapine to 300 mg daily because the ANC is less than 500
    D. Should make an appointment with the primary care provider for evaluation of the fever

(See answers next page.)

5. A) Abnormally large and dilated pupils

Mydriasis is abnormally large and dilated pupils. Miosis is excessive constriction of pupils. Amblyopia (also called "lazy eye") is poor vision that occurs in just one eye. Strabismus (also known as crossed eyes) presents as a misalignment of both eyes.

6. C) Lithium (Eskalith)

Lithium is the only medication that has acne as a possible side effect. Valproate, lamotrigine, and carbamazepine may have some of these side effects, but acne is not one of them.

7. C) Confusion, diplopia, flush, and delirium

Atropine is in the anticholinergic drug family and is present in a variety of medications. Atropine psychosis occurs with the combination of atropine and the anticholinergic effects of other drugs, particularly antipsychotic drugs and anti-Parkinson's drugs. Confusion, diplopia, flush, and delirium are signs of atropine psychosis. Oculogyric crisis, torticollis, restlessness, and opisthotonus are drug-induced acute dystonic reactions. Rigidity, myoclonus, and restlessness are signs of serotonin syndrome. Lead-pipe rigidity, hyperthermia, elevated creatine phosphokinase, and elevated WBC are signs of neuroleptic malignant syndrome.

8. C) Psychomotor agitation

Psychomotor agitation is one of nine symptoms listed as DSM-5 criteria A for major depressive disorder. It is exhibited through rubbing or pulling of the skin and/or clothing; pacing is a key manifestation, as is inability to be still or fidgeting. While restlessness is found in generalized anxiety disorder, worry and fatigue are key features, which are not present in this patient. Likewise, those with OCD have irritability and agitation, but this is due to an inability to control one's environment. Patients with obsessive—compulsive disorder will have obtrusive thoughts that involve rituals and/or numbers, such as washing hands a certain amount of times. Atypical features of depression include mood reactivity, significant weight gain/increase in appetite, leaden paralysis, hypersomnia, or interpersonal rejection.

9. B) Must discontinue the clozapine and be referred to hematology

An ANC less than 500 indicates severe neutropenia. Treatment must be interrupted. Referral to hematology is recommended. Myocarditis is a risk factor, but only in the first 6 weeks of treatment; this patient has been on clozapine for over a year. Decreasing the dosage is inappropriate with an ANC that low. Following up with the primary care provider (PCP) is an option; however, PCPs generally will not manage clozapine-induced neutropenia; a referral to hematology is indicated.

10. A patient's signs or symptoms to record under the perception component of the mental status examination during a clinical interview include:

    A. Ability to plan and execute a course of action after appraisal of a problem or situation
    B. Hallucinations, illusions, depersonalization, or derealization
    C. Level of alertness, memory, orientation, calculation, and fund of knowledge
    D. Capacity to appraise one's thoughts, feelings, and actions for appropriateness

11. During an initial psychiatric interview, a patient reports that this is their first time being evaluated for possible hospitalization and that they have no past history of psychiatric diagnosis, even after admitting to suicidal ideation. The psychiatric-mental health nurse practitioner has determined that the patient has not slept >2 hours at a time, has been told that they talk excessively by others, and has been easily distracted over the past week. Based on this evaluation, the nurse practitioner makes a diagnosis of bipolar I disorder over bipolar II disorder because there is:

    A. Evidence of mania
    B. History of suicide attempt
    C. At least one major depressive episode
    D. No history of psychiatric inpatient admissions

12. Auditory hallucinations are documented in the mental status examination under:

    A. Judgment
    B. Insight
    C. Perception
    D. Cognition

13. The psychiatric-mental health nurse practitioner is completing the developmental and social history portion of an initial psychiatric interview. The best way to gather this information is:

    A. Chronologically, working backward from the present
    B. Beginning with the patient's first contact with the mental health provider
    C. From the first developmental milestone the patient can recall
    D. Chronologically, working forward from birth

14. After determining the baseline functioning of a psychiatric patient, the next step would be to:

    A. Narrow the choices of psychiatric medications to prescribe
    B. Determine what psychosocial modality should be started immediately
    C. Predict the course of manic or depressive episodes to establish treatment
    D. Establish appropriate diagnosis and begin treatment planning

(See answers next page.)

10. B) Hallucinations, illusions, depersonalization, or derealization

Perceptual abnormalities recorded in the mental status examination include illusions, hallucinations, derealization, and depersonalization. Judgment is the ability to plan and execute a course of action after appraisal of a problem or situation. Cognition includes level of alertness, memory, orientation, calculation, and fund of knowledge. Insight is the individual's capacity to appraise one's thoughts, feelings, and actions for appropriateness.

11. A) Evidence of mania

Bipolar I disorder requires that the DSM-5 criterion for at least one manic episode must be met. This is the factor that differentiates bipolar I from bipolar II disorder. History of suicide attempt, psychiatric hospitalization, and episode(s) of depression do not distinguish bipolar I from bipolar II disorder.

12. C) Perception

Perceptual abnormalities recorded in the mental status examination include illusions, hallucinations, derealization, and depersonalization and would appear under the perception portion of the examination. Judgment is the ability to plan and execute a course of action after appraisal of a problem or situation. Insight is the capacity to appraise one's thoughts, feelings, and actions for appropriateness. Cognition includes level of alertness, memory, orientation, calculation, and fund of knowledge. Although judgment, insight, and cognition are components of the mental status examination, hallucinations would be documented under perception.

13. D) Chronologically, working forward from birth

Obtaining developmental and social history chronologically from birth to the present offers a natural flow of questions and helps to elicit a full history. Other approaches may prevent the psychiatric-mental health nurse practitioner from identifying pertinent causation and triggering factors for disorder/disease development because this should be a review of all stages of an individual's life.

14. D) Establish appropriate diagnosis and begin treatment planning

The goal of obtaining baseline functioning during the psychiatric interview is to determine the appropriate diagnosis and set treatment goals for the patient. Only after an appropriate diagnosis and partnering with the patient to develop an evidence-based treatment plan should decisions about medications and psychotherapy occur. Many variables contribute to the course of any psychiatric disorder, and predicting specific episodes cannot be done.

15. When performing an initial psychiatric evaluation, the psychiatric-mental health nurse practitioner completes the developmental and social history chronologically from birth to present to:

    A. Review all stages of an individual's life
    B. Assess the patient's memory
    C. Determine possible genetic causes of symptoms
    D. Decide what medications to prescribe

16. Conducting an initial psychiatric evaluation allows the psychiatric-mental health nurse practitioner to gather information to determine an appropriate diagnosis and set treatment goals. Information gained during this evaluation reveals:

    A. Appropriate types of psychotherapy to initiate
    B. Patient's baseline functioning
    C. Predictors of the disorder's course and prognosis
    D. Psychotropic medications that will work for the patient

17. The psychiatric-mental health nurse practitioner is evaluating a patient who has flight of ideas. This is documented in the mental status examination as:

    A. Thought content
    B. Thought process
    C. Patient mood
    D. Patient affect

18. The psychiatric-mental health nurse practitioner is evaluating a patient and asks them to interpret a proverb. The ability of a patient to correctly interpret a proverb indicates good:

    A. Abstract reasoning
    B. Thought content
    C. Judgment
    D. Insight

19. The psychiatric-mental health nurse practitioner is performing a mental status examination on a 6-year-old patient. The patient is not able to recall three objects after 5 minutes, repeat five digits forward, or add simple numbers. The nurse practitioner's next step is to:

    A. Continue with the examination; these are normal findings
    B. Suspect the child has an anxiety disorder
    C. Refer the child to a neurologist to assess for brain damage
    D. Suspect the child has a panic disorder

(See answers next page.)

15. A) Review all stages of an individual's life

Obtaining developmental and social history chronologically from birth to present offers a natural flow of questions, helps to elicit a full history, and is a review of all stages of an individual's life. Memory is assessed during the mental status examination. Family history assessment will elicit information to allow consideration of potential genetic correlations with symptoms. Multiple other factors are considered when determining appropriate medications for treating any disorder.

16. B) Patient's baseline functioning

The goal of the initial psychiatric evaluation is to assess baseline functioning to determine appropriate diagnosis and set treatment goals. After treatment strategies are developed, initiation of an evidence-based psychotherapy modality may be determined necessary. Factors such as compliance and treatment efficacy will impact a disorder's course. As all patients are individuals, psychotropic medications may or may not be indicated, and tolerability and efficacy can vary throughout medication classifications.

17. B) Thought process

Thought process describes how thoughts are formulated, organized, and expressed. A patient can have normal thought process with delusional thought content, or normal thought content with impaired thought process. Normal thought process is described as organized, linear, and goal directed. Impaired thought process can be described as a flight of ideas, circumstantiality, clang association, derailment, neologism, perseveration, tangentiality, or thought blocking. Thought content differs from thought process because it describes what types of thoughts are occurring to the patient, which are described during the context of the evaluation. Affect is the expression of mood that is reflected in the patient's appearance and what the nurse practitioner observes. Mood refers to the patient's internal and sustained emotional state; it is a subjective report of what the patient states they feel.

18. A) Abstract reasoning

Abstract reasoning is the ability to shift back and forth between general concepts and specific examples. This can be tested by asking the patient to interpret a proverb or identify similar objects or concepts. Thought content describes what types of thoughts are occurring to the patient, which are described during the evaluation. Judgment refers to the patient's ability to make well-reasoned decisions and act on them. Insight is the patient's understanding of how they feel, present, and function, as well as the potential cause of their psychiatric condition.

19. C) Refer the child to a neurologist to assess for brain damage

A school-age child should be able to recall three objects after 5 minutes, repeat up to five digits forward and three digits backward, and add simple numbers. These are assessments of memory. An inability to perform these tasks may indicate brain damage, intellectual disability, or a learning disability. Referring to a neurologist to assess for brain damage is the next best step. Although anxiety or a panic disorder may interfere with the child's ability to perform, the inability to do these simple tasks warrants attention.

20. The psychiatric-mental health nurse practitioner is assessing a patient who reports difficulty initiating and maintaining sleep 4 to 5 days per week, which affects the patient's ability to perform well at work. Before initiating a treatment plan, the nurse practitioner must first assess and educate the patient about:

    A. Sleep hygiene
    B. Mood record
    C. Patient Health Questionnaire (PHQ-9)
    D. General Anxiety Disorder-7 (GAD-7) screening tool

21. The psychiatric-mental health nurse practitioner is evaluating a patient who reports that they are sad. In the mental status examination, the nurse practitioner documents this finding as:

    A. Thought content
    B. Thought process
    C. Patient affect
    D. Patient mood

22. The psychiatric-mental health nurse practitioner has just prescribed phenelzine (Nardil) to a patient with treatment-resistant depression. To help the patient avoid a potentially life-threatening adverse effect, the nurse practitioner includes in the medication education that:

    A. A slow titration schedule for the medication is necessary
    B. The patient should take the medication at night to avoid sedation and prevent falls
    C. The medication must be tapered gradually when discontinuing
    D. The patient should avoid consuming foods that are high in tyramine

23. The psychiatric-mental health nurse practitioner is evaluating a patient who expresses delusional thoughts that are grandiose in nature. In the mental status examination, the nurse practitioner documents this finding as:

    A. Thought process
    B. Thought content
    C. Patient mood
    D. Patient affect

24. The psychiatric-mental health nurse practitioner is reviewing the treatment plan of an adolescent patient who was just diagnosed with major depressive disorder and placed on an antidepressant. When providing patient education, the nurse practitioner would prioritize including the information that:

    A. The medication will take 4 to 6 weeks to take effect
    B. The medication will be started at a low dose due to the patient's age
    C. The medication carries a risk of serotonin syndrome
    D. The medication may cause activation of suicidal thoughts

(See answers next page.)

20. A) Sleep hygiene
The patient is presenting with symptoms of insomnia. Before initiating treatment for insomnia, the nurse practitioner should assess and educate the patient regarding sleep hygiene practices and identify modifiable factors that may be affecting the patient's sleep. A mood record, PHQ-9, and GAD-7 screening tool would be important assessment tools and points of psychoeducation to use during an initial evaluation; however, the patient's primary report of symptoms should lead the nurse to suspect insomnia, so the priority is to assess sleep hygiene.

21. D) Patient mood
Mood is defined as the patient's internal and sustained emotional state. It is a subjective report of what the patient states they feel. Affect differs from mood in that it is the expression of mood that is reflected in the patient's appearance and what the nurse practitioner observes. Thought content is what type of thoughts are occurring to the patient, which are described during the context of the evaluation. Thought process differs from thought content because it describes how thoughts are formulated rather than what the person is thinking.

22. D) The patient should avoid consuming foods that are high in tyramine
Phenelzine is a monoamine oxidase inhibitor used in treatment-resistant depression. A life-threatening side effect of this medication is hypertensive crisis, which can occur when the patient consumes foods and drinks high in tyramine, such as smoked meats, fish, aged cheese, beer, red wine, and fermented foods. A slow titration is not necessary with phenelzine, and neither is a slow taper when discontinuing because the drug wears off slowly over 2 to 3 weeks. Although phenelzine may cause sedation, this side effect is rare because phenelzine is usually activating; moreover, increased sedation is not a life-threatening adverse effect.

23. B) Thought content
Thought content describes what type of thoughts are occurring to the patient, which are described during the context of the evaluation. These can be obsessional, suicidal, homicidal, or delusional thoughts. Thought process differs from thought content because it describes how thoughts are formulated rather than what the person is thinking. Affect is the expression of mood that is reflected in the patient's appearance and what the nurse practitioner observes. Mood refers to the patient's internal and sustained emotional state; it is a subjective report of what the patient states they feel.

24. D) The medication may cause activation of suicidal thoughts
Activation of suicidal thoughts is an FDA boxed warning on all antidepressants, indicating the increased risk of suicidal thoughts in children and adolescents. Although the other options are true and should be discussed, patient education on the possibility of suicidal thoughts takes precedence due to the high risk of death.

25. A 70-year-old patient with Parkinson's dementia has recently developed psychosis. The psychiatric-mental health nurse practitioner prescribes a low dose of quetiapine (Seroquel). When discussing the risk versus benefit of the medication, the nurse practitioner's first priority is educating the patient about:

    A. Activation of suicidal thoughts
    B. Increased risk of death
    C. Orthostatic hypotension
    D. Increased risk of falls

26. The psychiatric-mental health nurse practitioner is educating a patient regarding monoamine oxidase inhibitors (MAOIs), including that concurrent consumption of tyramine-containing foods will induce a hypertensive crisis. The nurse practitioner realizes the education was effective when the patient reports that they will not consume:

    A. Ripe bananas
    B. Smoked salmon
    C. Vodka tonic
    D. Chicken breast

27. The psychiatric-mental health nurse practitioner is evaluating a patient for symptoms of obsessive–compulsive disorder (OCD) using the Yale-Brown Obsessive–Compulsive Scale. The score that indicates moderate severity of symptoms is:

    A. 15
    B. 20
    C. 25
    D. 30

28. A clinician-administered scale that the psychiatric-mental health nurse practitioner uses to assess a patient's anxiety symptoms is the:

    A. General Anxiety Disorder-7 (GAD-7)
    B. Clinician-Administered PTSD Scale (CAPS)
    C. Patient Health Questionnaire (PHQ-9)
    D. Hamilton Anxiety Rating Scale (HAM-A)

29. The psychiatric-mental health nurse practitioner is assessing a 7-year-old child with reports of decreased concentration, hyperactivity, short attention span, and being easily distracted. The patient's parent reports that the child is not able to complete simple tasks at home such as bed making, and does not complete homework. The nurse practitioner decides that more information is needed and sends a screening tool home with the patient's parent, including one for the patient's teacher, to be filled out and brought back to the next visit. The screening tool the nurse practitioner uses is a:

    A. Young Mania Rating Scale
    B. Conners Rating Scale
    C. Hamilton Anxiety Rating Scale
    D. Brief Psychiatric Rating Scale

(See answers next page.)

25. B) Increased risk of death

Although quetiapine is one of the preferred antipsychotics to treat patients with psychosis who have Parkinson's disease, older adults with dementia-related psychosis who are given an antipsychotic are at increased risk of death, and this is noted as a boxed warning with all antipsychotics. The nurse practitioner should also educate the patient regarding the risk of increased falls and orthostatic hypotension, but the priority is to discuss the increased risk of death. Activation of suicidal thoughts is a boxed warning of antidepressant medications, not antipsychotics.

26. B) Smoked salmon

A hypertensive crisis occurs when MAOIs are taken with tyramine-containing foods such as smoked fish, aged cheeses, cured meats, organ meats, red wine, beer, and fermented foods such as sauerkraut. Ripe bananas, chicken breast, and vodka do not contain tyramine.

27. B) 20

The Yale-Brown Obsessive–Compulsive Scale is a standard instrument used to assess the severity of OCD symptoms. It is a 10-question scale that can be clinician administered or self-reported. Scores from 16 to 23 indicate moderate severity. Scores from 0 to 7 indicate subclinical severity, 9 to 15 mild, 24 to 31 severe, and 32 to 40 extreme.

28. D) Hamilton Anxiety Rating Scale (HAM-A)

The HAM-A is a 14-item clinician-rated anxiety scale used to assess both cognitive and somatic anxiety symptoms. A score of 14 is a threshold for clinically significant anxiety. The GAD-7 examines a patient's self-reported symptoms of anxiety. The CAPS is a 17-item scale used specifically to assess for posttraumatic stress disorder. The PHQ-9 is a nine-item patient-reported screening for symptoms of depression.

29. B) Conners rating scale

The patient is exhibiting signs and symptoms of attention deficit/hyperactivity disorder (ADHD). The Conners rating scale is used to help clinicians measure a range of childhood mental health disorders and is used most commonly to screen for ADHD symptoms. The Conners rating scale has parent, teacher, and self-report versions. The Young Mania Rating Scale is used to screen for bipolar disorder, the Hamilton Anxiety Rating Scale is used to screen for anxiety, and the Brief Psychiatric Rating Scale is used to assess for change or improvement in psychotic patients. Although it is important to screen for all possible mental health disorders, the Conners rating scale is the only scale that has both parent and teacher rating components; the other scales are clinician-administered screening tools.

30. The psychiatric-mental health nurse practitioner is evaluating a patient who is suspected to have a cognitive disorder. To further assess the patient's cognition, the nurse practitioner uses the:

   A. Beck Depression Inventory (BDI)
   B. Hamilton Rating Scale for Depression (HAM-D)
   C. Hamilton Anxiety Rating Scale (HAM-A)
   D. Mini-Mental State Exam (MMSE)

31. The psychiatric-mental health nurse practitioner is working in the psychiatric emergency department and wants to quickly screen a patient suspected of alcohol use disorder. The screening tool that best meets the needs of the nurse practitioner is the:

   A. CAGE questionnaire
   B. Michigan Alcoholism Screening Test (MAST) screening
   C. Addiction Severity Index (ASI) measure
   D. Panic Disorder Severity Scale (PDSS) scale

32. When educating the patient regarding the medication lamotrigine (Lamictal), the psychiatric-mental health nurse practitioner makes sure to discuss the rare adverse effect of Stevens–Johnson syndrome. The patient should immediately report:

   A. Maculopapular rash
   B. Elevated blood pressure
   C. Nausea and vomiting
   D. Severe headache

33. The psychiatric-mental health nurse practitioner is educating a patient regarding lithium toxicity. The nurse practitioner concludes that the patient has understood the education when the patient states that they will report:

   A. Persistent nausea and vomiting
   B. Constant diarrhea
   C. Hyperthermia
   D. Uncontrolled shivering

34. An older adult patient is brought into the hospital and involuntarily admitted for alcohol detoxification. After 72 hours, the hospital can no longer hold the patient involuntarily but recommends voluntary admission to an alcohol detox facility to further assist in recovery. This recommendation is supported by:

   A. A standard rule that all detox patients need further treatment in a facility
   B. A higher risk of adverse effects for older persons suffering from substance use disorder
   C. The appearance of a higher risk for relapse that means the patient does not seem competent to remain sober after discharge
   D. The patient's initial involuntary admission, which suggests they might resist change and therefore should go to a facility

(See answers next page.)

30. D) Mini-Mental State Exam (MMSE)

The MMSE is a 30-point cognitive test that is used to assess a broad array of cognitive functions, including attention, memory, cognition, and construction of language. The BDI and HAM-D would both be useful if the nurse practitioner suspects an underlying depressive symptomology that could co-occur or mimic a cognitive disorder. The HAM-A would be useful in evaluating a patient who is suspected of having an anxiety disorder.

31. A) CAGE questionnaire

The CAGE questionnaire is a quick screening tool for significant alcohol problems. CAGE is an acronym used to guide the clinician in the questioning, as follows: C: Have you ever felt you needed to cut down on your drinking? A: Have people annoyed you by criticizing your drinking? G: Have you ever felt guilty or bad about your drinking? E: Have you ever had a drink first thing in the morning to get rid of a hangover (eye-opener)? Each yes answer is scored as 1 point for a total of 4 points. A score of 1 needs further evaluation, and a score of 2 or more indicates significant alcohol problems. The MAST is a 22-item self-report. The ASI measure of symptoms, is a comprehensive quantitative tool used by clinicians to assess alcohol or drug disorders; it takes more than 1 hour in a structured interview to perform. The PDSS, is used to screen for panic disorder, not alcohol use disorder.

32. A) Maculopapular rash

Stevens–Johnson syndrome is a life-threatening adverse effect of lamotrigine. Symptoms include a maculopapular rash that develops all over the body and begins to necrotize. This may occur when lamotrigine is titrated too rapidly or combined with valproate (Depakote). Elevated blood pressure, nausea, vomiting, and severe headache are symptoms of hypertensive crisis, which occurs with the use of monoamine oxidase inhibitors along with tyramine-containing foods.

33. A) Persistent nausea and vomiting

Lithium toxicity can occur with lithium levels above 1.5 mEq/L. Toxicity ranges from mild to severe with symptoms including, but not limited to, persistent nausea and vomiting, abdominal pain, ataxia, tremors, blurred vision, delirium, syncope, and coma. Constant diarrhea, hyperthermia, and uncontrolled shivering are not signs of lithium toxicity but of serotonin syndrome, which may occur with concurrent use of lithium and an antidepressant.

34. B) A higher risk of adverse effects for older persons suffering from substance use disorder

Generally, older patients are more likely to have a higher risk of adverse effects due to coexisting medical or psychiatric conditions. They might have financial strain and a lack of care and support once discharged, which can also increase the risk for adverse effects. Continuous monitoring and collaboration with primary care providers and specialists can help minimize more severe adverse reactions and improve treatment outcomes. Although it is recommended that patients suffering from substance use disorder seek additional supportive services as a part of the recovery process to decrease the likelihood of relapse, there is no "standard rule," because not all patients require treatment in a specialized treatment facility to recover. That the patient is not competent to remain sober is an unfounded assumption, and more information is required. One of the most significant factors that impacts an individual's recovery is resistance to change. The first step in recovery with good outcomes is willingness to change. Therefore, forcing someone to go into treatment because they may resist change presents a decreased likelihood that they will experience overall benefits from the program.

35. A screening questionnaire used to identify adverse incidents that occurred during a patient's childhood and increase the patient's likelihood to suffer lifelong consequences is the:

   A. Scale of Adverse Childhood Experiences (ACE Scale)
   B. Mini-Mental Status Exam (MMSE)
   C. Child Attachment Interview (CAI)
   D. Young Mania Rating Scale (YMRS)

36. The psychiatric-mental health nurse practitioner is evaluating a 65-year-old patient with reports of low energy, poor concentration, and low mood. When conducting the geriatric depression scale (GDS) short form, the nurse determines the score to be 13. The action the nurse practitioner takes is to:

   A. Continue with the assessment as usual
   B. Perform a suicide risk assessment
   C. Start the patient on sertraline
   D. Call emergency medical services

37. If a patient presents for evaluation of posttraumatic stress disorder (PTSD), the assessment tool the psychiatric-mental health nurse practitioner would use to assess for the severity of the patient's symptoms is:

   A. Clinician-Administered PTSD Scale (CAPS)
   B. Panic Disorder Severity Scale (PDSS)
   C. Hamilton Anxiety Rating Scale (HAM-A)
   D. Hamilton Rating Scale for Depression (HAM-D)

38. A nontraditional method that helps improve brain function and cognition to further assist with building resilience is:

   A. Attending weekly psychotherapy sessions with a counselor
   B. Practicing mindfulness and journaling
   C. Joining a trauma support group offered at school
   D. Engaging in regular physical exercise

39. A factor that enhances resilience in individuals recovering from a traumatic event is:

   A. Presence of supportive relationships and purpose
   B. Avoidance of things that might trigger memories of trauma
   C. Regarding of past trauma as a negative event
   D. Feeling anger at the event or person that caused trauma

(See answers next page.)

35. A) Scale of Adverse Childhood Experiences (ACE Scale)

The ACE Scale can play a role in identifying a patient's likelihood of suffering from diseases, mental health issues, and poorer outcomes. Recognizing the score early on helps guide implementation of healthy interventions into the treatment plan to improve patient outcomes and assist with the development of resilience and recovery from these adverse experiences. The MMSE assesses patients' cognition and overall cognitive abilities to look for any signs of dementia. It is usually performed in the older adult population. The CAI looks into what things are like in a family from a patient's point of view to help the interviewer better understand the patient. The YMRS is used to assess the patient's severity of manic symptoms.

36. B) Perform a suicide risk assessment

A score of 13 on the GDS is a positive screen for severe depressive symptoms. A patient who is experiencing severe depressive symptoms should be assessed for safety as a priority intervention; therefore, performing a suicide risk assessment is the next step. To continue with the assessment as usual would not address safety, and safety is the priority. The patient may be started on medication or may need emergency medical services depending on the outcome of the suicide risk assessment.

37. A) Clinician-Administered PTSD Scale (CAPS)

The CAPS is a 17-item scale that clinicians may use to diagnose PTSD. The items can also be used to generate a total PTSD severity score, which is obtained by summing the frequency and intensity scales for each item. The PDSS can be useful in determining severity of panic attacks, which may or may not be present in someone with PTSD. The HAM-A is used to assess for generalized anxiety disorder, which may be comorbid with PTSD. However, it does not measure PTSD symptom severity. The HAM-D is used to assess for major depression in patients, which too may be comorbid in some patients with PTSD; however, the HAM-D does not measure PTSD symptoms severity.

38. D) Engaging in regular physical exercise

Several scientific studies indicate that physical exercise helps improve brain function and cognitive abilities, including thinking and memory. It can also help reduce the rates of cortisol released from stress. Exercise as a whole can help elevate moods and calm anxiety, thereby assisting in the healing process toward recovery and building resilience. Attending weekly psychotherapy sessions, practicing mindfulness and journaling, and joining a trauma support group are forms of traditional therapy.

39. A) Presence of supportive relationships and purpose

Studies have shown that supportive relationships, attachments, and a sense of purpose can help enhance an individual's resilience and recovery. Avoiding things that may trigger a response is not always the best option. While it is a protective measure, it does not allow the individual to work through trauma, process, and attempt to heal. Working with a skilled therapist who can safely help the patient process the trauma and manage triggers can further facilitate healing. Looking back at the traumatic event as solely negative may negate the recovery process, whereas reframing the incident and looking at it from a more positive mindset may assist with building resilience and helping the patent cope. Feeling hurt or angry at the person or situation is an emotion and a normal part of the grieving and processing portion of healing; however, it does not explicitly enhance resilience on its own.

40. A young adult patient calls the office and reports diarrhea, heavy sweating, goosebumps, shivering, and pupils that look slightly dilated as noted by the patient's parent. The symptoms began a few hours ago after the patient started paroxetine (Paxil) 20 mg for depression. The nurse practitioner will:

    A. Have the nurse contact the patient regarding the side effects with assurances of gradual improvement after a week or so
    B. Inform the patient to reduce the dosage of paroxetine to 10 mg for a few days and see if that improves the side effects
    C. Immediately discontinue the paroxetine and start the patient on fluoxetine (Prozac) 20 mg
    D. Refer the patient to the emergency department with instructions to discontinue the paroxetine immediately

41. The psychiatric-mental health nurse practitioner is screening a patient for alcohol use disorder using the CAGE questionnaire. To assess the "A" in CAGE, the nurse asks:

    A. "Have you felt anxious about your drinking?"
    B. "Have people felt alarmed by your drinking?"
    C. "Have people annoyed you by criticizing your drinking?"
    D. "Have you felt you needed to drink to feel awake?"

42. A young adult patient was discharged from a drug and alcohol program after spending 12 weeks detoxing from alcohol and opioids. After discharge, the patient understood the need to make lifestyle changes to continue supporting progress. An example of a healthy change the patient can make to support recovery is to:

    A. Return to employment at the local distillery
    B. Spend time at home reflecting on what was learned in recovery
    C. Enroll in a psychology course at the local community college
    D. Apply for a position as a receptionist at the pain clinic near home

43. When meeting for the first time a patient suffering from trauma, the psychiatric-mental health nurse practitioner would first:

    A. Introduce self and provide background
    B. Briefly discuss the therapeutic process
    C. Ensure that the patient feels safe and secure
    D. Obtain history and discuss treatment options

44. An older adult patient presents to the psychiatric-mental health nurse practitioner's office for an initial intake for depression. During the history-taking process, the patient admits to previously being in rehab for alcohol use disorder and having relapsed several times. The screening tool to administer to assess the patient for alcoholism is the:

    A. CAGE questionnaire
    B. Clinical Institute Withdrawal Assessment (CIWA) scale
    C. Hamilton Scale for Depression
    D. DSM-5 to assess the criteria for alcoholism

(See answers next page.)

40. D) Refer the patient to the emergency department with instructions to discontinue the paroxetine immediately

The patient reports symptoms consistent with the development of serotonin syndrome, which is considered a medical emergency and requires a higher-level evaluation of the symptoms. Other symptoms of serotonin syndrome include confusion, agitation, loss of muscle control, rapid heart rate, restlessness, changes in blood pressure, tremor, high fever, and seizures. While cutting back a medication or teaching the patient about side effects may be appropriate interventions for mild side effects, they do not appropriately address the patient's concerns about their symptoms. Starting the patient on fluoxetine does not address the problem; it poses additional risks to the patient's safety, considering that fluoxetine is also a selective serotonin reuptake inhibitor and increases serotonin at the synapse level.

41. C) "Have people annoyed you by criticizing your drinking?"

The CAGE questionnaire is a brief screening tool for significant alcohol problems. CAGE is an acronym used to guide the clinician in the questioning, as follows: C: Have you ever felt you needed to **cut down** on your drinking? A: Have people **annoyed** you by criticizing your drinking? G: Have you ever felt **guilty** or bad about your drinking? E: Have you ever had a drink first thing in the morning to get rid of a hangover (**eye-opener**)? Each yes answer is scored as 1 point for a total of 4 points. A score of 1 needs further evaluation, and a score of 2 or more indicates significant alcohol problems.

42. C) Enroll in a psychology course at the local community college

Part of recovery is to make healthy choices and lifestyle changes that help an individual to reach their highest potential. Enrolling in a course is a step toward making positive changes. While it is a good idea to reflect, an essential part of recovery is to make changes, and too much time spent reflecting misses a crucial element of the recovery process. While obtaining a job is a positive step forward, a position at a distillery or a pain clinic poses a risk for relapse due to the high likelihood of being exposed to alcohol or pain medication.

43. C) Ensure that the patient feels safe and secure

The healing process and interactions with the patient should start by building rapport and ensuring that the patient feels safe to assist with the stabilization process, to be followed by assessment of the need for further crisis interventions. A patient is more likely to be open and honest when they feel safe and trust their practitioner. The nurse practitioner might later provide background, discuss the therapeutic process, obtain history, and discuss treatment options, and each practitioner performs their care differently, but assessing safety must come before anything else.

44. A) CAGE questionnaire

The CAGE questionnaire is a quick screening tool that can assess alcoholism in a patient. A positive response to two or more of the questions increases the likelihood that the patient might struggle with alcoholism, and the nurse practitioner should then perform a further evaluation. The CIWA scale is a tool that is used to assess a patient who is experiencing alcohol withdrawal. The Hamilton Rating Scale for Depression is a tool used to evaluate a patient's depression complaints and is not specific to alcohol usage. Referring to the DSM-5 can help target the reported findings and assist with questioning, but it is not a specific screening tool for alcoholism and instead assists with determining if the patient meets the criteria for a particular mental illness.

45. A patient reports being 3 months sober from opioids. The psychiatric-mental health nurse practitioner will consider performing a toxicology screening upon noting that the patient:

A. Appears tired but is easily arousable
B. Has pinpoint pupils
C. Appears disheveled
D. Reports feeling constipated

46. A medication to reduce the risk of adverse reactions and further complications in cases of suspected opioid overdose is:

A. Naloxone
B. Naltrexone
C. Carbamazepine
D. Acamprosate

47. The psychiatric-mental health nurse practitioner follows up with an adult male patient regarding a CAGE questionnaire and notices that the patient reports frequently feeling like he should cut back on his alcohol usage. He admits to becoming annoyed by others around him when they "nag" him about his drinking and says he feels guilty at times but cannot stop using alcohol despite trying in the past. He denies that he feels the need to drink first thing in the morning and describes himself as a functional alcoholic. Based on these answers, the nurse practitioner diagnoses the patient with:

A. Alcohol abuse
B. Suspected alcoholism
C. Substance use disorder
D. Alcohol use disorder

48. A 16-year-old patient presents to the clinic with her parent for an evaluation. The patient reports feeling depressed and hopeless. She says her mind is always racing, and she has often felt anxious for no reason over the past 3 months. After further discussion, the nurse practitioner discovers that the patient is engaged in binging and purging activities. Per the parent, the patient recently had a comprehensive physical examination with an ECG and lab work, and everything was normal. The patient has never seen a therapist or any other specialist to manage her condition. The nurse practitioner's next best step is to:

A. Start the patient on bupropion (Wellbutrin) 150 mg XR to address low energy and motivation
B. Admit the patient into an intensive outpatient program for eating issues
C. Start the patient on escitalopram (Lexapro) 10 mg and refer the patient to therapy
D. Refer the patient to a dietitian to address the binging and purging issues

(See answers next page.)

45. B) Has pinpoint pupils

Patients who are acutely intoxicated with opioids may have pinpoint pupils, display slurred speech, be sedated, and, if recently injected, may have track marks or new injection sites that are noticeable during the assessment. Although sedation can be present with opioid intoxication, the patient appearing tired but easily arousable would not, by itself, warrant a toxicology screening. Similarly, a disheveled appearance is insufficient grounds for a toxicology screening; there may be many reasons for the appearance that are unrelated to substance use. Long-term opioid usage, in general, can lead to the development of constipation; however, there are several other reasons that the patient might be reporting constipation. The nurse practitioner would require more information and further assessment to determine if the constipation is caused by opioid usage.

46. A) Naloxone

Naloxone is an opioid antagonist that can rapidly reverse and quickly restore normal breathing in the case of opioid overdose, reducing the risks of further complications. Naltrexone is a Mu opioid receptor antagonist used to reduce cravings and the rewarding effects of alcohol. Carbamazepine is an anticonvulsant medication that is used in the treatment of seizures and chronic neuropathic pain. Acamprosate is used for the treatment of alcohol dependence.

47. B) Suspected alcoholism

The CAGE questionnaire is a screening tool to assess for alcoholism. Two or more positive responses indicate that a person may suffer from alcoholism. Although the patient responded positively to three out of the four questions in the CAGE questionnaire, the nurse practitioner can give no formal diagnosis without further evaluation and assessment. The patient does not meet the criteria for substance or alcohol use disorder per DSM-5 criteria. Alcohol abuse is no longer an approved DSM-5 diagnosis, and therefore the nurse practitioner would not use this diagnosis.

48. C) Start the patient on escitalopram (Lexapro) 10 mg and refer the patient to therapy

The nurse practitioner will initiate a low dose of escitalopram and refer the patient to therapy. Due to reported symptoms, duration of symptoms, and an unremarkable medical history, starting the patient on a selective reuptake inhibitor such as escitalopram is the recommendation as a front-line treatment for depression and anxiety. Referral to therapy services is also beneficial to help address the root cause of her depression, anxiety, and eating issues to further assist the patient in developing healthy coping mechanisms and managing her symptoms more effectively. While bupropion effectively improves low motivation, drive, and energy levels in individuals suffering from depression, its use is contraindicated in individuals who are actively or previously engaged in binging/purging activities due to the risk of seizures and cardiovascular complications. Bupropion is also an activating medication and can often cause more anxiety in individuals who struggle with anxiety. The patient might require admission to an inpatient program later for her depression, anxiety, and eating disorder; however, the patient does not meet the criteria at this time. Referral to a dietitian would not address the patient's depression or anxiety.

49. A description of serotonin syndrome includes:

A. Development of a headache, appetite changes, and sleep disruption that begin shortly after starting escitalopram (Lexapro) and subside and improve after a week

B. Decrease in sexual drive and libido, increase in irritability, and mild gastrointestinal upset that improves a few days after starting sertraline (Zoloft)

C. Rapid onset of agitation, confusion, muscle rigidity, fever, and elevated blood pressure hours after starting sertraline (Zoloft)

D. Increase in sweating, diarrhea, agitation, and headaches that develops 2 days after starting paroxetine (Paxil)

50. A patient has been triaged by the medical assistant, and before entering the room, the psychiatric-mental health nurse practitioner briefly reviews the results of the patient's CAGE questionnaire from 1 year ago and the responses completed today. The results indicate that the patient has alcoholism. To gather more information about how the patient is feeling since the appointment a year ago, the nurse practitioner would:

A. Use the Michigan Alcohol Screening Test (MAST)

B. Analyze aspartate aminotransferase (AST) and alanine transaminase (ALT)

C. Perform a blood pressure check

D. Readminister the CAGE for accuracy

51. An older adult patient makes an appointment with a psychiatric-mental health nurse practitioner to address depression and anxiety symptoms that have been getting progressively worse after a myocardial infarction 3 months ago. When considering medication choices, the nurse practitioner will avoid prescribing:

A. Amitriptyline (Elavil)

B. Sertraline (Zoloft)

C. Fluoxetine (Prozac)

D. Lamotrigine (Lamictal)

52. The G in the CAGE questionnaire indicates:

A. Gluttony

B. Guilt

C. Greed

D. Gauge

53. Patients with anorexia nervosa have an increased rate of:

A. Job loss

B. Suicide

C. Drug usage

D. Domestic violence

(See answers next page.)

49. C) Rapid onset of agitation, confusion, muscle rigidity, fever, and elevated blood pressure hours after starting sertraline (Zoloft)

Serotonin syndrome is a medical emergency that requires prompt intervention and is a risk associated with starting selective serotonin reuptake inhibitors (SSRIs). It is characterized by a sudden onset of increased agitation, confusion, muscle rigidity, sweating, fever, extreme diarrhea, and elevated blood pressure. These issues occur shortly after starting medication with serotonergic properties; the risk of developing these issues is increased if the patient takes other drugs or supplements, such as St. John's wort, that also work on serotonin. Headache, appetite change, sleep disruption, decreased libido, and mild gastro-intestinal upset are all common side effects that can occur after initiating an SSRI and that generally subside after about a week. The risk of the development of side effects can be decreased by starting at a lower dosage. If symptoms are already occurring, reduce the dosage and continue monitoring the side effects and assessing for improvement.

50. A) Use the Michigan Alcohol Screening Test (MAST)

The MAST is a screening tool used to assess how a patient has felt and if they have experienced any issues in the past 12 months due to their drinking. While an AST, ALT, and blood pressure check are all typically part of a wellness check, none of them are concerned with how the patient is "feeling" concerning their drinking. Since the CAGE was administered today, there is no need to readminister it unless the practitioner suspects it was not completed correctly.

51. A) Amitriptyline (Elavil)

Amitriptyline is contraindicated in patients who recently experienced myocardial infarction due to the risk of developing cardiovascular arrhythmias, heart failure, QT prolongation, and other serious cardiovascular complications. Sertraline and fluoxetine have proven cardiovascular safety in patients suffering from depression following a myocardial infarction. While there is limited information on cardiovascular complications, lamotrigine is not contraindicated, although it should be used with caution. As with all other medications, careful consideration of the patient's history and current medicines, as well as knowledge of the risks, benefits, indications, and contraindications of drugs, is essential in the prescriptive process.

52. B) Guilt

The G in CAGE stands for Guilt and asks the patient if they have ever felt guilty about their drinking. Gluttony, greed, and gauge are not aspects of the CAGE questionnaire.

53. B) Suicide

Suicide rates are elevated in patients with anorexia nervosa. Therefore, a comprehensive assessment of suicidality and any reports of self-harm or other risk factors for suicide should be completed by the practitioner. There are no specific indications that a person with anorexia nervosa is at higher risk for losing their job, using drugs, or enduring domestic violence outside of the average population. However, any healthcare professional should always consider safety first, and these factors should be ruled out or mediated further.

54. On mental status examination, a patient's thoughts reveal a lack of directedness, excessive and often irrelevant details, and difficulty getting to the point of closure. This pattern is called:

    A. Tangentiality
    B. Circumstantiality
    C. Perseveration
    D. Thought blocking

55. When using the CAGE questionnaire, the psychiatric-mental health nurse practitioner will ask the patient:

    A. "Do you enjoy drinking?"
    B. "Do you ever feel you should cut down on your drinking?"
    C. "What made you decide to cut down on your drinking?"
    D. "Do you think you have a drinking problem?"

56. After being caught binge drinking on several occasions by their parents, a young adult patient responds to a CAGE screening after presenting to the office. After reviewing the screening, the psychiatric-mental health nurse practitioner determines that the patient may be suffering from alcoholism based on the patient saying:

    A. "I sometimes drink with my friends, but everyone does it, and it is not a huge deal."
    B. "I often feel guilty and think that I need to cut back on how often I drink."
    C. "Although I socially drink, I only have one or two drinks a few times a month, if that."
    D. "My dad was a functioning alcoholic, so I grew up around it."

57. A 75-year-old patient presents in the emergency department and is diagnosed with Wernicke encephalopathy. While performing a mental status examination, the psychiatric-mental health nurse practitioner expects ophthalmoplegia and other symptoms, including:

    A. Abnormal motor activity, sensorium, and cognitive ability
    B. Disturbances to perception and motor activity
    C. Abnormality in thought processes and impulse control
    D. Perceptual disturbances and abnormal thought processes

58. A 5-year-old is referred by his pediatrician for evaluation. The patient is withdrawn, has been drawing pictures with dark themes, has nightmares, and has nocturnal enuresis. The psychiatric-mental health nurse practitioner plans to interview the child and perform a mental status exam. The nurse practitioner proceeds:

    A. With the parent/caregiver present to complete Achenbach's Youth Self Report (YSR)
    B. To contact social services. Based on the patient's history, abuse is suspected
    C. With the parent/caregiver present to offer the child crayons and paper or age-appropriate toys
    D. Without the parent/caregiver present to ask the child close-ended questions

(See answers next page.)

54. B) Circumstantiality

Circumstantiality is a speech pattern characterized by roundabout irrelevant details, often unrelated, before the speaker gets to the main point. Tangentiality is a speech pattern that is characterized by unimportant, nonessential information but does not lose the main point. Perseveration occurs when a person continuously repeats the same thing abnormally (sound, word, or phrase). Thought blocking occurs when a person loses their train of thought and stops speaking. They are unable to complete an idea or conversation due to constant pauses.

55. B) "Do you ever feel you should cut down on your drinking?"

The "C" in the CAGE mnemonic asks if the patient ever feels the need to cut down on their drinking. This question is used during screening as an initial nonthreatening inquiry. Asking if the patient enjoys drinking is not included in the CAGE mnemonic. Asking about the decision to cut down or if the patient thinks they have a drinking problem are good follow-up questions that can be useful after the initial screening but are not included in the CAGE mnemonic.

56. B) "I often feel guilty and think that I need to cut back on how often I drink"

Two elements of the CAGE questionnaire are if the patient ever feels the need to "cut back," or if they ever feel "bad or guilty" about drinking habits. Having a positive response to two or more of the screening questions may indicate that the person is suffering from alcoholism or alcohol abuse. Occasional social drinking and growing up with a functional alcoholic may provide more information about the patient's drinking habits, but an element of the CAGE questionnaire would be needed to determine alcoholism.

57. A) Abnormal motor activity, sensorium, and cognitive ability

Wernicke encephalopathy is diagnosed with a triad of acute mental confusion, ataxia, and ophthalmoplegia. The nurse practitioner should expect to find a deficit in sensorium and cognitive ability, evidenced by confusion or memory loss. Motor activity is abnormal with the presence of an ataxic gait. Perceptual disturbances (such as hallucinations, illusions, depersonalization, or derealization) are not present in the triad of symptoms. Abnormality in thought processes (the content of thought) such as delusions, suicidal/homicidal ideas, obsessions, or paranoia is not present in the triad of symptoms.

58. C) With the parent/caregiver present to offer the child crayons and paper or age-appropriate toys

Preschool-aged children should always have a parent/caregiver present. Very young children show their feelings during play. Bringing toys or allowing them to draw will facilitate a comfortable environment. Children often share more when engaged in play while answering questions from an adult stranger. The YSR is a 112-item self-report designed for children and adolescents ages 11 to 17; it is inappropriate for a 5-year-old child. Contacting social services is premature. Asking a child direct questions is appropriate; however, open-ended questions are the preferred communication technique in all psychiatric interviews.

59. The psychiatric-mental health nurse practitioner will perform an alcohol and drug screening assessment on a patient who is 18 weeks pregnant and suspected of using drugs and alcohol using:

   A. The Michigan Alcohol Screening Test (MAST)
   B. The used, neglected, cut down, objected preoccupied, emotional discomfort (UNCOPE)
   C. The Clinical Institute Withdrawal Assessment (CIWA)
   D. CAGE

60. In the mental status examination, the psychiatric-mental health nurse practitioner documents that a patient is using imitative behavior and copies the gestures that other people in the room are using. This is an example of:

   A. Neologism
   B. Catatonia
   C. Echolalia
   D. Echopraxia

61. A 23-year-old patient visits a psychiatric-mental health nurse practitioner accompanied by a close friend. The nurse practitioner observes that the patient's face is pale and bruised. The patient shares that she got married 3 months ago and that her spouse is a binge drinker. She states that she is not allowed to work or to participate in activities according to her free will, and that attempts to do so usually result in verbal or physical abuse. During the interview, the nurse practitioner observes that the patient is not maintaining direct eye contact while speaking and that her hands are trembling. When the nurse practitioner tries to move closer to the patient and examine the bruises, the patient jumps up and asks the nurse to stay away from her. The nurse practitioner should:

   A. Ask whether the patient is forced to do things without her consent
   B. Perform a physical examination even if the patient is resistant
   C. Avoid validation and judgmental responses
   D. Ask the friend of the patient to stay in the room during the interview

62. The portion of the medical history addressing familial, occupational, and recreational aspects of the patient's personal life that have the potential to be clinically significant is the history known as:

   A. Personal/social
   B. Surgical
   C. Past
   D. Family

(See answers next page.)

59. B) The used, neglected, cut down, objected preoccupied, emotional discomfort (UNCOPE)

The UNCOPE is a tool used to screen for alcohol and drug use in pregnant patients. The MAST is a screening tool used to assess how a patient has felt or if they have experienced any issues in the past 12 months due to drinking. The CIWA scale is used to assess the severity of alcohol withdrawal. The CAGE test is used to screen for alcohol dependence in all adults, not just pregnant patients, and it does not address drug use.

60. D) Echopraxia

Echopraxia refers to a pathological automatic or semi-automatic imitation or mimicking of movement. Neologism is the invention of words that are meaningless to others but understood by the patient. Catatonia is a psychomotor disorder and would not be part of the mental status examination. Echolalia is repeating or mimicking what others say repetitively.

61. A) Ask whether the patient is forced to do things without her consent

In cases of domestic abuse, sexual abuse is also commonly observed. Therefore, a nurse practitioner needs to ask the patient if she was ever sexually abused or forced into acts without her consent. It is necessary to perform a physical assessment, in order to check for signs of vaginal laceration or bruises on other parts of the body resulting from sexual or physical abuse. However, if the patient does not give her consent, then her decision should be respected, and the nurse practitioner should not conduct the physical assessment. Giving judgmental responses should be strictly avoided because it is not an approach of a skilled interviewer. However, an empathetic approach and validation are necessary because they help to make a patient feel comfortable. For a patient who has experienced abuse or trauma, it is highly recommended to conduct the interview process privately and not in others' presence.

62. A) Personal/social

The personal and social history includes information about life events, social class, race, religion, and occupation. It describes the patient's education level and relationships. Surgical history is the history of the surgeries that the patient has had, past history involves the past illness or surgeries that the patient might have had. Family history includes any condition that a family member has or once had.

63. A 60-year-old patient with chronic schizophrenia is waiting for an initial assessment in the psychiatric-mental health nurse practitioner's office. The nurse practitioner asks the patient to "hop over here to this chair." The patient hops to the adjacent chair. The nurse practitioner asks the patient, "What brought you to the clinic today?" The patient answers, "The van." As the evaluation continues, the nurse practitioner decides to include the Mini-Mental Status Exam (MMSE) and asks, "What does it mean when someone says a rolling stone gathers no moss?" The patient responds, "The stone is moving, so no moss gets on it." The patient's behavior and responses are examples of:

A. Psychosis

B. Concrete thinking

C. Anxiety

D. Oppositional behavior

64. A 15-year-old patient presents for evaluation in the emergency department for a severe headache. The patient reports sudden-onset chest pain, nausea, difficulty concentrating, heart palpitations, and shortness of breath. The patient denies any previous history of these symptoms or any recent trauma. Complete blood count, complete metabolic panel, urinalysis, thyroid-stimulating hormone test, and ECG are normal. Vital signs are normal. The medical team has cleared the patient, and psychiatry has been consulted. The psychiatric-mental health nurse practitioner's diagnosis is:

A. Generalized anxiety disorder

B. Posttraumatic stress disorder

C. Panic attack

D. Panic disorder

65. A 75-year-old patient reports memory and mood problems, stating, "I find myself forgetting what I am going to say a lot. I feel sad and embarrassed." The psychiatric-mental health nurse practitioner asks the following set of questions: (1) What is today's date? (2) I will ask you to remember three things: a pen, a book, and a chair. Please repeat these three things. (3) Spell WORLD backward. (4) Beginning with 100, subtract 7. (5) Here is a blank piece of paper. Please write a sentence. (6) I am going to draw three shapes. Please copy the shapes. The patient scores a 20. The test used by the nurse practitioner is the:

A. Mini-Cog Instrument

B. Mini-Mental State Examination (MME)

C. Geriatric Depression Scale (GDS)

D. Beck Depression Inventory-II (BDI II)

66. A 35-year-old patient visits the clinic. She reports that during the last few months she has felt alone and sad and has burst into tears at unexpected times. She has sudden outbursts of anger, has lost interest in her relationship, and has insomnia. The screening tool the nurse practitioner will use for this patient is the:

A. Patient Health Questionnaire (PHQ-9)

B. Columbia Suicidal Severity Rating Scale

C. Montreal Cognitive Assessment

D. Insomnia Severity Index

(See answers next page.)

63. B) Concrete thinking
Concrete thinking is defined as the inability to engage in abstract thought. Chronic schizophrenics are limited in their understanding of nonliteral expressions, such as proverbs. Their reasoning is literal. The patient processes communication with exact interpretations. There is no evidence of active psychosis, which presents with delusions, hallucinations, and disorganized speech. The ability to think abstractly related to concentration may be affected by anxiety, but patients with anxiety can interpret proverbs and can abstractly reason. The patient is not resistant, defiant, or uncooperative, so there is no evidence of oppositional behavior.

64. C) Panic attack
In children, anxiety manifests with multiple somatic complaints. A panic attack is the first symptom that may lead to the diagnosis of panic disorder; an isolated attack does not meet the criteria for panic disorder. Generalized anxiety disorder is a chronic condition characterized by frequent, persistent worry and anxiety. Although the patient's symptoms can occur with post-traumatic stress disorder, diagnosis requires symptoms to have been present for at least a month. Panic disorder is a chronic condition requiring a history of panic attacks and persistent concern about having additional attacks that have lasted more than a month with significant changes in behavior.

65. B) Mini-Mental State Examination (MME)
The MME is a rating scale that is used to screen for cognitive deficits/dementia. It measures the severity of symptoms and is meant to track changes over time. A score of 20 indicates mild depression. The Mini-Cog instrument is used to screen for cognitive impairment in older adults in various settings. The Mini-Cog uses a three-item recall test for memory and a simply scored clock-drawing test. A score of 1 or 2 indicates a positive screen for dementia. The GDS is a screening measure for depression in older adults. Scores between 20 and 32 indicate that severe depression is present. The BDI-II is a 21-question multiple-choice self-report inventory. Moderate depression is scored between 20 and 28.

66. A) Patient Health Questionnaire (PHQ-9)
Symptoms of depression include sadness, tearfulness, angry outbursts, loss of interest or pleasure in most or all normal activities, and insomnia. The Patient Health Questionnaire is used to screen for depressive and other mental disorders. It is a self-administered version of the PRIME-MD diagnostic instrument for common mental disorders. A PHQ-9 score of 10 has a sensitivity of 88% and a specificity of 88% for major depression. PHQ-9 scores of 5, 10, 15, and 20 represent mild, moderate, moderately severe, and severe depression, respectively. The Columbia Suicidal Severity Rating scale is used to assess suicidal behavior. The Montreal Cognitive Assessment is used for cognitive disorders such as Alzheimer's disease. The Insomnia Severity Index is used to assess insomnia only.

67. A parent brings a 2-year-old to the clinic. The child has a small head and an excitable demeanor, with frequent smiling, laughter, and hand-flapping movements. During the clinical interview, the psychiatric-mental health nurse practitioner asks:

    A. "When did your child first sit up without assistance?"
    B. "Have you noticed your child struggling to form words?"
    C. "Does your child have difficulty chewing and swallowing foods?"
    D. "Has your child shown difficulty holding their head upright?"

68. At 8:00 p.m., the psychiatric-mental health nurse practitioner evaluates a patient who has been using heroin and morphine for over a year. The patient reports last use was "around lunchtime." The nurse practitioner can anticipate that the patient will exhibit signs of physical withdrawal, such as:

    A. Increased lacrimation, rhinorrhea, and piloerection
    B. Pinpoint pupils and bradycardia
    C. Tonic-clonic seizures and tremors
    D. Dysthymia; vivid, unpleasant dreams; and insomnia

69. The number of domains listed in the DSM-5 Self-Rated Level 1 Cross-Cutting Symptom Measure adult tool are:

    A. 6
    B. 8
    C. 12
    D. 13

70. The skilled interview technique demonstrated when the psychiatric-mental health nurse practitioner repeats a patient's last words is referred to as:

    A. Taking notes
    B. Nonverbal communication
    C. Facilitation
    D. Echoing

(See answers next page.)

67. B) "Have you noticed your child struggling to form words?"

Angelman syndrome results from the loss of function of a gene called UBE3A. The characteristics of Angelman syndrome are delayed development, intellectual disability, severe speech impairment, and problems with movement and balance (ataxia). Most affected children also have recurrent seizures (epilepsy) and a small head size. Children with Angelman syndrome typically have a happy, excitable demeanor with frequent smiling, laughter, and hand-flapping movements. Hyperactivity, a short attention span, insomnia, and a fascination with water are common. Klinefelter syndrome, affecting males, is a collection of characteristics that occurs as a result of two or more X chromosomes and affects many parts of the body. In infancy, this condition is characterized by weak muscle tone (hypotonic), feeding difficulties, poor growth, and delayed development. Beginning in childhood, Prader-Willi patients develop an insatiable appetite, which leads to chronic overeating (hyperphagia) and obesity. These children also are delayed in sitting upright without assistance and do not walk until 2 years of age or even older. Down syndrome is caused due to trisomy, and the children have typical features like flattened face and almond shaped eyes with delayed development. These children often have difficulty forming words or chewing foods at this age.

68. A) Increased lacrimation, rhinorrhea, and piloerection

Increased lacrimation, rhinorrhea, and piloerection are signs of early withdrawal. Typically, a patient experiencing withdrawal from short-term opioids such as heroin and morphine becomes symptomatic within 6 to 24 hours from the last dose. Withdrawal peaks within 48 to 72 hours and subsides after 7 to 10 days. Pinpoint pupils and bradycardia are signs of life-threatening opioid overdose. Tonic-clonic seizures and tremors present in alcohol withdrawal. Patients withdrawing from cocaine and amphetamines experience dysthymia; vivid, unpleasant dreams; and insomnia.

69. D) 13

There are 13 psychiatric domains. On the adult self-rated version of the measure, each item is rated on a 5-point scale (0 = none or not at all; 1 = slight or rare, less than a day or two; 2 = mild or several days; 3 = moderate or more than half the days; and 4 = severe or nearly every day). The score on each item within a domain should be reviewed. The rating of mild (i.e., 2) or greater on any item within a domain, except for substance use, suicidal ideation, and psychosis, serves as a guide for additional inquiry and follow-up to determine if a more detailed assessment is required.

70. D) Echoing

Repeating the patient's last words is known as echoing. It encourages the patient to elaborate on details and feelings. Echoing also demonstrates careful listening and a subtle connection with the patient by using the patient's words. Taking notes is creating a detailed record of the patient interview. Detailed notes help the practitioner to collect appropriate records. Nonverbal communication is the interview technique that includes creating eye contact with the patient and observing facial expressions. Facilitation is an interview technique that encourages the patient to talk.

71. A patient reports nausea and vomiting, tremors, dry mouth, sweating, and increased thirst, with onset 7 hours ago. The screening tool the psychiatric-mental health nurse practitioner uses is the:

    A. CAGE Questionnaire
    B. Patient Health Questionnaire (PHQ-9)
    C. Insomnia Severity Index Tool
    D. General Anxiety Disorder-7 (GAD-7)

72. A 23-year-old patient visits a psychiatric-mental health nurse practitioner accompanied by a close friend. The nurse practitioner observes that the patient's face is pale and bruised. The patient shares that she got married 3 months ago and that her spouse is a binge drinker. She states that she is not allowed to work or to participate in activities according to her free will, and that attempts to do so usually result in verbal or physical abuse. During the interview, the nurse practitioner observes that the patient is not maintaining direct eye contact while speaking and that her hands are trembling. When the nurse practitioner tries to move closer to the patient and examine the bruises, the patient jumps up and asks the nurse to stay away from her. The nurse practitioner should:

    A. Ask whether the patient is forced to do things without her consent
    B. Perform a physical examination even if the patient is resistant
    C. Avoid validation and judgmental responses
    D. Ask the friend of the patient to stay in the room during the interview

73. A 70-year-old patient is brought to the clinic by his son, who reports that his father has memory trouble, mood swings, and difficulty speaking. The son also reports that the patient has been losing track of dates and is often unable to identify people. The screening test the nurse practitioner will use is the:

    A. Insomnia Severity Index
    B. Montreal Cognitive Assessment (MoCA)
    C. Patient Health Questionnaire (PHQ-9)
    D. Columbia Suicidal Severity Rating scale

74. A patient displaying aggressive behaviors has been referred to the psychiatric-mental health nurse practitioner. In order to determine if the patient has any risk of violence, during the clinical interview the nurse practitioner should be aware of the:

    A. Impulsive nature of the patient
    B. Body language of the patient
    C. Problem-solving skills of the patient
    D. Patience level of the patient

75. A 16-year-old patient visits a psychiatric-mental health nurse practitioner with their parents. The parents reported that the patient has an older sibling who has bipolar I disorder. The nurse practitioner will assess for:

    A. Schizotypal personality disorder
    B. Narcissistic personality disorder
    C. Cyclothymic disorder
    D. Conduct disorder

(See answers next page.)

71. A) CAGE questionnaire

The patient's symptoms and their duration lead the nurse practitioner to suspect alcohol withdrawal. The CAGE questionnaire is a tool used to screen for suspected alcohol abuse. It is administered by healthcare professionals. Item responses are scored 0 or 1, with the higher score being indicative of alcohol abuse. A total score of 2 or greater is considered clinically significant. If the screen is positive, the nurse practitioner can further screen with quantity and frequency questions. The Patient Health Questionnaire is a self-administered instrument for common mental disorders. The Insomnia Severity Index tool is used for assessing the nature, severity, and impact of insomnia, and the General Anxiety Disorder-7 is used to assess anxiety disorders.

72. A) Ask whether the patient is forced to do things without her consent

In cases of domestic abuse, sexual abuse is also commonly observed. Therefore, a nurse practitioner needs to ask the patient if she was ever sexually abused or forced into acts without her consent. It is necessary to perform a physical assessment, in order to check for signs of vaginal laceration or bruises on other parts of the body resulting from sexual or physical abuse. However, if the patient does not give her consent, then her decision should be respected, and the nurse practitioner should not conduct the physical assessment. Giving judgmental responses should be strictly avoided because it is not an approach of a skilled interviewer. However, an empathetic approach and validation are necessary because they help to make a patient feel comfortable. For a patient who has experienced abuse or trauma, it is highly recommended to conduct the interview process privately and not in others' presence.

73. A) Insomnia Severity Index

The MoCA is a 30-question screening tool. It evaluates different types of cognitive abilities, such as orientation, short-term memory, executive function, and visuospatial ability. Scores on the MoCA range from 0 to 30. The MoCA's advantages include its brevity, simplicity, and reliability as a screening test for Alzheimer's disease. MoCA is available in more than 35 languages, and the MoCA Test Blind allows cognitive testing for those who are visually impaired. The Insomnia Severity Index is used to determine the severity of insomnia while examining the various components of insomnia. The Patient Health Questionnaire is used to detect depression and its severity. The Columbia Suicidal Severity Rating scale is used to detect suicide risk.

74. B) Body language of the patient

Several types of body language, including rigid posture and tendency to clench fists, can indicate that the patient is at risk of violence. Impulsivity denotes the risk of suicide. Low problem-solving skills indicate impaired coping, and being impatient denotes overloaded stress.

75. C) Cyclothymic disorder

Having a sibling with bipolar I disorder is a risk factor for cyclothymic disorder, a rare type of mood disorder. The risk factor of schizotypal personality disorder is having a relative with schizophrenia. Patients with narcissistic personality disorder generally have relatives with the same disorder. The risk factors for developing conduct disorder involve being rejected or neglected by parents, living in a large family, and consuming alcohol or other substances at home.

76. A patient states that their father passed away a week ago. The first response by the psychiatric-mental health nurse practitioner is to:

A. Ask about the patient's feelings regarding the loss

B. State that the loss is upsetting and ask the patient to share further

C. Express that they are sorry for the loss and show interest in knowing the story

D. Reassure the patient that this phase will soon pass

77. An 18-month-old patient is brought to the clinic by his parent. His parent has noticed that the patient does not react to others or smile. The screening test that the nurse practitioner will administer is:

A. Checklist for Autism in Toddlers

B. Denver Development Screening Test

C. Child Behavior Checklist

D. Montreal Cognitive Assessment Scale

78. The screening tool is used to assess the development of a child from age 1 month to 6 years is the:

A. Denver Developmental Screening Test (DDST)

B. Weber's test

C. Children's Depression Inventory (CDI)

D. TORCH test

79. A 12-year-old patient comes to the psychiatric-mental health nurse practitioner with their parents. During a one-on-one conversation, the patient says that although their parents are very loving, it often feels like they are overly controlling. The nurse practitioner's priority is to assess the patient for the disorder known as:

A. Dissociative

B. Reactive attachment

C. Disinhibited social engagement

D. Posttraumatic stress

80. A 24-year-old patient visits a psychiatric-mental health nurse practitioner. The patient is extremely extroverted and loves to spend time with people. The patient claims to be extremely reliant on a close friend and feels helpless when that friend is not around. The patient lacks confidence at work when the friend is not there. The patient states that friendships in the past have ended abruptly. The nurse practitioner should ask if the patient:

A. Faced any chronic physical disorder in childhood

B. Feels inferior regarding their own self

C. Has an extreme focus on perfectionism

D. Has some beliefs that others regard as strange

(See answers next page.)

76. C) Express that they are sorry for the loss and show interest in knowing the story

The nurse practitioner should take an empathetic approach when a patient describes a loss. Responses that involve feeling sorry about the loss and showing interest in knowing the story express empathy and help the patient to clarify their feelings. In certain cases, the loss of a parent or family member may not be upsetting; in fact, it might be a relief for the patient, so it is preferable not to state that the loss is upsetting when asking the patient to share further. Rather than asking specifically about the patient's feelings, the nurse practitioner should ask about the whole situation or story as a means to better understand the patient's feelings. The nurse practitioner's approach should be empathetic first, and after the end of the interview, the patient may be given reassurance as appropriate.

77. A) Checklist for Autism in Toddlers

Lack of response to others and lack of appropriate facial expressions may be early signs of autism. The Checklist for Autism in Toddlers (CHAT) is a psychological questionnaire designed to evaluate risk for autism spectrum disorder in children ages 18 to 24 months. The purpose of an autism screening is to identify common early signs of autism. The first nine questions (part A) of the CHAT identify common play habits and behaviors, while the last five questions (part B) concern the child's behavior and reaction to certain stimuli initiated by the provider. The Denver Developmental Screening Test assesses child development at different ages. The Child Behavior Checklist is used to detect behavioral or emotional problems in children and adolescents. The Montreal Cognitive Assessment is a cognitive screening tool for conditions such as Alzheimer's and Parkinson's diseases.

78. A) Denver Developmental Screening Test (DDST)

The DDST is used to test the development of a child from age 1 month to 6 years. A child's personal and social skills, facility with language, fine motor skills, and gross motor skills are tested with this tool. Additionally, the test administrator asks the parents a series of questions to collect more information about how the child behaves at home. If a child doesn't perform at the desired levels, then the child is at risk for developmental issues. The Weber's test is used on the ear to test for hearing loss. The CDI is used to check the level of depression. TORCH is the screening test for toxoplasmosis, rubella, cytomegalovirus, and herpes simplex virus to help determine small-for-gestational-age and intrauterine-growth-restricted neonates.

79. D) Posttraumatic stress

Having overly controlling parents is a risk factor for posttraumatic stress disorder; it brings detrimental effects whenever the patient faces any stress. The risk factor of dissociative disorder is not an overly controlling parent but a neglectful parent. Disinhibited social engagement disorder and reactive attachment disorder are types of attachment disorders. Attachment disorders occur in patients with abusive parents.

80. A) Faced any chronic physical disorder in childhood

The patient's symptoms indicate a dependent personality disorder. A risk factor of this disorder is having a chronic physical disorder in childhood; by seeking this information, the nurse practitioner can proceed a step ahead toward an accurate diagnosis. None of the patient's symptoms indicates histrionic personality disorder or avoidant personality disorder, so it is not mandatory to ask if the patient has an inferiority complex. The patient has no symptoms of obsessive–compulsive personality disorder, so it is not crucial to ask about a focus on perfectionism. The problem of having odd beliefs comes with schizotypal personality disorder, which has no similarity with the patient's symptoms. Therefore, the nurse practitioner does not need to ask this question.

81. A 77-year-old patient visits the psychiatric-mental health nurse practitioner with their adult son. The son says that the patient has recently spent some days in the intensive care unit after experiencing a stroke. After being discharged from the hospital, the patient talks constantly about the fear of dying. In the clinical interview, the nurse practitioner should:

A. First greet the patient by stating their name and then asking the patient's name
B. Address the patient politely by their first name so that the patient becomes comfortable
C. Ask the son to stay for the interview because of the patient's age, even if the patient disagrees
D. Ask sensitive questions only when the patient is alone

82. A risk factor for anxiety disorder in older adults is:

A. Having more than one child
B. Being of female sex
C. Having a spouse
D. Having high socioeconomic status

83. A 28-year-old patient has an appointment with a psychiatric-mental health nurse practitioner for the first time. The nurse practitioner reviews the patient's history and finds that she experienced three miscarriages within the last 2 years and is recently divorced. On the initial encounter, the nurse practitioner greets the patient, makes her comfortable, and begins taking notes. The next approach of the nurse practitioner should be:

A. Inviting the patient to share her story
B. Examining the patient's point of view
C. Recognizing the patient's emotional cues
D. Creating the agenda

84. A patient visits a psychiatric-mental health nurse practitioner. The clinical record shows that the patient visited frequently a year ago for depression due to the loss of their youngest child. During the interview, the patient states that the therapies were of little effect and that they still experience difficulty in managing everyday activity. The patient reports ongoing insomnia for 2 months and the inability to take care of their other children. The patient expresses self-blame throughout the interview for the loss of the youngest child. The nurse practitioner should:

A. Tell the patient to be grateful for the moments spent with the youngest child
B. Tell the patient that their youngest child is with God now
C. Share a long personal story about the loss of a family member
D. Express that it is difficult to understand the feelings of the patient at present

(See answers next page.)

81. D) Ask sensitive questions only when the patient is alone

The family member of a patient can stay with the patient while interviewing, but the nurse practitioner should ask sensitive questions only when the patient is alone. The nurse practitioner should first greet the patient taking the patient's name, and then introduce themselves. The nurse practitioner should never address any patient by their first name unless the patient is a child or adolescent. The nurse practitioner should ask if the patient wants to allow their son to stay during the interview and act accordingly.

82. B) Being of female sex

Many older adults experience anxiety disorders, and most remain undiagnosed. In the case of older adults, women experience anxiety more than men do. Single, not married, older adults are mainly seen to be suffering from anxiety. Having more than one child is not a risk factor for anxiety. Older adults of lower socioeconomic status have a higher chance of anxiety compared with those of higher economic status.

83. D) Creating the agenda

Once rapport is established with the patient, the nurse practitioner should listen to the chief complaints of the patient. This helps in identifying the patient's concerns and prioritizing the agenda based on the concerns. After the agenda is established, the patient should be encouraged to share her story. This can be done by initiating an open-ended approach. The next step involves the evaluation of the patient's point of view toward the complaints. This can be done by asking about any fear related to the complaints, any ideas related to the complaints, the effect of the complaints on the patient's life, and any expectations due to previous experience. Afterward, when the patient's emotional cue is identified, the nurse practitioner should respond to it.

84. D) Express that it is difficult to understand the feelings of the patient at present

In cases where a patient is experiencing a complex or persistent feeling of grief even after therapies, it is important to acknowledge that the feeling of loss or grief must have been devastating and that it is very difficult for the nurse practitioner to understand what the patient must be currently feeling. Telling the patient to be grateful implies that the patient is ungrateful; instead, the nurse practitioner should show the positive side of the situation, which is that the patient has other children who need to be taken care of. Telling a patient that their child is with God may imply that the child's death is God's punishment. Instead, the nurse practitioner should express an understanding of how much the patient misses their youngest child. Sharing a long story about a loss in the nurse practitioner's own family is not helpful. Instead, the shared story should be concise and used only for helping the patient understand the feelings others experience with the loss of a loved one and how they overcome those feelings after the acute grief period.

85. A psychiatric-mental health nurse practitioner has received the case study of a severely withdrawn patient. While interviewing the patient, the nurse practitioner should:

   A. Never speak of anything regarding suicide in front of the patient
   B. Speak with the patient in very simple terms
   C. Console the patient by saying that everyone goes through this phase
   D. Not talk until the patient breaks the silence

86. A 12-year-old patient visits a psychiatric-mental health nurse practitioner with parents. The parents report that the patient is reluctant to talk with others and has no friends. The patient often faces ridicule at school and receives poor grades. The parents have noticed that the patient has a habit of talking with shadows or pictures, although they have confirmed that the patient does not experience any hallucinations or delusions. During the clinical interview with the patient, the nurse practitioner should ask questions:

   A. That are personal, to help the patient come out of isolation
   B. To check if the patient is having suicidal thoughts
   C. That will help the patient to talk about anxiety
   D. To check if anything is bringing exaggerated feelings to the patient their own self

87. The strongest risk factor for cognitive impairment is:

   A. Advanced age
   B. Having never been married
   C. Alcohol misuse
   D. Low education level

88. A 22-year-old patient visits a psychiatric-mental health nurse practitioner. The patient states that they have extreme mood swings and an impulsive nature. The patient also shares that despite behaving oddly during the mood swings, the patient never has any intention of harming people or seeking attention. The mood swings mainly occur when a patient feels that a situation is getting out of control. The patient feels ashamed and trusts that the nurse practitioner can help the patient. The nurse practitioner asks if the patient:

   A. Often feels jealous of people and finds difficulty in forgiving
   B. Receives pleasure by self-destructive activities like cutting
   C. Feels extremely anxious when in the middle of a crowd of people
   D. Thinks they have extraordinary talent or beauty that others hardly notice

(*See answers next page.*)

85. B) Speak with the patient in very simple terms

Severely withdrawn patients take time to comprehend because their thinking capacity is slowed. They also face issues with concentrating. Therefore, the nurse practitioner should talk to the patient in very simple language. Suicide is a sensitive topic, but it often needs to be discussed so that the patient does not feel isolated and can overcome such thoughts. Consolation can make the patient feel guilty. The nurse practitioner can break the silence by expressing simple observations.

86. C) That will help the patient to talk about anxiety

The symptoms of the patient signify that the patient has schizoid personality disorder. To address this disorder, the nurse practitioner should ask the patient questions that will make the patient feel comfortable discussing the anxieties the patient faces. The nurse practitioner should avoid being overfriendly with patients who have schizoid personality disorder by not asking personal questions and by respecting the patient's need for isolation. Schizoid personality disorder does not bring suicidal thoughts, so it is not mandatory for the nurse practitioner to ask questions regarding them. The sources of exaggerated feelings are identified in patients with narcissistic personality disorder, which the patient shows no sign of having.

87. A) Advanced age

Cognitive impairment disrupts mental health by causing issues related to the person's ability to recall, solve problems, pay attention, and make plans. The strongest risk factor for the occurrence of cognitive impairment is advanced age. Remaining unmarried throughout life, alcohol misuse, and low education level are also considered risk factors for cognitive impairment, but advanced age is the strongest risk factor.

88. B) Receives pleasure by self-destructive activities like cutting

The symptoms indicate that the patient has borderline personality disorder. In this disorder, patients experiences extreme mood swings and difficulty controlling their emotions. They may also engage in self-destructive behaviors like promiscuous sexual activity or cutting, so the nurse practitioner should ask about any such activities. Feeling jealous often and struggling to forgive are symptoms of histrionic personality disorder. Feeling anxious in front of other people is a symptom of avoidant personality disorder. A person having exaggerated beliefs regarding their own talent and beauty is narcissistic personality disorder.

Diagnosis and Treatment

3

1. An 11-year-old patient comes to the office for an initial visit with the psychiatric-mental health nurse practitioner accompanied by parents. Teachers have noticed the patient's careless mistakes on math assignments, difficulty keeping school supplies in order, lack of interest in lengthy assignments, and distractibility in the classroom. The patient's parents have noticed that he loses his eyeglasses often and forgets to do assigned chores. Based on DSM-5 criteria, the nurse practitioner realizes that the patient meets the criteria for:

   A. Attention deficit disorder, predominantly hyperactive/impulsive presentation
   B. Attention deficit disorder, combined presentation
   C. Attention deficit disorder, predominantly inattentive presentation
   D. A learning disorder

2. A 24-year-old patient is admitted to a psychiatric unit. The patient studies at a university, lives in a dormitory, and has been an excellent student. Friends describe the patient as amiable and socially active. However, for the last few months, the patient has lost interest in studies, self-care, and hygiene and has spent most time alone. For the past 2 days, he has locked himself in his room and has not eaten, stating that the food has been poisoned. The patient whispers to the nurse practitioner that someone is looking at them and asking them not to share this personal information. The nurse practitioner will probably:

   A. Administer haloperidol (Haldol) and order an ECG
   B. Prescribe perphenazine (Trilafon) and order a test for anticholinergic toxicity
   C. Prescribe olanzapine (Zyprexa) and order a test for metabolic syndrome diagnosis
   D. Administer loxapine (Loxitane) and a order test for diagnosis of neuroleptic malignant syndrome

3. A patient comes into the office with a prior diagnosis of opioid use disorder, but states that she has not used opioids or experienced any cravings within the past 2 months. The psychiatric-mental health nurse practitioner understands that the patient is in:

   A. Withdrawal from opioid use
   B. Early remission
   C. Sustained remission
   D. No remission

1. C) Attention deficit disorder, predominantly inattentive presentation
Careless mistakes, difficulty keeping things in order, lack of interest in activities that require mental effort, being easily distracted, losing things easily, and being forgetful are all symptoms of inattention. No hyperactive/impulsive symptoms are noted. A learning disorder would indicate difficulty with reading, spelling, mastering number facts, or written expression, or lack of understanding around reading and mathematical reasoning.

2. C) Prescribe olanzapine (Zyprexa) and order a test for metabolic syndrome diagnosis
The patient is reflecting all the signs and symptoms of paranoid schizophrenia: The patient is socializing less, is not studying, is declining self-care, and is experiencing hallucinations and delusions. This type of schizophrenia is treated with a second-generation antipsychotic drug, olanzapine (Zyprexa). Second-generation drugs can treat both the positive and the negative symptoms of schizophrenia. The risk associated with this drug is metabolic syndrome; therefore, the priority nursing order would be to send blood samples for testing to detect metabolic syndrome. Haloperidol (Haldol), perphenazine (Trilafon), and loxapine (Loxitane) are all first-generation antipsychotic drugs and are used in the case of treatment of either positive or negative symptoms of schizophrenia, but an ECG or testing for antcholinergic toxicity or neuroleptic malignant syndrome would not be a priority at this time.

3. D) No remission
The patient is currently not in remission due to the limited time (2 months) without diagnostic criteria for opioid use disorder. According to the DSM-5, early remission is defined as the patient being without diagnostic criteria for opioid use disorder for at least 3 months and no more than 12 months. Sustained remission is defined as 12 months or longer. There are no clinical indicators that the patient is in a withdrawal state from opioid use.

4. An ambulance brings a 50-year-old patient to the emergency department (ED) at 10 a.m. The patient is having difficulty breathing and reports dizziness, chest pain, and palpitations. The patient is trembling and diaphoretic. The vitals at the time of admission are blood pressure of 180/96 mmHg, heart rate of 108 beats per minute, respirations at 26 breaths per minute, and a temperature of 98.7°F. The patient states that the symptoms began early in the morning and became worse during a meeting at around 9:30 a.m. The patient admits to having stress at home and work. Full medical work in the ED reveals that all parameters are normal. ECG results and other laboratory reports are also within normal limits. Based on the information, the psychiatric-mental health nurse practitioner would consider prescribing:

A. Lorazepam (Ativan) 1 mg stat

B. Modafinil (Provigil) 200 mg oral dose

C. Donepezil (Aricept) 10 mg once daily

D. Carbamazepine (Carbatrol) 200 mg oral

5. A 68-year-old patient comes into the office of a psychiatric-mental health nurse practitioner for an initial visit accompanied by his spouse. The spouse is concerned that the patient has developed patterns of alcohol misuse since he stopped working over the past year. The nurse practitioner demonstrates understanding and can diagnose mild alcohol use disorder if the patient:

A. Drinks alcohol in larger amounts, is unsuccessful in cutting down, and develops cravings for alcohol

B. Continues to use alcohol in situations in which it is physically hazardous to do so

C. Starts to avoid his favorite recreational activities in order to spend the time drinking alcohol

D. Continues alcohol use despite the effect on his relationships, develops cravings for alcohol, continues use despite health concerns, and desires to drink more than anything else

6. The psychiatric-mental health nurse practitioner sees a patient with major depressive disorder for a follow-up visit. The patient has a medical history of epilepsy. The patient has had a limited efficacious response to sertraline (Zoloft), and the nurse practitioner is planning to adjust the patient's treatment. The medication that would be contraindicated for this patient would be:

A. Fluoxetine

B. Bupropion

C. Venlafaxine

D. Aripiprazole

(See answers next page.)

4. A) Lorazepam (Ativan) 1 mg stat

Lorazepam (Ativan) is used in treating anxiety disorder and trouble sleeping, as well as regulating breathlessness. It works by enhancing the release of gamma-aminobutyric acid and producing a calming effect. Modafinil (Provigil) is a psychostimulant used to treat drowsiness and sleepiness. Donepezil (Aricept) is a cholinesterase inhibitor used to treat dementia-causing brain disorders such as Alzheimer's disease. Carbamazepine (Carbatrol) belongs to a class of mood stabilizers and is used in the treatment of convulsions and seizures.

5. A) Drinks alcohol in larger amounts, is unsuccessful in cutting down, and develops cravings for alcohol

The patient meets the criteria for alcohol use disorder due to a problematic pattern within a 12-month period. Mild alcohol use disorder is classified as the presence of two or three symptoms, such as drinking larger amounts, being unsuccessful in cutting down, and developing cravings for alcohol. Moderate alcohol use disorder is indicated with the presence of four or five symptoms, such as using alcohol despite is effects on relationships, developing cravings for alcohol, continuing alcohol use despite health problems, and wanting to drink more than anything else.

6. B) Bupropion

Bupropion (Wellbutrin) is associated with increased risk of seizures. Due to the patient's history of epilepsy, bupropion is contraindicated for treatment of this patient's depression. Fluoxetine (Prozac) and venlafaxine (Effexor) are options for treatment. Aripiprazole (Abilify) is also indicated for severe depression.

7. A psychiatric-mental health nurse practitioner in the health center of a college campus has been working with a first-year student for a few weeks. The nurse practitioner notes that the patient feels significantly uncomfortable in social situations. The student describes using alcohol to "calm my nerves" by having two or three drinks before socializing. According to the DSM-5, the patient appears to have:

   A. Alcohol use disorder, mild
   B. Alcohol use disorder, moderate
   C. Personality disorder
   D. No mental disorder

8. The intervention strategy for patients with severe mental illness is based on:

   A. Reduction in severity of symptoms
   B. Holistic improvement of patients
   C. Elimination of the impact of the disorder on day-to-day life
   D. Education of patients about their illness and recovery

9. A patient is evaluated in the emergency department with symptoms of being easily distracted and hyperverbal with fast speech. The patient has had no sleep in the past 3 days and has experienced significant irritability for the past 3 days. According to the DSM-5, the patient's symptoms are consistent with:

   A. Anxiety
   B. Depression
   C. Attention deficit/hyperactivity disorder (ADHD)
   D. Hypomania

10. The first-line treatment for attention deficit/hyperactivity disorder (ADHD) includes:

    A. Psychostimulants
    B. Second-generation antipsychotics
    C. First-generation antipsychotics
    D. Anticonvulsant medications

11. Evidence-based practice suggests that cognitive enhancement therapy is best suited to:

    A. Shape the behavior and cognition of the patient positively
    B. Strengthen attention span, retention, and recall of information
    C. Help the patient manage and solve problems step by step
    D. Enhance employment or financial support for attaining employment

12. An advanced practice related to evidence-based treatment for use by nurse practitioners is:

    A. Prescriptive authority
    B. Milieu therapy
    C. Counseling
    D. Cultural assessment

(*See answers next page.*)

7. D) No mental disorder

The patient does not currently meet the criteria for a mental disorder. Alcohol use disorder would entail a problematic pattern of alcohol use leading to clinically significant impairment or distress within a 12-month period. The patient appears to be using alcohol sparingly and without evidence of significant impairment. The patient's alcohol use and discomfort in social situations are not sufficient to diagnose a personality disorder or any other mental disorder.

8. B) Holistic improvement of patients

According to the evidence-based approach, the best treatment strategy is planning intervention for the holistic improvement of patients. Patients learn how to cope with their mental illness more healthily when a holistic approach is considered. Therapy, which eliminates the impact of the disorder on day-to-day life, or drugs, which reduce the severity of symptoms alone, are more likely to cause relapse. Educating patients about their illness helps in raising awareness of their condition and dispels misconceptions about the recovery process, but it is not the basis for the best treatment strategy.

9. D) Hypomania

Symptoms of hypomania include increased self-esteem, decreased need for sleep, being more talkative than usual, flight of ideas, distractibility, increased goal-directed behavior, and excessive involvement in activities with high consequences. While irritability may be a common symptom of depression and anxiety, all other symptoms are not consistent with depression or anxiety. Although the symptom of easy distractibility is consistent with ADHD, the rest of the patient's symptoms are not.

10. A) Psychostimulants

Psychostimulants are used for first-line treatment of ADHD because they function through blockage and reuptake of dopamine as well as norepinephrine. First- and second-generation antipsychotics are used for treating schizophrenia by lowering the activity of dopamine. Anticonvulsant medications change the electrical conductivity inside the membranes and, therefore, help in treating bipolar disorder.

11. B) Strengthen attention span, retention, and recall of information

Lengthy and structured cognitive enhancement therapy sessions strengthen attention span, information retention, and remembrance. This therapy is based on the concept of neuroplasticity. Cognitive—behavioral therapy helps in shaping the behavior of the patients positively. Social skills training helps in managing and solving problems step by step. Vocational rehabilitation helps in enhancing employment and financial support for attaining employment.

12. A) Prescriptive authority

Prescribing is a part of evidence-based treatment in an advanced practice role because it requires experience. Milieu therapy is all about providing a secure environment for proper recovery. Nurse practitioners use counseling interventions to help patients in the process of recovery. Cultural assessments are performed to evaluate the patient before treatment.

13. In community health settings, the introduction of evidence-based practice is slower than in other settings because of less understanding:

    A. About the patients
    B. Of health-related research
    C. Of influences of the family
    D. About self-care among patients

14. The cholinesterase inhibitor used to treat both Alzheimer's disease and Parkinson's disease is:

    A. Donepezil
    B. Rivastigmine
    C. Galantamine
    D. Paraoxon

15. The potential long-term adverse effects of lithium include:

    A. Hypothyroidism
    B. Thrombocytopenia
    C. Hepatic failure
    D. Pancreatitis

16. A patient calls the clinic reporting symptoms that include lack of sleep, irritation, and increased weight. The patient gave birth 12 weeks ago. The psychiatric-mental health nurse practitioner would consider prescribing:

    A. Esketamine (Spravato)
    B. Lithium
    C. Valproate (Depakote)
    D. Brexanolone (Zulresso)

17. Emergency services brings an unconscious patient to the hospital with a femoral fracture and head injuries following a motor vehicle crash. After surgery, the patient is stable. The patient's medication administration record includes alprazolam (Xanax), morphine, acetaminophen, and ibuprofen. The patient regains consciousness and asks about alprazolam, and the psychiatric-mental health nurse practitioner replies that alprazolam is used to:

    A. Treat anxiety
    B. Treat oversleeping
    C. Prevent inflammation
    D. Relieve pain

18. The monoamine oxidase inhibitor (MAOI) found as a transdermal patch is:

    A. Phenelzine (Nardil)
    B. Selegiline (Eldepryl)
    C. Isocarboxazid (Marplan)
    D. Tranylcypromine (Parnate)

(See answers next page.)

13. B) Of health-related research

In community health, the introduction of evidence-based practice can be slower if people fail to understand the research related to it. Research is a crucial part of introducing evidence-based practice in the right manner because the evidence and observation of research are introduced in practice. Nurses take patient data before treatment to assess their condition, which gives them a clear understanding of the patient. Familial influence on the patient improves the use of counseling of the family and does not slow down evidence-based practice. Patients receive ideas for self-care from nurses to help them recover faster.

14. B) Rivastigmine

Alzheimer's disease is usually treated with drugs that target acetylcholine or glutamate. Cholinesterase inhibitors are used for treating Alzheimer's disease because they function by slowing down the memory loss rate. Rivastigmine is the cholinesterase inhibitor approved for treating mild to severe Alzheimer's disease as well as Parkinson's disease because it focuses on the improvement of the function of the brain's nerve cells. Donepezil and galantamine are used only for treating Alzheimer's disease. Paraoxon is used in the treatment of Alzheimer's disease and can also be used for treating glaucoma.

15. A) Hypothyroidism

Lithium has adverse effects on endocrine function by lowering the secretion of thyroid hormones, potentially causing hypothyroidism. Thrombocytopenia, liver failure, and pancreatitis do not occur as a result of lithium but can occur due to the adverse effects of an anticonvulsant medicine.

16. D) Brexanolone (Zulresso)

Brexanolone is an antidepressant that can be used for treating postpartum depression due to its similarities to allopregnanolone, which is produced by the female hormone progesterone. Esketamine is an antidepressant found as an intranasal spray, but it is not FDA approved for postpartum depression. Lithium is used for treating bipolar disorder; valproate is also used for bipolar disorder and is an anticonvulsant drug.

17. A) Treat anxiety

Alprazolam is effective in preventing anxiety attacks. It is a tranquilizer and would therefore also help the patient fall asleep. Ibuprofen is an anti-inflammatory drug. Acetaminophen is used in case of fever and pain. Morphine is used to remove the sensation of severe or mild pain.

18. B) Selegiline (Eldepryl)

The only antidepressant medicine found as a transdermal patch is selegiline. Phenelzine, isocarboxazid, and tranylcypromine are MAOIs used for treating depression, but none are available as a patch.

19. A patient with bipolar disorder has been prescribed lithium and several other medications. The patient asks the psychiatric-mental health nurse practitioner about the side effects of lithium. The nurse practitioner informs the patient about lithium toxicity to help with self-assessment. The nurse practitioner mentions symptoms such as:

    A. Weight loss
    B. High blood pressure
    C. Insomnia
    D. Blurred vision

20. A neuroleptic that has not been found to be associated with weight gain is:

    A. Ziprasidone (Geodon)
    B. Clozapine (Clozaril)
    C. Olanzapine (Zyprexa)
    D. Chlorpromazine (Thorazine)

21. An older patient who recently lost a spouse consults a psychiatric-mental health nurse practitioner. The patient has a liver disorder as well as depression. The nurse practitioner prescribes escitalopram. The patient does not respond well to this drug and has side effects like diarrhea and restlessness. The nurse practitioner changes the medication and prescribes:

    A. Tricyclic antidepressants
    B. Electroconvulsive therapy (ECT)
    C. Selective serotonin reuptake inhibitor (SSRI) antidepressants
    D. Atypical antidepressants

22. A 60-year-old patient visits a mental health clinic accompanied by his adult son, who explains that the patient experiences tremors and involuntary muscle movements. The psychiatric-mental health nurse practitioner diagnoses the patient, and the reports suggest that there is a degeneration of the neurons of the basal ganglia. The patient's son informs the nurse practitioner that the patient had treatment of depression and epilepsy involving fluoxetine and phenytoin. The nurse practitioner informs the patient's son that his father has:

    A. Pick's disease
    B. Huntington's disease
    C. Alzheimer's disease
    D. Parkinson's disease

23. Ramelteon (Rozerem) regulates:

    A. Sleep paralysis
    B. Anxiety
    C. Insomnia
    D. Sleep apnea

(See answers next page.)

19. D) Blurred vision

Lithium is used to manage symptoms of mania in a bipolar patient. Lithium toxicity has symptoms like dry mouth, vomiting, blurred vision, headache, diarrhea, dizziness, and hypothyroidism. It can cause weight gain, not weight loss. Hypotension, rather than hypertension, is another side effect of lithium toxicity. Insomnia is not a side effect of lithium administration.

20. A) Ziprasidone (Geodon)

Neuroleptics are used to regulate psychotic behavior and are often associated with weight gain. Ziprasidone is not associated with weight gain. The weight gain risk is high with clozapine and olanzapine, whereas the risk is high to medium with chlorpromazine.

21. D) Atypical antidepressants

When an SSRI such as escitalopram does not work, an atypical antidepressant is preferred. Atypical antidepressants can inhibit the uptake of serotonin, dopamine, and norepinephrine. Tricyclic antidepressants are contraindicated in patients with liver issues. Cyclic antidepressants are not a preferred choice for an older adult due to their side effects. ECT is not preferred for older patients and is considered the last resort when a patient is suicidal and there is no time to wait for drugs to have healing effects on the patient.

22. D) Parkinson's disease

Loss of neurons of the basal ganglia is a major symptom of Parkinson's disease. Excessive use of strong antidepressant medicines can induce this disease. Damage to the frontal and temporal lobes of the brain occurs in Pick's disease. Huntington's disease is a cognitive disease in which enlargement of the ventricles of the brain can occur. Loss of speech and loss of motor functioning are characteristic of Alzheimer's disease.

23. C) Insomnia

Ramelteon (Rozerem) is a drug that has been approved by the FDA to treat insomnia, in which the patient faces difficulty in staying asleep. It does so by binding to the melatonin receptor sites, either MT1 or MT2. Based on the receptor the drug binds to, it helps with either regulating sleep or regulating the circadian rhythm. Sleep paralysis is a side effect of orexin receptor antagonists, which promote wakefulness. The hormone melatonin helps in naturally regulating the sleep pattern and circadian rhythm in the body, but the drug binding to either of its receptors does not have any effect on anxiety. Lifestyle changes and use of a CPAP machine can help in the case of sleep apnea.

24. The antidepressant drug paroxetine (Paxil) belongs to the group of:

    A. Benzodiazepines
    B. Beta blockers
    C. Serotonin-norepinephrine reuptake inhibitors
    D. Serotonin reuptake inhibitors

25. Short-acting sedative-hypnotics, or Z-hypnotics, are reportedly a better choice than benzodiazepines because they:

    A. Have muscle relaxant effects
    B. Cause fewer substance dependency issues
    C. Do not cause slowed-down reflexes
    D. Help the patient to stay asleep

26. The actions of antiepileptic drugs such as carbamazepine and phenytoin include:

    A. Ensuring the sodium channels remain inactive for a longer duration
    B. Making the patient unconscious and thus inhibiting the reflexes
    C. Blocking the peripheral nerves to ease the pain
    D. Inhibiting acetylcholine breakdown at the synapse

27. The mesocortical pathway of dopamine shows second-generation antipsychotic response by:

    A. Blocking D2
    B. Increasing prolactin levels
    C. Blocking serotonin receptors
    D. Blocking D3 and D4

28. Typical antipsychotics help in alleviating:

    A. Delusions and hallucinations in schizophrenia
    B. Mixed episodes of bipolar disorder
    C. Manic episodes of bipolar disorder
    D. Difficulty staying asleep in insomnia

29. The neurotransmitter gamma-aminobutyric acid shows control in:

    A. Mood regulation
    B. Anxiety reduction
    C. Fear conditioning
    D. Appetite

(See answers next page.)

24. D) Serotonin reuptake inhibitors

Serotonin reuptake inhibitors such as paroxetine (Paxil) are mostly used as the first line of defense against anxiety disorders. Benzodiazepine compositions are used only after the intensity of anxiety is reduced. Beta-blockers can treat generalized anxiety issues. Serotonin—norepinephrine reuptake inhibitors help in treating severe as well as generalized anxiety disorders, but paroxetine is not one of them.

25. B) Cause fewer substance dependency issues

Z-hypnotics, also known as short-acting sedative-hypnotics, selectively bind to the gamma-aminobutyric acid-A receptor complex. This selective binding helps in lowering the number of side effects and in lowering tolerance and dependency issues. Z-hypnotics do not possess antianxiety and muscle relaxant effects. Both benzodiazepines and Z-hypnotics cause ataxia and slow down reflexes. If a patient needs help in falling asleep, Z-hypnotics are useful because they are mostly used for their hypnotic and amnestic effects, which last for a shorter period compared with benzodiazepines; however, if a patient needs help in staying asleep, benzodiazepines are of more use.

26. A) Ensuring the sodium channels remain inactive for a longer duration

Antiepileptic drugs act on the sodium channels and prolong their inactivated state. Anesthetic drug administration leads to loss of consciousness and inhibition of autonomic and sensory reflexes. Analgesic drugs block peripheral nerves and prevent pain. Anticholinesterase drugs act as acetylcholine breakdown inhibitors.

27. C) Blocking serotonin receptors

The second-generation antipsychotic (SGA) response of the mesocortical dopaminergic pathway mainly performs by blocking the 5HT (serotonin) receptors in this area. The first-generation antipsychotic drugs generally block the D2 receptors. The tuberoinfundibular pathway controls the regulation of the prolactin hormone. The other dopamine pathway carries out the SGA response by blocking D3 and D4.

28. A) Delusions and hallucinations in schizophrenia

The symptoms of schizophrenia occur due to the overactivity of dopamine in the mesolimbic system, which causes hallucinations and delusions. First-generation antipsychotics act as antagonists of dopamine in the central nervous system. They bind to the D2 receptors and decrease the binding of dopamine, which helps in reducing dopaminergic stimulation. This ultimately reduces the delusions and hallucinations in schizophrenia patients. Bipolar disorder is treated by the use of anticonvulsant medication, and insomnia is treated with benzodiazepines, not antipsychotics.

29. B) Anxiety reduction

Gamma-aminobutyric acid slows neuronal activity to reduce anxiety and regulate memory. Serotonin helps to regulate mood. Norepinephrine plays a major role in fear conditioning and stress response. Serotonin controls appetite, sexual desire, and sleep and inhibits pain.

30. The antidepressant drug used to treat insomnia is:

   A. Bupropion (Wellbutrin)
   B. Mirtazapine (Remeron)
   C. Fluoxetine (Prozac)
   D. Tricarboxylic acid (Cymbalta)

31. The drug that acts as a norepinephrine and serotonin-specific antidepressant is:

   A. Paroxetine (Paxil)
   B. Mirtazapine (Remeron)
   C. Bupropion (Wellbutrin)
   D. Vortioxetine (Trintellix)

32. The single element that is widely regarded as the gold standard among mood stabilizers used to treat patients with bipolar disorder is:

   A. Sodium
   B. Potassium
   C. Lithium
   D. Monoamine oxidase

33. The type of medication used for Alzheimer's disease is:

   A. Muscle blockers
   B. Cholinesterase inhibitors
   C. Antipsychotics
   D. Lithium

34. A reduced level of serotonin is believed to cause:

   A. Parkinson's disease
   B. Mania
   C. Schizophrenia
   D. Depression

35. MRI is used for the detection of:

   A. Cortical atrophy
   B. Brain lesions
   C. Reduction in the temporal lobe
   D. Mood disorders

36. Antianxiety medications help to increase the effectiveness of:

   A. Acetylcholine
   B. Gamma-aminobutyric acid (GABA)
   C. Dopamine
   D. Glutamate

(See answers next page.)

30. B) Mirtazapine (Remeron)

Insomnia can be treated with mirtazapine, which belongs to the category of noradrenergic and serotonergic antidepressants. Bupropion is used for treating sexual dysfunction and fatigue. Fluoxetine is an antidepressant that is not used to treat insomnia. Tricarboxylic acids help in reducing pain.

31. B) Mirtazapine (Remeron)

Mirtazapine acts as a norepinephrine and serotonin-specific antidepressant. Patients with weight loss and severe appetite loss or insomnia often receive this treatment. Mirtazapine binds as an antagonist with the postsynaptic serotonin receptor. Paroxetine is a selective serotonin reuptake inhibitor. Bupropion is a norepinephrine and dopamine reuptake inhibitor. Vortioxetine is a serotonin modulator and stimulant.

32. C) Lithium

Lithium is considered the gold standard among mood stabilizers to treat patients with bipolar disorder. Lithium interacts in a complex manner to stabilize the electrical activity in the neurons. Sodium and potassium directly take part in the process of neurotransmission; hence, they do not affect the patient. Introducing them in excess will only lead to ionic imbalance in the body. Monoamine oxidase degrades neurotransmitters.

33. B) Cholinesterase inhibitors

The use of cholinesterase inhibitors slows down the effects of Alzheimer's disease. As the cholinesterase is inhibited, the effect of acetylcholine increases, which inhibits the breakdown of cholinergic neurons. Muscle blockers are used in the process of anesthesia. Antipsychotics reduce and control many psychotic symptoms but do not control degradation due to Alzheimer's disease. Lithium acts as a mood stabilizer, but it does not affect Alzheimer's disease because it affects the serotonergic neurons.

34. D) Depression

Depression is believed to be caused by a decreased level of the neurotransmitter serotonin. Parkinson's disease is caused by a reduced level of dopamine. Mania and schizophrenia are both caused by an increased level of dopamine.

35. C) Reduction in the temporal lobe

MRI is used to detect several neurological disorders such as schizophrenia, brain edema, ischemia, and reduction in the temporal and prefrontal lobes. CT scan is used for the detection of cortical atrophy and lesions in the brain. PET helps to detect mood disorders.

36. B) Gamma-aminobutyric acid (GABA)

Antianxiety medications increase the activity and secretion of GABA. Excessive acetylcholine causes muscarinic and nicotinic toxicity. Dopamine has a role in increasing the probability of schizophrenia with excessive secretion. Glutamate has a direct influence on dopamine-releasing cells, so it can also increase the probability of schizophrenia.

37. Pharmacokinetics is the study of the:

    A. Effect of a drug on the body
    B. Absorption, distribution, transformation, and removal of a drug from the body
    C. Influence of genetic factors on a person's response to medications
    D. Prevention of the adverse effects of medications or drugs

38. Chlorpromazine (Thorazine) was the first pharmacotherapeutic:

    A. Antipsychotic
    B. Analgesic
    C. Antipyretic
    D. Antispasmodic

39. A melatonin receptor agonist used to treat insomnia is:

    A. Doxepin (Silenor)
    B. Ramelteon (Rozerem)
    C. Suvorexant (Belsomra)
    D. Lemborexant (Davvigo)

40. Prior to starting a patient suspected of having bipolar with mania on a mood stabi-
    lizer, the nurse practitioner orders a thyroid panel to rule out a disorder based on the
    patient's symptoms, which include tremor, tachycardia, profuse sweating, and:

    A. Weight gain
    B. Abdominal pain
    C. Dry mouth
    D. Weight loss

41. Atomoxetine (Straterra) is used to treat children with:

    A. Attention deficit/hyperactivity disorder
    B. Schizophrenia
    C. Depression
    D. Bipolar disorder

42. The disorder consistent with a patient's decreased free thyroxine (T4) and elevated
    thyroid-stimulating hormone (TSH) level is:

    A. Primary hypothyroidism
    B. Hyperthyroidism
    C. Acute thyroiditis
    D. Secondary hypothyroidism

(See answers next page.)

37. B) Absorption, distribution, transformation, and removal of a drug from the body

Pharmacokinetics is the study of how a drug is absorbed and distributed in the patient's body. It also studies the transformation of the drug for use and how it is excreted from the body. Pharmacodynamics is the study of the effect of a drug on the body. Pharmacogenetics studies the effect of genetic factors in determining a person's metabolic response to a particular drug or medication. Pharmacovigilance is the study of prevention of the adverse effects of medications or drugs.

38. A) Antipsychotic

Chlorpromazine was the first antipsychotic drug that functioned by blocking the D2 receptors of the post-synaptic neurons in the mesolimbic pathway. Analgesics are painkillers, antipyretic drugs reduce fever, and antispasmodic medications relieve muscle spasms.

39. B) Ramelteon (Rozerem)

Ramelteon is the significant melatonin agonist that binds to the melatonin receptor and generates sleepiness. Doxepin is a low-dose formulation of antidepressant that acts on the histamine level in the body. Suvorexant and lemborexant are orexin receptor antagonists that block orexin receptors to suppress wakefulness.

40. D) Weight loss

The symptoms of hyperthyroidism may mimic signs and symptoms of a manic episode or severe anxiety. These symptoms include increased pulse, fine tremor, heat intolerance with excessive sweating, weight loss, hyperverbal speech, exaggerated startle response, menstrual irregularities, muscle weakness, and exophthalmos. Weight gain can be seen in hypothyroidism, which often mimics symptoms of depression. Abdominal pain and dry mouth are not specific to hyperthyroidism, but they may be seen in lithium toxicity, which could be present if the patient has been taking lithium. However, patient treatment has not yet been initiated.

41. A) Attention deficit/hyperactivity disorder

Straterra is prescribed for adult and childhood attention deficit/hyperactivity disorder. This medication is a good choice for people who experience anxiety while taking stimulants and can also be used for comorbid anxiety. Medications like haloperidol (Haldol) are used to treat schizophrenia. Lithium has been used to treat severe agitation in bipolar disorders. Duloxetine or tricyclic antidepressants are used for treating depression.

42. A) Primary hypothyroidism

Primary hypothyroidism occurs when free T4 is decreased and TSH levels are elevated in response to the low T4. It occurs due to destruction of the thyroid gland, as in autoimmune disease, surgery, and radioiodine or radiation therapy. It can also occur as a result of low intake of iodine; however, that is now rare due to the addition of iodine to table salt. In secondary hypothyroidism, the pituitary gland fails and both TSH and free T4 are low. Hyperthyroidism and acute thyroiditis both present with elevated free T4 levels.

43. A 15-year-old patient is seen in the psychiatric emergency department with reports of uncontrolled shivering, tremors, and diarrhea. The patient recently started fluoxetine (Prozac) for depression. After the patient experienced anxiety earlier in the day, the patient's parent gave the patient an over-the-counter supplement to help calm the patient down. The psychiatric-mental health nurse practitioner suspects that the patient's symptoms are caused by the supplement:

A. St. John's wort
B. Valerian root
C. Chamomile extract
D. Passionflower

44. The complementary alternative treatment used in psychiatric care that is considered a mind-body intervention is:

A. Meditation
B. Massage therapy
C. Acupressure
D. Reflexology

45. Prior to starting a patient on an antidepressant for major depressive disorder, the nurse practitioner orders a thyroid panel to rule out a disorder based on the patient's symptoms, which include low mood, lethargy, weight gain, and:

A. Tachycardia
B. Cold intolerance
C. Difficulty sleeping
D. Pruritis

46. The psychiatric-mental health nurse practitioner is evaluating an older adult patient with recent onset of confusion and reports of decreased appetite and low mood. The nurse practitioner suspects pernicious anemia as the cause for the recent presentation of symptoms. Upon confirmation of pernicious anemia, the nurse practitioner will prescribe:

A. Folic acid
B. Thiamine
C. Cobalamin
D. Niacin

47. A patient presents to the psychiatric emergency department with a history of bipolar disorder. The patient reports dizziness and abdominal pain. The patient's lithium level is 1.8 mEq/L. Other symptoms the nurse practitioner expects to see include:

A. Vomiting and dry mouth
B. Profuse sweating and weight loss
C. Blurred vision and syncope
D. Lethargy and weight gain

(See answers next page.)

43. A) St. John's wort

The patient is displaying signs and symptoms of serotonin syndrome. Although many over-the-counter supplements may be used to treat anxiety, only St. John's wort is contraindicated for use with antidepressants such as selective serotonin reuptake inhibitors and monoamine oxidase inhibitors. Fluoxetine is a common SSRI used in the treatment of depression in children and is FDA approved for ages 8 and older. Along with its sedative and anxiolytic affects, St. John's wort is also used for its antidepressant effects and acts by increasing levels of serotonin; therefore, it is contraindicated with concomitant use of other medications that increase serotonin.

44. A) Meditation

Meditation is a technique that involves focusing on a mantra or object while practicing being present in a state of calm. Meditation has physiological effects, such as decreasing heart and respiratory rates and blood pressure, increasing alpha brain waves, and reducing anxiety. Other examples of mind-body interventions include art therapy, yoga, dance therapy, guided imagery, biofeedback, prayer, and counseling. Massage therapy, reflexology, and acupressure are categorized as manipulative and body-based interventions.

45. B) Cold intolerance

The symptoms of hypothyroidism are commonly mistaken for depression. Symptoms of hypothyroidism include apathy, weight gain, thin and dry hair, cold intolerance, facial puffiness, and slowed thinking. Therefore, it is important for the nurse to rule this out prior to starting a patient on an antidepressant. Tachycardia is commonly seen in hyperthyroidism, which often mimics anxiety or mania. Difficulty sleeping and pruritis are also associated with hyperthyroidism.

46. C) Cobalamin

Pernicious anemia, a deficiency in cobalamin (vitamin B12), presents with apathy, malaise, depressed mood, confusion, and memory deficits. It is often seen in older adults, patients who have had gastric bypass surgery, and malnourished patients. Cobalamin deficiency is a common cause of reversible dementia and should be evaluated and ruled out in all patients with suspected dementia. Folic acid is Vitamin B9 and is used in treatment of folate deficiencies. Thiamine, or Vitamin B1, deficiency is associated with Korsakoff syndrome. Niacin, or Vitamin B3, deficiency is associated with a condition known as pellagra.

47. A) Vomiting and dry mouth

Mild to moderate lithium toxicity is seen in patients with lithium levels between 1.5 and 2.0 mEq/L. Signs of mild to moderate lithium toxicity include vomiting, abdominal pain, dry mouth, ataxia, dizziness, slurred speech, nystagmus, lethargy or excitement, and muscle weakness. Profuse sweating and weight loss are symptoms of hyperthyroidism. Blurred vision and syncope are symptoms of moderate to severe lithium toxicity. Lethargy and weight gain are symptoms of hypothyroidism.

48. Alprazolam (Xanax) is a benzodiazepine that functions by enhancing the effects of:

A. Serotonin

B. Dopamine

C. Gamma-aminobutyric acid (GABA)

D. Melatonin

49. The complementary alternative treatment considered a type of energy approach is:

A. Massage

B. Acupressure

C. Reiki

D. Reflexology

50. The psychiatric-mental health nurse practitioner is evaluating a 12-year-old patient for attention deficit/hyperactivity disorder (ADHD). The nurse practitioner is reviewing the patient's ECG and notes a short PR interval and a delta wave, or upstroke of the QRS complex. Keeping this information in mind, the nurse practitioner decides to treat the patient's ADHD with:

A. Methylphenidate (Ritalin)

B. Atomoxetine (Strattera)

C. Amphetamine (Adderall)

D. Nortriptyline (Pamelor)

51. Primary hypothyroidism is indicated by laboratory values of:

A. Free T4 0.5 ng/dL and TSH 12 mU/L

B. Free T4 0.8 ng/dL and TSH 8 mU/L

C. Free T4 2.8 ng/dL and TSH 11 mU/L

D. Free T4 3.0 ng/dL and TSH 13mU/L

52. The psychiatric-mental health nurse practitioner is assessing a 3-year-old child who has short palpebral fissures, a smooth philtrum with a thin upper lip, and some learning disabilities. The nurse practitioner would assess for a central nervous system (CNS) manifestation of:

A. Microphthalmia

B. Midface hypoplasia

C. Microcephaly

D. Growth restriction

53. When monitoring a patient on lithium, the laboratory value that would warrant the psychiatric-mental health nurse practitioner's immediate attention is:

A. Glomerular filtration rate of 90

B. Serum creatinine of 2.0 mg/dL

C. Free thyroxine of 0.8 ng/dL

D. Thyroid-stimulating hormone of 5.0 mU/L

(See answers next page.)

48. C) Gamma-aminobutyric acid (GABA)
Benzodiazepines like alprazolam have antianxiety and anticonvulsant properties. These bind to the GABA receptor complex, enhance the activity of the neurotransmitter GABA, and produce a calming effect. Many medications for mood disorders target serotonin. Excessive dopamine has been associated with schizophrenia. Thus, many antipsychotic drugs have a high affinity for dopamine receptors. The pineal gland secretes melatonin as a part of the normal sleep cycle. A drug called ramelteon (Rozerem) targets melatonin receptors and is prescribed for insomnia patients.

49. C) Reiki
Reiki practitioners use light and nonmanipulative touch to the head and torso to precipitate a flow of healing energy into the patient. Reiki treatment is said to produce a feeling of relaxation, which may reduce the biochemical effects of prolonged stress. Other energy approaches include blue light treatment, electroacupuncture, electromagnetic field therapy, and electro stimulation or neuromagnetic stimulation. Acupressure, massage, and reflexology are all forms of manipulative and body-based practices.

50. B) Atomoxetine (Strattera)
Atomoxetine is a nonstimulant medication that is FDA approved for adults and children older than 6 years. It does not pose a risk of cardiac side effects and would be the safest choice for this patient. The patient's ECG is descriptive of Wolff-Parkinson-White syndrome (WPW), a type of congenital heart condition that causes rapid heart rate or palpitations. Patients with known congenital heart disease or any type of cardiac arrhythmias should avoid use of stimulant medications due to adverse cardiac effects such as tachycardia and arrhythmias. Methylphenidate and amphetamine are stimulants that may cause adverse cardiovascular effects. Nortriptyline is a nonstimulant medication, a tricyclic antidepressant (TCA) that may be used as second-or third-line off-label treatment for ADHD. However, TCAs also have the potential to produce cardiac arrhythmias and tachycardia, which would be contraindicated for a patient with WPW.

51. A) Free T4 0.5 ng/dL and TSH 12 mU/L
Normal free T4 levels are 0.8 to 2.8 ng/dL. Normal TSH values are 2 to 10 mU/L. Primary hypothyroidism occurs when free T4 is decreased and thyroid-stimulating hormone (TSH) levels are elevated in response to the low T4. In secondary hypothyroidism, the pituitary gland fails and TSH and free T4 will be low. Acute thyroiditis would present with elevated free T4 and TSH levels.

52. C) Microcephaly
The nurse practitioner would assess for the CNS manifestation of microcephaly. The sequelae that this child presents with is seen in fetal alcohol syndrome. The characteristics of fetal alcohol syndrome include growth restriction, microphthalmia, midface hypoplasia, short palpebral fissures, a smooth philtrum, and a thin upper lip. The CNS manifestations include microcephaly, attention deficits, hyperactivity, and a history of delayed development with learning disabilities and even seizures.

53. B) Serum creatinine of 2.0 mg/dL
A rare adverse effect of long-term lithium use is nephrotoxicity. This is indicated by serum creatinine of greater than 1.3 mg/dL (normal levels are 0.6 to 1.3 mg/dL) and a glomerular filtration rate of less than 60. A glomerular filtration rate of 90 is normal, as is free thyroxine of 0.8 ng/dL and thyroid-stimulating hormone of 5.0 mU/L.

54. For the psychiatric-mental health nurse practitioner to diagnose a patient with general-ized anxiety disorder (GAD), the patient must have experienced the symptoms of GAD for at least:

    A. 3 months
    B. 2 weeks
    C. 6 months
    D. 1 year

55. A patient presents with being easily distracted, having rapid speech, and expressing a flight of ideas. The patient states, "The voices tell me I am God." The patient's friend reports that prior to this, the patient was severely depressed for months with feelings of guilt, worthlessness, and hypersomnia, but now the patient can't seem to sleep and has been up for 4 days straight. The psychiatric-mental health nurse practitioner admits the patient to the hospital with a diagnosis of:

    A. Major depressive disorder
    B. Bipolar I disorder
    C. Bipolar II disorder
    D. Brief psychotic episode

56. Characteristic ECG changes seen in patients with severe bulimia nervosa include:

    A. Elevated T waves
    B. Widened QRS complex
    C. ST-segment depression
    D. Shortened QT interval

57. To differentiate bipolar disorder from attention deficit/hyperactivity disorder (ADHD), the psychiatric-mental health nurse practitioner asks:

    A. "Do your symptoms occur episodically?"
    B. "Are you easily distracted?"
    C. "Do your friends say you talk fast?"
    D. "Would you say your symptoms are troubling?"

58. To be considered for diagnosis, major depressive symptoms must be present for at least:

    A. 1 year
    B. 2 weeks
    C. 6 months
    D. 3 months

(See answers next page.)

54. C) 6 months

A patient with GAD must present with anxiety and worry and experience at least three of the following symptoms for at least 6 months to be diagnosed with GAD: excess worry, restlessness, fatigue, muscle tension, and decreased sleep and concentration.

55. B) Bipolar I disorder

The patient is exhibiting signs consistent with a manic episode of a bipolar I presentation. To differentiate between bipolar I and bipolar II disorders is to differentiate between a manic and a hypomanic episode. This is typically differentiated by the duration of the symptoms. Bipolar I would indicate manic symptoms that last for 7 days or longer, whereas bipolar II (hypomanic) symptoms last 4 to 6 days. However, a manic episode can also be characterized by the presence of psychosis, such as hearing voices, or of symptoms so severe the patient requires hospitalization, regardless of the duration of symptoms. Both bipolar I and bipolar II diagnostic criteria must also meet the criteria for major depressive disorder; however, the addition of the manic symptoms justifies a bipolar I diagnosis. A brief psychotic episode is a period of psychosis that lasts less than 30 days but that cannot be better explained by a major depressive episode or bipolar disorder.

56. C) ST-segment depression

A patient with severe bulimia nervosa will have severe hypokalemia due to vomiting, abuse of laxatives, and/or use of diuretics. Characteristic ECG findings that occur with hypokalemia include U waves, flattened T waves, and ST-segment depression and lengthening of the QT interval. Elevated T waves, widened QRS complex, and shortened QT interval are seen in hyperkalemia, and depressed T waves may be seen with acute coronary ischemia or pulmonary embolism.

57. A) "Do your symptoms occur episodically?"

Bipolar disorder and ADHD share common traits such as rapid speech, racing thoughts, distractibility, and reduced need for sleep. In order to differentiate these symptoms as a bipolar or ADHD symptomology, the nurse practitioner must ask if the presenting symptoms occur episodically. With bipolar disorder, the symptoms would be present only periodically during the manic episode, and when the patient switches to a depressed or euthymic state, the manic symptoms would resolve. In the case of a comorbid presentation, the nurse practitioner may ask if the symptoms worsen during a distinct period of time, which may indicate that the symptoms are presenting during a manic episode. The questions "Are you easily distracted?" "Do your friends say you talk fast?" and "Would you say your symptoms are troubling?" would not differentiate bipolar disorder from ADHD because these symptoms are present in both disorders.

58. B) 2 weeks

Although the symptoms of major depression can last for years, to meet the criteria for a diagnosis of major depressive disorder, a patient must have five of the following symptoms for at least 2 weeks: depressed mood, lack of interest or pleasure (anhedonia), weight loss or weight gain, increased or decreased activity, feelings of hopelessness/worthlessness or guilt, fatigue/loss of energy, insomnia or hypersomnia, diminished ability to think or concentrate, and/or recurring thoughts of death or suicide. At least one of those symptoms must be depressed mood or anhedonia.

59. An older adult presents with chronic confusion and depressed mood. The patient's spouse reports that the patient has a history of excessive drinking as a younger adult. To determine whether the symptoms stem from Alzheimer's dementia or a common chronic condition associated with alcohol use, the psychiatric-mental health nurse practitioner orders a:

A. Complete blood count
B. Thiamine level
C. Basic metabolic panel
D. Folic acid level

60. A patient has recently given birth and reports feelings of low mood, tearfulness, and inability to sleep due to worrying about the baby. Prior to diagnosing the patient with postpartum depression (PPD), the psychiatric-mental health nurse practitioner must assess:

A. Time of onset of symptoms
B. Type of support system
C. Significant weight loss
D. Change in appetite

61. To differentiate between bipolar I and bipolar II disorders, the psychiatric-mental health nurse practitioner asks a patient who presents with rapid speech, distractibility, and decreased need for sleep:

A. "Do you feel you are unstoppable?"
B. "How long do your symptoms last?"
C. "Are you easily distracted?"
D. "Do you feel depressed?"

62. A 72-year-old patient visits the hospital with his adult son. The son reports that some time ago, the patient suddenly fell, but did not get hurt. He also says that the patient reports not being able to smell food and having difficulty while swallowing. The psychiatric-mental health nurse practitioner notes that the patient is drooling and that his right hand is severely trembling even when it is put on rest. The patient answers several questions and does not have any issue remembering details. History includes a head injury 6 years ago. The nurse practitioner notes an initial diagnosis of:

A. Huntington's disease
B. Amyotrophic lateral sclerosis (ALS)
C. Parkinson's disease
D. Alzheimer's disease

(See answers next page.)

59. B) Thiamine level
Wernicke-Korsakoff syndrome is a condition resulting from depleted thiamine related to chronic alcohol abuse. Wernicke's encephalopathy is an acute presentation, whereas Korsakoff syndrome is a chronic impairment in memory and anterograde amnesia in an alert and responsive patient. Alcohol abuse should be assessed in all older adults presenting with dementia. Complete blood count, basic metabolic panel, and folic acid level tests are appropriate for a patient presenting with confusion; however, only a thiamine level would assess for the chronic condition of Korsakoff syndrome.

60. A) Time of onset of symptoms
Prior to diagnosing a patient with PPD, the nurse practitioner must rule out if the patient is experiencing "baby blues." Baby blues will occur in 30% to 75% of those who give birth. It can be differentiated from PPD by time of onset and duration. Baby blues typically occur 3 to 5 days after delivery, while PPD occurs within 3 to 6 months after delivery. Duration of baby blues is days to weeks, whereas PPD can last months to years if left untreated. The nurse practitioner will also assess type of support system, weight changes, and appetite changes; however, these factors will not differentiate PPD from baby blues.

61. B) "How long do your symptoms last?"
To differentiate between bipolar I and bipolar II disorders is to differentiate between a manic and a hypomanic episode. This is determined by the duration of the symptoms. Bipolar I would indicate manic symptoms that last for 7 days or longer, whereas bipolar II (hypomanic) symptoms last 4 to 6 days. A manic episode can also be characterized by the presence of psychosis or of symptoms so severe the patient requires hospitalization, regardless of the duration of symptoms. Asking if the patient feels unstoppable, if they are easily distracted, or if they feel depressed would not differentiate between bipolar I and bipolar II because these symptoms are found in both disorders.

62. C) Parkinson's disease
In a patient with Parkinson's disease, symptoms like difficulty swallowing, drooling, not being able to smell food, and trembling of a limb can be seen. The person can fall due to being lightheaded because this condition can lower the blood pressure suddenly. Additionally, this disease is quite common in men older than 70 years, and head injury can lead to it. It is less likely that the patient is suffering from Huntington's disease. Although most of the symptoms match with this disease, in general, people age 30 to 50 years suffer from this disease. Also, it is a genetic disease, so it will not be caused by a head injury. The patient also has a smaller chance of suffering from ALS, as it does not hamper one's sense of smell. Because the patient is not facing any issue regarding memory, Alzheimer's disease is an unlikely diagnosis.

63. When screening a patient for depression, the psychiatric-mental health nurse practitioner also performs screening for medical conditions that may potentiate the patient's symptoms. The nurse practitioner understands that up to 10% of patients who have symptoms of depression may also have:

    A. Anxiety
    B. Diabetes mellitus
    C. Hypothyroidism
    D. Hypertension

64. The psychiatric-mental health nurse practitioner interviews a 10-year-old patient, accompanied by their parents, with concerns of being irritable and overwhelmed easily, with excessive worrying and difficulty concentrating. Based on the patient's symptoms, the nurse practitioner prescribes:

    A. Lorazepam
    B. Escitalopram
    C. Buspirone
    D. Diphenhydramine

65. When treating a patient with antipsychotics, it is important for the psychiatric-mental health nurse practitioner to know that the peak plasma concentration after an oral dose is reached in:

    A. 1 to 2 hours
    B. 2 to 3 hours
    C. 6 to 8 hours
    D. 12 to 16 hours

66. According to the DSM-5, diagnostic criteria for major depressive disorder (MDD) includes:

    A. Three symptoms of depression for the same 2-week period
    B. Fatigue or loss of energy nearly every day for 2 weeks
    C. Marked disinterest in activities for most of the day, every day for 1 week
    D. Restlessness or feeling on edge for 2 weeks

67. A 70-year-old patient comes into the office of a psychiatric-mental health nurse practitioner, accompanied by his adult daughter, for an initial visit with concerns around worsening symptoms of memory loss over the past 6 months. The nurse practitioner suspects that the patient may be showing early signs of Alzheimer's disease. For an accurate diagnosis, according to the DSM-5, the patient must also show signs of:

    A. Progressive decline in cognition, with no evidence of any other neurological or mental disorder
    B. Inconsistent decline in cognition, with no evidence of any other neurological or mental disorder
    C. Evidence of a cerebrovascular accident and ataxia and poor speech
    D. Visual field cuts and increased irritability

(See answers next page.)

63. C) Hypothyroidism

Symptoms of depression can be attributed to hypothyroidism in up to 10% of patients; there-fore, screening for this medical condition is necessary. There is no identifiable link between diabetes mellitus or hypertension and overlapping symptoms of depression. While anxiety may coexist with depression, it is not a medical condition.

64. B) Escitalopram

The presenting symptoms are consistent with generalized anxiety disorder. Selective sero-tonin reuptake inhibitors like escitalopram (Lexapro) are the first line of treatment for anxi-ety disorders in children. While benzodiazepines such as lorazepam (Ativan) and other anxiolytics such as buspirone (Buspar) may be used, they are not the first line of treatment for anxiety in this population. Antihistamines such as diphenhydramine (Benadryl) are occasionally used for pediatric patients with sleep disturbances.

65. B) 2 to 3 hours

Antipsychotics are metabolized primarily in the liver, with metabolites excreted primarily in urine. Many metabolites are active, and peak plasma concentration usually is reached 2 to 3 hours after an oral dose.

66. B) Fatigue or loss of energy nearly every day for 2 weeks

According to the DSM-5, five or more symptoms of depression should be present for the same 2-week period, inclusive of fatigue or loss of energy, to meet diagnostic criteria for MDD. Three symptoms of depression over 2 weeks do not meet diagnostic criteria for MDD. While marked disinterest in activities for most of the day is a symptom of depres-sion, symptoms must be present for at least 2 weeks to meet diagnostic criteria. Restlessness or feeling on edge is a symptom of generalized anxiety disorder, not MDD.

67. A) Progressive decline in cognition, with no evidence of any other neurologi-cal or mental disorder

According to the DSM-5, diagnosis for Alzheimer's disease must include clear evidence of a decline in memory or learning, a progressive and gradual decline in cognition, and no evidence of mixed etiology. Evidence of a cerebrovascular accident (CVA) is an example of mixed etiology. Accompanying symptoms of a CVA are ataxia, poor speech, and visual field cuts. While irritability may be present with Alzheimer's disease, it is not a marker for diagnostic criteria.

68. When adjusting valproate (Depakote) for treatment of mania in bipolar disorder, the target serum level is between:

    A. 350 and 450 ng/mL
    B. 50 and 125 mcg/mL
    C. 0.8 and 1.2 mEq/L
    D. 0.1 and 1.5 mEq/L

69. A symptom of generalized anxiety disorder is:

    A. Excessive worry
    B. Feelings of hopelessness
    C. Inflated self-esteem
    D. Decreased need for sleep

70. The psychiatric-mental health nurse practitioner evaluates a patient who presents to the emergency department with symptoms of hypomania. The nurse practitioner obtains the patient's history and identifies that the patient has a history of amphetamine use, although the patient denies any recent use. The nurse practitioner plans to do a urine drug screen with the understanding that last use of amphetamines can be detected in urine for up to:

    A. 12 hours
    B. 24 hours
    C. 48 hours
    D. 3 days

71. A 75-year-old patient who has been diagnosed with Alzheimer's dementia is evaluated by the psychiatric-mental health nurse practitioner for changes in behavior and severe psychosis that causes significant distress. After thorough assessment and review of response to non-drug interventions, risks and benefits of the chosen drug, and other treatment options, the nurse practitioner prescribes a low dose of:

    A. Lithium
    B. Aripiprazole
    C. Sertraline
    D. Clonazepam

72. The psychiatric-mental health nurse practitioner sees a high-functioning, active 65-year-old male patient with a history of hypertension and anxiety in the emergency department with a suspected diagnosis of delirium. Predisposing risk factors for this patient include:

    A. Male sex
    B. High level of activity
    C. Anxiety
    D. Treatment with anti-hypertensive medication

(See answers next page.)

68. B) 50 and 125 mcg/mL

The target serum level for valproate is 50 to 125 mcg/mL. The range 350 to 450 ng/mL is the target serum level for clozapine (Clozaril). The therapeutic range for lithium is 0.8 to 1.2 mEq/L. The range 0.1 to 1.5 mEq/L is not a specific target range for any psychotropic medication.

69. A) Excessive worry

According to the DSM-5, key symptoms of generalized anxiety disorder are excessive worrying, difficulty concentrating, restlessness or feeling on edge, being easily fatigued, irritability, muscle tension, and sleep disturbance. Feelings of hopelessness are a symptom of depression. Inflated self-esteem and a decreased need for sleep are symptoms of hypomania or mania, indicative of bipolar disorder.

70. C) 48 hours

Amphetamines can be detected in urine up to 48 hours after last use. Alcohol may be detected between 7 and 12 hours after last use. Barbiturates may be detected up to 24 hours after last use. Benzodiazepines and methadone may be detected 3 days after last use.

71. B) Aripiprazole

Alzheimer's dementia may be treated with low-dose antipsychotics, such as aripiprazole (Abilify), in older adults with severe agitation and psychosis that pose danger and significant distress to the patient. Lithium is a mood stabilizer and is most often used to treat mania in bipolar disorder, while sertraline is a selective serotonin reuptake inhibitor used to treat depression and anxiety. Clonazepam is a benzodiazepine used to treat anxiety.

72. A) Male sex

Predisposing risk factors for delirium include male sex and age 65 years and older. Low level of activity and depression are also additional risk factors. While anxiety may coexist with signs and symptoms of delirium, it is not a direct predisposing factor for delirium. There is no correlation between treatment with anti-hypertensive medication and delirium; there is a correlation with treatment with psychoactive drugs or drugs with anticholinergic properties.

73. The psychiatric-mental health nurse practitioner sees an older adult patient for an initial visit and suspects a diagnosis of dementia. Prior to diagnosis, the nurse practitioner must evaluate for treatment with a/an:

    A. Statin for cholesterolemia
    B. Corticosteroid for swelling
    C. Antihistamine for allergic reaction
    D. Proton pump inhibitor for gastroesophageal reflux disease

74. According to the DSM-5, based on diagnostic criteria for obsessive-compulsive disorder (OCD), obsessions are defined as:

    A. Behaviors that are aimed at preventing anxiety
    B. Repetitive behaviors that the individual feels driven to perform
    C. Recurrent thoughts, urges, or images that are intrusive and unwanted
    D. Mental acts that the individual is able to suppress

75. One of the core features of delirium is:

    A. Altered consciousness
    B. Unsteady gait
    C. Stable mood
    D. Slow onset of symptoms

76. Treatment with lithium, a mood stabilizer used to treat mania in bipolar disorder, must include:

    A. Urine drug screen
    B. Complete metabolic panel
    C. Valproic acid level
    D. EEG

77. The psychiatric-mental health nurse practitioner has an initial visit with a 17-year-old patient accompanied by his parents. The patient's parents report concern for the patient's sudden onset of inattention, distractibility, fidgetiness in the classroom, and difficulty completing homework. With some symptoms consistent with attention deficit/hyperactivity disorder (ADHD), the nurse practitioner understands that further screening is required if:

    A. There were no noticeable concerns or symptoms in early childhood
    B. The patient is male
    C. The patient is a teenager
    D. There is a family history of depression

78. The psychiatric-mental health nurse practitioner plans to start a patient on clozapine (Clozaril). The results of the patient's complete blood count are abnormal, with an absolute neutrophil count (ANC) of 1,000 per mm^3 and a white blood cell count (WBC) of 2,500 per mm^3. The appropriate action for the nurse practitioner to take is to:

    A. Not start the medication and order a hematology consult
    B. Start the medication with daily ANC levels
    C. Start the medication at the lowest dose
    D. Admit the patient to the hospital and start medication in a controlled setting

(See answers next page.)

73. B) Corticosteroid for swelling

Treatment with corticosteroids may resemble signs and symptoms of dementia. Additional medications that may potentiate symptoms of dementia are anticholinergic agents, antihypertensives, antipsychotics, digitalis, opioids, nonsteroidal anti-inflammatory agents, phenytoin, and sedative hypnotics. Treatment with statins, antihistamines, or proton pump inhibitors does not directly potentiate effects of dementia.

74. C) Recurrent thoughts, urges, or images that are intrusive and unwanted

According to the DSM-5, obsessions are recurrent and persistent thoughts, urges, or images that are often intrusive and unwanted, leading to marked distress or anxiety. Individuals with OCD attempt to suppress such thoughts by neutralizing them with another thought or action. Compulsions are behaviors that are repetitive in nature that the individual feels driven to perform, aimed at preventing anxiety. While obsessions are mental acts, the individual is not able to suppress them.

75. A) Altered consciousness

The core features of delirium are altered consciousness, decreased memory, disorganized thoughts, perceptual disturbances, sundowning, disruption of sleep—wake cycle, altered neurological function, and mood alteration. Although patients with delirium may be at risk for falls, unsteady gait is not a core feature of delirium. Delirium has a rapid onset of symptoms that are short-lived (usually days to weeks).

76. B) Complete metabolic panel

Lithium must be accompanied by baseline labs including complete metabolic panel, complete blood count, ECG, thyroid function tests, and liver function tests. A urine drug screen is not a standard of treatment with lithium unless substance abuse is suspected or is being treated. Valproic acid levels are specific to treatment with Depakote. An EEG would be ordered with concerns for seizures or other neurologic conditions.

77. A) There were no noticeable concerns or symptoms in early childhood

According to the DSM-5, patients should show symptoms of ADHD before age 12 years. Given the patient's age, with no concerns prior to his current age, ADHD is not a probable diagnosis. Additional factors, including that the patient is male and a teenager, or if he has a family history of depression, would not be the most important predictors of a diagnosis of ADHD.

78. A) Not start the medication and order a hematology consult

Medication cannot be started because the guidelines for initiation of clozapine require the baseline WBC to be at least 3,500 per mm3, and the absolute neutrophil count (ANC) must be at least 2,000 per mm3. A hematology consult is appropriate for determining the cause of patients' neutropenia. The medication cannot be started at any dose, regardless of the monitoring schedule, in any setting, until minimum ANC is reached.

79. An 8-year-old patient is brought to the emergency department by his parent, who reports that he lost consciousness an hour earlier and that his body stiffened prior to "jerking." Upon examination in the emergency department, the patient appears pale, confused, and lethargic. Upon evaluation, a bite on the tongue and blood-stained teeth are noticed, along with urine-stained pants. The type of seizure the nurse practitioner would diagnose is:

A. Absence
B. Simple focal
C. Tonic-clonic
D. Myoclonic

80. Patients diagnosed with bipolar disorder are most commonly treated with:

A. Antidepressants
B. Benzodiazepines
C. Methadone
D. Mood stabilizers

81. A 17-year-old patient comes into the office of a psychiatric-mental health nurse practitioner accompanied by parents for an initial visit. The patient reports worsening symptoms from a traumatic brain injury (TBI) since being involved in a car crash 3 months ago. The nurse practitioner is concerned that the patient may have a mild neurocognitive disorder due to the TBI. According to the DSM-5, this diagnosis involves having one or more symptoms, including:

A. Headaches
B. Poor concentration
C. Amnesia
D. Anxiety

82. According to the DSM-5, borderline personality disorder is categorized in cluster:

A. A
B. B
C. C
D. Other

83. A 32-year-old patient who has been treated with lithium for bipolar disorder for more than 3 years comes to the office because she has felt weak and has experienced cold intolerance, constipation, and weight gain during the past 6 months. Physical examination shows dry, coarse skin and bradycardia, hypothermia, and swelling of the hands and feet. The most appropriate diagnostic study to check is:

A. Blood alcohol level
B. Serum thyroid-stimulating hormone
C. Liver function testing
D. ECG

(See answers next page.)

79. C) Tonic-clonic

Patients who experience a tonic-clonic, or grand mal, seizure often lose consciousness suddenly, with a stiffening of the body followed by the clonic jerking of the muscles lasting 3 or more minutes. Tongue biting and urinary incontinence are often noted. The patient has a state of drowsiness and lethargy afterward. An absence seizure is a sudden brief lapse of consciousness accompanied by staring or movements of the lips or hands. It lasts for less than 10 seconds and is followed by no postictal state. Simple focal seizures are similar to absence seizures and present as twitching of muscles and staring off into space, but there is no loss of consciousness. Myoclonic seizure increases the patient's muscle tone suddenly, as if hit by a bolt of lightning, but it is not continuous and appears as more of a spasm.

80. D) Mood stabilizers

The most common treatment for bipolar disorder is mood stabilizers. While antidepressants and benzodiazepines may be used to augment treatment, they are not the primary treatment. Methadone is used only in the setting of opiate use disorder.

81. C) Amnesia

According to the DSM-5, diagnosis for a neurocognitive disorder includes a TBI with one or more of the following: loss of consciousness, posttraumatic amnesia, disorientation and confusion, and neurological signs. Although anxiety, poor concentration, and headaches may exist with a TBI, these particular symptoms do not meet the criteria for a mild neurocognitive disorder.

82. B) B

According to the DSM-5, cluster B personality disorders are borderline personality disorder, antisocial personality disorder, histrionic personality disorder, and narcissistic personality disorder. Cluster A disorders are paranoid personality disorder, schizoid personality disorder, and schizotypal personality disorder. Cluster C disorders are avoidant personality disorder, dependent personality disorder, and obsessive–compulsive personality disorder. Other personality disorders show a persistent personality disturbance but do not otherwise meet criteria of any other identified personality disorder.

83. B) Serum thyroid-stimulating hormone

The patient's reported symptoms suggest a thyroid disorder. Serum thyroid-stimulating hormone (TSH) measures the amount of TSH produced by the pituitary gland, which regulates hormones released by the thyroid. It is appropriate to order a medical workup when physical causes are suspected; however, there is no correlation with abnormal blood alcohol level, liver function tests, or ECG changes with the patient's symptoms.

84. The main U.S. governmental agency for investigating nontraditional treatments for mental illness and other conditions is the:

A. National Center for Complementary and Integrative Health (NCCIH)
B. National Institute of Mental Health (NIMH)
C. National Alliance on Mental Illness (NAMI)
D. Food and Drug Administration (FDA)

85. An adult patient is brought to the emergency department (ED) for erratic behavior. Previous ED history includes serious headaches, fatigue, and transient blurry vision 3 months ago. The patient was prescribed 40 to 60 mg per day of prednisone for approximately 1 month; then the dose was tapered. Anxiety and poor sleep were reported during that time, and depressive episode was denied. The patient has not slept for >3 hours a night for over a week. Mood is irritable, with no cognitive deficits. Although affect is labile, it is appropriate to the content of his speech (e.g., he becomes tearful when reporting pending divorce). Speech is loud, pressured, and over-elaborative. No perceptual disturbances are reported or observed. Exhibited mental status exam abnormalities include flight of ideas, racing thoughts, increased energy, and being easily distractible. The patient is oriented to time and place and convincingly denies suicidal and homicidal ideation. The patient exhibits poor judgment, and insight is absent. Based on medical and psychiatric history and current mental status findings, the nurse practitioner diagnoses:

A. Adjustment disorder with mixed anxiety and depressed mood
B. Bipolar II
C. Bipolar I
D. Steroid psychosis

86. The psychiatric-mental health nurse practitioner sees a 20-year-old patient with presenting symptoms of acute and recurrent angry outbursts and irritability, occurring about three times per week. She lives with her parents, and this has become a major disruption to their living environment. The nurse practitioner has concerns for disruptive mood dysregulation disorder. This can be ruled out due to the patient's:

A. Outbursts and irritability
B. Symptoms occurring three times a week
C. Sex
D. Age

87. The study to determine the effectiveness of an intervention is a:

A. Case study
B. Cross-sectional study
C. Randomized control trial
D. Cohort study

88. Brexanolone (Zulresso) is the first FDA-approved medication for:

A. Postpartum depression
B. Bipolar disorder
C. Schizophrenia
D. Alzheimer's disease

(See answers next page.)

84. A) National Center for Complementary and Integrative Health (NCCIH)

The NCCIH is 1 of 27 institutes and centers at the National Institutes of Health. Its responsibility is to oversee nontraditional treatments for mental illness. The NIMH is the leading federal agency for research on mental disorders. The NAMI is the nation's largest grassroots mental health organization dedicated to building better lives for the millions of Americans affected by mental illness. The FDA is the United States' regulatory agency for food, medicines, and medical supplies.

85. C) Bipolar I

The patient's most likely diagnosis is bipolar I. Their mental status abnormalities meet the Diagnostic and Statistical Manual of Mental Disorders (DSM-5) criteria for bipolar I disorder (has inflated self-esteem, requires less sleep, is overtalkative, has a history of functional impairment, and has an increase in goal-directed activity). Manic symptoms have lasted for over a week. Patients with an adjustment disorder with mixed anxiety and depressed mood do not experience the severity of symptoms and loss of function described. Although there is a history of stressful events, symptoms preceded these events. Steroid psychosis is categorized by DSM-5 as a form of substance/medication-induced psychotic disorder. The patient did not experience delusions or hallucinations after taking prednisone, and the exposure was 3 months ago. Bipolar II involves periods of hypomania; there is no history of mania. A bipolar II diagnosis requires a patient to experience at least one major depressive episode, which the patient has not experienced.

86. D) Age

Disruptive mood dysregulation disorder (DMDD) is characterized by recurrent angry outbursts and irritability relative to developmental age, occurring at least three times a week. However, DMDD is diagnosed only between the ages of 6 and 18 years. The patient's sex is not relevant to the diagnosis.

87. C) Randomized control trial

The gold standard for an intervention to be effective is a randomized control trial. Results from a randomized control trial are essential for determining if nursing care or intervention is effective for patients. Focusing on a specific patient will not determine the practices suitable for multiple patients; therefore, a case study would not determine effectiveness well. A cross-sectional study is very specific for a given time and a given population, which can limit the efficacy to a specific population only. Determining the changes of a specific patient due to treatment for a specific period is a cohort study. This is a time-dependent process with only specific people as a part of the treatment and is not suitable to detect efficacy.

88. A) Postpartum depression

Breaxanolone is the first FDA-approved drug for postpartum depression. It appears to function by interacting with gamma-aminobutyric acid (GABA) receptors. Drugs like valproate (Depakote) are mood stabilizers that have been approved for bipolar disorder. Antipsychotic medications are commonly used to target the negative and positive symptoms of schizophrenia. Drugs used for Alzheimer's disease, like donepezil (Aricept), function by inhibiting cholinesterase.

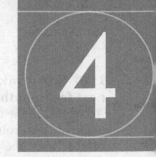

Psychotherapy and Related Theories

1. The psychiatric-mental health nurse practitioner sees a patient for an initial visit with concern for alcohol use disorder. The statement that identifies that the patient is in the contemplation stage of change is:

   A. "My drinking is not a problem for me at all. That's not the reason why I am here today."
   B. "My drinking is a problem, and I'm thinking about how to improve in the next few months."
   C. "My drinking has always been a problem, but I'm not sure if it can get better at this point."
   D. "My alcohol use is not something I need any help with at this time."

2. After working with a family with significantly dysfunctional patterns, the psychiatric–mental health nurse practitioner observes that the 16-year-old daughter begins to show signs of self-differentiation. This would be observed by:

   A. The patient continuing to feel enmeshed in family boundaries
   B. The patient feeling she has self-worth despite her family relationships
   C. The patient feeling that she has continued low self-worth
   D. The patient showing that she is developing self-identity

3. Social practice theory analyzes the behavior of a person based on the use and consumption of energy. The element of the theory that refers to images and concepts concerning a particular behavior is called:

   A. Materials
   B. Meanings
   C. Procedure
   D. Contemplation

4. The family system has reached homeostasis when the family:

   A. Continues with maladaptive communication
   B. Returns to stability despite continuing dysfunction
   C. Continues with the same behaviors as previously
   D. Communicates less effectively among its members

5. Multisystemic therapy involves:

   A. Patient treatment in home and community
   B. Patient placement in custody
   C. Patient hospitalization
   D. Patient placement in remand home

1. B) "My drinking is a problem, and I'm thinking about how to improve in the next few months."

According to the transtheoretical model of change, in the contemplation phase, the individual identifies problematic behavior and intends to make changes to the behavior in the near future. When the patient acknowledges alcohol misuse and wants to make changes within the next few months, it demonstrates readiness, which is indicative of the contemplation stage. Lack of acknowledgment of alcohol misuse, vague planning around treatment, and refusal of treatment are actions that indicate lack or readiness, indicative of the precontemplation stage.

2. B) The patient feeling she has self-worth despite her family relationships

Self-differentiation is the level at which an individual's self-worth is not dependent on external relationships. Enmeshment in family boundaries demonstrates lack of self-differentiation due to the value external relationships hold in such patterns. Continued low self-worth demonstrates lack of self-differentiation. Self-identity is not a factor when determining self-differentiation.

3. B) Meanings

The social practice theory is based on a three-element model. Meanings, the second element of the model, are symbolic gestures like images and concepts that facilitate a particular behavior. Materials, the first element of the model, are the physical or material objects that allow a particular behavior. The procedure, the third element of the model, refers to the skills or competencies of a person that allows certain behavior. Contemplation is one of the stages of the transtheoretical change model and is not a part of the three-element model of social practice theory.

4. B) Returns to stability despite continuing dysfunction

Homeostasis indicates the family's achievement of stability, despite dysfunction. Continuing with maladaptive communication and previous behavior patterns of family members suggests no change in the family system, with continuing negative outcomes. Less effective communication between family members demonstrates a worsening outcome for the family system, which is not congruent with achievement of homeostasis/stability.

5. A) Patient treatment in home and community

Multisystemic therapy (MST) is an intensive home- and community-based treatment for adolescents who engage in severe willful misconduct that places them at risk for out-of-home placement. MST has been used for adolescents presenting with a wide range of serious clinical problems, including chronic and violent juvenile offenders, adolescent sexual offenders, those in psychiatric crisis (homicidal, suicidal, and psychotic), and those with maltreating families. A custody-based model includes the imprisonment of the patient, which is not part of MST. MST is home and community based, so hospitals and child remand homes are not part of the therapy.

6. A parent has been experiencing and displaying ongoing anger at a work colleague due to the colleague's dishonesty. The parent's preschool-aged child is not happy with the current expressed behavior of the parent. The bioecological system of the child that has become hampered is:

    A. Mesosystem
    B. Exosystem
    C. Macrosystem
    D. Chronosystem

7. A teenage patient expresses confidence in their ability to avoid smoking and exercise regularly to prevent pulmonary disease. This statement is an example of:

    A. Self-efficacy
    B. Unrealistic optimism
    C. Self-liberation
    D. Dramatic relief

8. A nonprofit organization is planning an initiative to assist older adults in leading a more healthy and active lifestyle. The initiative will last 6 months and includes monthly counseling sessions, seminars, and collaboration with a top healthcare facility. The planned long-term outcome of this project is:

    A. To collaborate with a well-regarded hospital
    B. To assess the number of patients treated
    C. To help patients achieve a healthier lifestyle
    D. To create detailed literature about the project

9. The behavioral framework that involves the identification of several noncoercive influences affecting an individual's behavior is the model known as:

    A. Four E's
    B. MINDSPACE
    C. Energy culture
    D. Behavior change wheel

10. At a boarding school, the curfew for entering the boys' dormitory is 10 p.m., and the curfew for the girls' dormitory is 8 p.m. A protest is held by residents of the girls' dormitory to remove this social inequity, and the school principal is approached. Without discussion with other panel members or student council, the principal extends the curfew time for the girls' dormitory to 9 p.m. This change is not accepted by the student council. The principal's method for dealing with the situation is an example of the theory of:

    A. Conflict
    B. Functionalism
    C. Symbolic interactionism
    D. Family systems

(See answers next page.)

6. B) Exosystem

Because the relationship between the parent and the workplace is hampered, the exosystem of the child is affected. The child has no connection with the workplace, so the affected system is the exosystem and not the mesosystem. The dishonesty of the parent's colleagues has no connection with any cultural value or belief, so it is not a macrosystem issue. The chronosystem of the child is not altered because drastic changes have not occurred in the child.

7. A) Self-efficacy

Self-efficacy is the ability of a person to perform any behavior with dedication. The teenage patient is confident in their ability to perform certain behaviors (smoking avoidance, regular exercise), which is an example of self-efficacy. Unrealistic optimism is predicting an outcome that is not relevant or realistic; in this case, it is not unrealistic to expect to reduce the likelihood of pulmonary disease if smoking is avoided and regular exercise is performed. Self-liberation is decision making after a process has happened. Dramatic relief refers to expressing one's feelings about a particular problem or solution.

8. C) To help patients achieve a healthier lifestyle

Helping older adults achieve a healthier, more active lifestyle is the long-term outcome for this nonprofit. The long-term outcome is the intended result of the intervention, which can be achieved by guiding older adults to participate in a healthy, active lifestyle. For the outcome to be achieved, the nonprofit includes an external condition of collaboration with a well-regarded hospital. This component is an assumption of what is needed to achieve the goal and is not the overall outcome. The number of treated patients is one of the indicators of progress toward the goal. Creating literature and spreading information about the initiative can help in reaching the goal.

9. B) MINDSPACE

The MINDSPACE model involves the identification of noncoercive influences of a particular behavior. The four E's model deals with the consumer behavior of an individual and analyzes behavioral change under four conditions: enable, encourage, engage, and exemplify. The energy culture model involves understanding behavior based on cognitive norms like education, energy practice like social marketing, and material culture like efficiency rating schemes. The behavioral change wheel model involves three conditions: capability, opportunity, and motivation to understand the outcome of behavior.

10. C) Symbolic interactionism

Symbolic interactionism theory deals with individual interpretation, not thinking of the whole society as a system. Hence, the principal making a decision without consulting others is an example of symbolic interactionism theory. Functionalism theory regards society as a whole and talks about a family's contribution to society. It faces criticism because it has failed to account for social change properly and considers a sudden change in society to be undesirable. Conflict theory regards a sudden social change as a solution to social inequality. The family systems theory includes the concept of boundaries.

11. The criterion that the psychiatric-mental health nurse practitioner uses to determine if a child is in the preoperational stage of cognitive development is that the child:

    A. Can think about theoretical and abstract concepts and use logic to draw solutions
    B. Can remember things is not able to describe them properly
    C. Can draw pictures to represent objects
    D. Does not consider other people's thoughts as different from the child's

12. A couple married for 15 years visits a psychiatric-mental health nurse practitioner to consult about their deteriorating relationship. Both patients are attracted to others romantically, but they feel guilty and depressed. The couple wants to attempt to save their marriage and also to alleviate depression. The nurse practitioner treats them using symbolic interactionism theory and tells them that the therapy will continue for 18 to 20 weeks. The common therapy that the nurse will use is:

    A. System desensitization
    B. Interpersonal
    C. Behavioral
    D. Psychodynamic

13. An older adult has recently developed negative feelings toward his son. The father thinks that the son is avoiding him and not caring for him properly. This is a recent thought pattern for the father, and he has not experienced any previous mental disturbance. The son brings the father to the psychiatric-mental health nurse practitioner to help improve their relationship. The nurse practitioner finds that the father's feelings and expectations have developed due to excessive watching of movies. The therapy that can be used by the nurse practitioner is:

    A. Humanistic
    B. Cognitive behavioral
    C. Interpersonal
    D. Psychodynamic

14. A person takes care of others and is highly aware of social rules. The person possesses the determination to maintain all the rules and never judge whether the rules are beneficial or not. According to Lawrence Kohlberg's stages of moral development, the person belongs to the stage of moral reasoning known as:

    A. 3
    B. 4
    C. 5
    D. 6

15. A child with academic issues is presented to the psychiatric-mental health nurse practitioner. The child does not want to study mathematics because he scored low on previous tests. The child is also not interested in attending his guitar and drawing lessons. The crisis the nurse practitioner must resolve for the advancement of the child is:

    A. Trust versus mistrust
    B. Autonomy versus shame and doubt
    C. Initiation versus guilt
    D. Industry versus inferiority

(See answers next page.)

11. B) Can remember things is not able to describe them properly

A child in a preoperational stage can remember things but cannot describe them properly. A child in the sensorimotor stage can draw pictures to represent objects. During the concrete operational stage, a child learns about the concept of volume and can address other people's thoughts. A child in the formal operational stage knows about abstract and theoretical concepts.

12. B) Interpersonal

Interpersonal therapy is a short-term therapy of 12 to 20 weeks that is intended to improve current interpersonal relationships. Its goal is to find the role of relationships in one's life and find ways to resolve it issues. System desensitization therapy mainly treats phobia. Behavioral therapy focuses on changing the behavior of a person, which then affects an emotion. Psychodynamic therapy generally takes more than 20 sessions and is used when a conflict occurred in childhood and has remained unresolved for a long time.

13. B) Cognitive behavioral

The nurse practitioner will use cognitive behavioral therapy in this situation. This therapy addresses both the behavior and the negative thoughts of the patient. Humanistic therapy is used where self-concept is important. Interpersonal therapy is a short-term therapy of 12 to 20 weeks that is used to make current interpersonal relationships better. It works well when both participating people are ready to improve the relationship. Psychodynamic therapy is used when the past of the patient is involved.

14. B) 4

The person belongs to Stage 4 of the conventional level of Kohlberg's theory of moral development. This stage is present in the age group of later years and is characterized by following all the rules to avoid punishment. A person in Stage 3 relates rightness or wrongness to motivations. A person in Stage 5 believes that social rules must be beneficial enough to be followed and should be changed if corrupt. People in Stage 6 believe that unjust laws should be broken down, which will create justice for everyone.

15. D) Industry versus inferiority

The child has unresolved industry versus inferiority because the child is having a sense of inferiority and difficulty in working and learning. The resolution would help the child in feeling confident that he is improving in his abilities. Unsuccessful resolution of trust versus mistrust leads to general issues relating to suspicion of people. Unsuccessful resolution of autonomy versus shame and doubt leads to fear of conflict and self-doubt. Unsuccessful resolution of initiative versus guilt leads to aggression and a sense of inadequacy.

16. A patient with a fear of dogs comes to the clinic and reports increasing obsession about the phobia. The patient has started to feel extremely anxious whenever leaving home. The psychiatric-mental health nurse practitioner will recommend possible treatment with the therapy referred to as:

    A. Psychoanalytical
    B. Exposure
    C. Dream analysis
    D. Aversion

17. Dream analysis is a primary technique used in the therapy known as:

    A. Interpersonal
    B. Psychoanalytical
    C. Behavioral
    D. Humanistic

18. A patient reports feeling depressed due to stress at work and describes how the stress causes body aches and general malaise. The psychiatric-mental health nurse practitioner asks the patient to monitor and record heart rate and blood pressure when experiencing stress. The patient is also instructed to perform certain stretching exercises to reduce the muscle pain. This type of behavior therapy is called:

    A. Exposure
    B. Aversion
    C. Biofeedback
    D. Modeling

19. Nursing theorist Patricia Benner's major contribution is the:

    A. Goal of promoting self-care in the patient through nursing interventions
    B. Theory of caring as a foundation for nursing by emphasizing nurse-patient relations
    C. Continual need for the patient to adapt physically, psychologically, and socially
    D. Focus on nursing interventions that can help a patient use stress-reducing strategies

20. At the beginning of the psychodynamic therapy session, the patient and the psychotherapist decide to work on an issue mutually. This is appropriate for a patient:

    A. With borderline personality disorder
    B. Experiencing psychosis
    C. With severe personality disorder
    D. Experiencing clinical depression

21. The common cognitive distortion that emphasizes the negative view and invalidates the positive view is known as:

    A. All-or-nothing thinking
    B. Labeling
    C. Disqualifying the positive
    D. Mind reading

(See answers next page.)

16. B) Exposure

The patient should be treated with exposure therapy in cases of phobia. This will slowly eliminate the patient's fear and will also help reduce the anxiety. Psychoanalytical therapy is a classical theory that is not valid in many cases today. It involves looking at the dreams and childhood traumas of the patient; similarly, dream analysis would not be considered a valid therapy. Aversion therapy applies when there is substance abuse or when the patient is required to avoid a certain stimulus or element that has been causing harm.

17. B) Psychoanalytical

Dream analysis is a key part of psychoanalytical theory, wherein dreams are considered projections of the unconscious awareness of the patient. Interpersonal therapy focuses on the deficit of social interaction and attempts to resolve interpersonal conflicts to treat a mental issue. Behavioral therapy is focused on the behavior of the patient and how it can be changed with reinforcement and punishment. Humanistic therapy is an insightful therapy that focuses on the overall subjective experiences of the patient, but dream analysis is not a primary technique of this therapy.

18. C) Biofeedback

Biofeedback therapy involves the use of technology and exercise that can help the patient. It can include using smart watches to monitor changes in vital signs or doing exercises to reduce pain. Exposure therapy is used to help a patient become accustomed to a certain situation. This therapy is used for phobias and for stopping the abuse of drugs or alcohol. Aversion therapy is chosen when other measures fail to help a patient react in a certain way, and it can be used for behaviors like nail-biting. Modeling therapy involves providing a role model to the patient so that imitation can help a patient adopt the desired change.

19. B) Theory of caring as a foundation for nursing by emphasizing nurse-patient relations

Patricia Benner mainly focused on the theory of caring as the foundation of nursing. The goal of self-care as an integral part of nursing is the major contribution of Dorothea Orem. The continuous need for adaptations is the major contribution of theorist Sister Callista Roy. Betty Neuman described the role of stressors in the equilibrium of the system.

20. D) Experiencing clinical depression

Psychodynamic therapy is most suited to patients who are functional and are psychologically sound or intelligent enough to understand that they have an issue, such as those experiencing clinical depression. At the beginning of the treatment in psychodynamic therapy, the goal of the therapy is discussed. This is not a suitable technique for borderline personality disorder, personality disorder, or psychosis because patients with these conditions may not understand that they have issues to be addressed.

21. C) Disqualifying the positive

Disqualifying the positive is the distortion that focuses on maintaining the negative view and disqualifying the positive view by marking it as irrelevant or inaccurate. All or nothing makes the mind think in a black-and-white manner by reducing all complex outcomes. Labeling is a form of generalization and results in an overly harsh label for self or others. Mind reading is a type of distortion for jumping into the negative interpretation.

22. According to Maslow's hierarchy, the safety needs are:

    A. Affiliation and love
    B. Security, protection, and stability
    C. Food, water, oxygen, and rest
    D. Self-esteem and esteem from others

23. In trauma-focused cognitive behavioral theory, a child tends to:

    A. Focus on suicidal thoughts
    B. Avoid reminders about past problems
    C. Incorporate self-injury
    D. Draw a conclusion based on an emotional state

24. The theory of cognitive development was developed by:

    A. Jean Piaget
    B. Lawrence Kohlberg
    C. Carl Rogers
    D. Viktor Frankl

25. A 7-year-old child shows a sense of being lesser than others. The child finds it difficult to learn and work. The psychological crisis exhibited is:

    A. Trust versus mistrust
    B. Autonomy versus shame and doubt
    C. Industry versus inferiority
    D. Intimacy versus isolation

26. A patient is admitted to a hospital after suffering a fracture in the right leg. The patient is advised to take bed rest for a month. The patient is a top manager and is visited by several friends and family members. The psychiatric-mental health nurse practitioner hears the patient lament having achieved nothing in life and having no one by their side. The nurse practitioner needs to resolve the psychological crisis of:

    A. Trust versus mistrust
    B. Initiative versus guilt
    C. Identity versus role confusion
    D. Integrity versus despair

27. The stage of cognitive development during which a child learns to comprehend other's viewpoints and can think logically is the stage known as:

    A. Preoperational
    B. Formal operational
    C. Sensorimotor
    D. Concrete operational

(See answers next page.)

22. B) Security, protection, and stability

The safety needs are security, protection, stability, structure, order, and limits. Love and belonging needs are affiliations, affectionate relationships, and love. Physiological needs are food, water, oxygen, elimination, rest, and sex. Self-esteem is related to competency, achievement, and esteem from other people.

23. B) Avoid reminders about past problems

A traumatized child tends to avoid reminders of incidents that caused trauma in the first place and avoids talking about those incidents. This type of child becomes more isolated, alone, and numb. The dialectal cognitive behavior makes the child or adolescent suicidal. Women usually try to incorporate self-injury, which can be cured through dialectal cognitive therapy. The cognitive distortion of emotional reasoning makes a child or any other person draw a conclusion based on an emotional state.

24. A) Jean Piaget

Jean Piaget developed the theory of cognitive development, which was a significant contribution to the field of psychiatric-mental health. Lawrence Kohlberg proposed the theory of moral development. Carl Rogers is known for proposing the theory of humanism. Viktor Frankl has contributed significantly to the development of existentialism.

25. C) Industry versus inferiority

Ages 6 to 12 are characterized by developing social and physical skills and the ability to do work efficiently. The child who is unable to develop these skills finds it difficult to learn and work and forms an inferiority complex, exhibiting the industry versus inferiority crisis. Trust versus mistrust is a psychological crisis that occurs in the age group of 0 to 18 months. Autonomy versus shame is characterized in the age group of 18 months to 3 years. Intimacy versus isolation is characterized in the age group of 20 to 35 years.

26. D) Integrity versus despair

The patient is facing the psychological crisis of integrity versus despair, which occurs when an unresolved issue causes a person to live in despair and be unsatisfied. Trust versus mistrust is characterized by not trusting anyone. Initiative versus guilt is characterized by aggression. Identity versus role confusion is characterized by self-doubt.

27. D) Concrete operational

During the concrete operational stage, a child learns to understand others' viewpoints and develops logical thinking. The preoperational stage is characterized by the inability of the child to think abstractly. The sensorimotor stage is characterized by the development of simple reflexes and spatial abilities. The formal operational stage is characterized by the development of the ability to think abstractly.

28. According to the theory of object relations, a child becomes independent by:

    A. Securing a base of support during the initial years
    B. Exhibiting basic control over oneself
    C. Being egocentric
    D. Transitioning from childhood to adulthood

29. During adolescence, the development of interest in learning new skills and taking initiatives is a part of the type of development referred to as:

    A. Psychological
    B. Physical
    C. Social
    D. Cognitive

30. A child enrolls in a dance class is unable to learn the steps. One day, the child trips, becomes very self-conscious, and has still more difficulty learning the steps. Eventually the child stops going to the class. The probable unresolved crisis is:

    A. Integrity versus despair
    B. Autonomy versus shame and doubt
    C. Trust versus mistrust
    D. Intimacy versus isolation

31. According to Freud's stages of development, the stage at which the child derives pleasure from the genital region and normal sexual behavior is developed is the stage called:

    A. Oral
    B. Anal
    C. Phallic
    D. Latency

32. The period of development in which one develops the ability to classify different objects, people, and situations is the stage called:

    A. Toddlerhood
    B. Childhood
    C. Adolescence
    D. Adulthood

33. The developmental crisis of generativity versus stagnation occurs at the developmental stage of:

    A. Adolescence
    B. Early adulthood
    C. Middle adulthood
    D. Late adulthood

(See answers next page.)

28. A) Securing a base of support during the initial years

A secure base of support up till the age of 3 years builds up confidence in a child. Gaining basic control over self builds up willpower. Egocentric thinking makes a child expect others to view things from their viewpoint. The transition from childhood to adulthood is marked by the building up of self-identity.

29. A) Psychological

Psychological development involves the ability to take new initiatives and learn new skills with great interest. Physical development involves changes in growth rate, height, weight, bones, and muscle development. Social development involves the influence of peer groups. Cognitive development involves the development of reasoning skills and logical thinking.

30. B) Autonomy versus shame and doubt

The child is exhibiting an unresolved crisis of autonomy versus shame and doubt, generating self-doubt. Integrity versus despair is characterized by a dissatisfied sense of life. Trust versus mistrust refers to a sense of suspiciousness when it comes to trusting others. Intimacy versus isolation is characterized by emotional isolation.

31. C) Phallic

In the phallic stage, the child derives pleasure from the genital region and many of the sexual behaviors. Any kind of reproductive issue is generally resolved in this stage. In the oral stage, the primary pleasure-giving organ is the mouth via various activities like feeding, crying, biting, and teething. In the anal stage, the child gets pleasure if they can withhold and expel feces in a correct fashion. In the latency stage, there is no sexual development, but the child starts learning new skills, and this is the period of calmness.

32. B) Childhood

In the childhood stage, the child develops the ability to classify people, situations, and objects. This is an example of cognitive development. In the toddlerhood stage, the child starts developing creativity and socialization. In adolescence, reasoning skills and abstract thinking develop. In adulthood, the person uses all experiences and skills to develop recognition.

33. C) Middle adulthood

Generativity versus stagnation is a crisis found in middle adulthood. The main challenge is productive as well as nurturant for the upcoming generation. In adolescence, the crisis is identity versus role. The challenge is in deciding who they are and what occupation suits them. In early adulthood, the crisis is intimacy versus isolation. The challenge is to develop an intimate relationship by expressing true feelings. In late adulthood, the crisis is ego integrity versus despair.

34. The developmental theory, proposed by Bowlby, that focuses on the early relationships of a child and the development of social relationships is the theory called:

    A. Behavioral child development
    B. Cognitive-developmental
    C. Attachment
    D. Social learning

35. According to Piaget's cognitive development theory, the stage where a child develops symbolic thinking and learns to use words for representing an object is the stage called:

    A. Preoperational
    B. Sensorimotor
    C. Formal operational
    D. Concrete operational

36. A preteen has poor ego strength and early issues of trauma and primarily uses immature defenses. The likely step the psychiatric-mental health nurse practitioner takes is to:

    A. Advise avoidance of emotional pain through returning to an earlier level of development
    B. Suggest avoidance of the painful reality of trauma by ignoring or refusing to acknowledge it
    C. Support defenses that are adaptive and use a longer period of stabilization
    D. Advise use of an altered state of consciousness to avoid emotional distress

37. The psychiatric-mental health nurse practitioner evaluates a older adult patient who believes life is meaningless. The nurse practitioner helps the patient in resolving life's existential themes through psychotherapy. The goal of this therapy is to:

    A. Decrease the use of secondary and instrumental emotions
    B. Help the patient move toward wholeness and self-actualization
    C. Help the patient visualize how they want their life to be different
    D. Help the patient take responsibility for their choices

38. According to Bronfenbrenner, the system that involves the influence of attitude and cultural ideology on an individual's life is called:

    A. Microsystem
    B. Mesosystem
    C. Exosystem
    D. Macrosystem

39. The key concept in gestalt psychotherapy is:

    A. Organismic self-regulation
    B. Self-concept
    C. Actualizing tendency
    D. Full functioning

(See answers next page.)

34. C) Attachment

The attachment theory is proposed by Bowlby and focuses on the development of social relationships throughout life. The behavioral child development theory is proposed by Watson and Skinner, who state that learning occurs purely through association and reinforcement. The cognitive-developmental theory, by Piaget, deals with the development of the thought process of an individual. The social learning theory is proposed by Bandura and states that behavior is influenced by observation, listening, and modeling.

35. A) Preoperational

The development of symbolic thinking and learning of language is a part of the preoperational stage. During this stage, the child starts to learn communication and to think logically. The sensorimotor stage involves the development of movement and sensations. The formal operational stage involves thinking abstractly and starting to think more about moral, ethical, and political issues. The concrete operational stage involves thinking in a very specific way but also beginning to use logic and reasoning.

36. C) Support defenses that are adaptive and use a longer period of stabilization

Someone who primarily uses immature defenses most likely has poor ego strength and early issues of trauma. This may indicate that a longer period of stabilization in psychotherapy is indicated. The therapist supports the defenses that are adaptive and helps the person to develop higher-level defenses, if needed. This can be accomplished through clarification and exploration so that the person's awareness of their defenses is enhanced. Avoiding emotional pain through returning to an earlier level of development and avoiding the painful reality of trauma by ignoring or refusing to acknowledge it are immature defenses. Avoiding emotional distress through an altered state of consciousness is a neurotic defense.

37. D) Help the patient take responsibility for their choices

The nurse practitioner places the patient on existential psychotherapy. The goals of existential psychotherapy center on the given themes of existence and helping patients face the anxieties of life, freely choose their life direction, take responsibility for their choices, and create a meaningful existence. The goal in emotion-focused therapy (EFT) is to help patients move toward wholeness and self-actualization by helping them develop emotional awareness and adaptive emotional processing. Another goal of EFT is to decrease the use of secondary and instrumental emotions so that patients are not encumbered by them. The two key therapeutic goals of solution-focused therapy are to determine (a) how the patient wants their life to be different, and (b) what it will take to make it happen.

38. D) Macrosystem

Macrosystem includes the influence of attitude and ideologies of culture on individual behavior. Microsystem involves the influence of living settings like family, peers, neighbors, and school. Mesosystem involves the influence of relationships between different microsystems, like relationships with family and neighbors. Exosystem involves influences of an external setting in which the individual has no active role.

39. A) Organismic self-regulation

The key concept of gestalt psychotherapy is organismic self-regulation. Self-concept, actualizing tendency, and full functioning are key concepts in person-centered psychotherapy.

40. The psychiatric-mental health nurse practitioner places an older adult patient with alcoholism in therapy that does not necessitate processing problems in order to resolve them. The goal of such therapy is to:

    A. Enable the patient to see how they want their life to be different
    B. Help the patient move toward wholeness and self-actualization
    C. Help the patient develop emotional awareness and adaptive emotional processing
    D. Decrease the patient's use of secondary and instrumental emotions

41. The family therapy that operates on the belief that a person's problematic behavior may serve a function or purpose for the family was originated by:

    A. Salvador Minuchin
    B. Virginia Satir
    C. Jay Haley
    D. Murray Bowen

42. A preteen evaluated by a psychiatric-mental health nurse practitioner was found to have a core sense of abandonment, worthlessness, and shame. After therapy, the patient was able to develop the ability to access the important information that emotions provide and use that information to live a full, vital life. The marker for therapy used by the psychiatric-mental health nurse practitioner is:

    A. Conflict splits
    B. Self-concept
    C. Actualizing tendency
    D. Interruptions

43. The psychiatric-mental health nurse practitioner decides to take an approach of psychotherapy with a family based on strategic therapy and gives each family member a task to perform by the next visit, with an expectation of compliance. This is an example of:

    A. Reframing
    B. Paradoxical intervention
    C. Directive
    D. Emotional cutoff

44. Boundaries, as emphasized in structural family therapy, can be defined as:

    A. A negative task that is assigned when a family member is resistant
    B. Problematic behaviors that are relabeled to have more positive meaning
    C. Physical or psychological barriers that protect the integrity of family systems
    D. Dyads that decrease stress

45. The psychiatric-mental health nurse practitioner uses reflective statements in an approach to psychotherapy with a family who comes in for a follow-up visit. This is an intervention used in the family therapy called:

    A. Family systems
    B. Emotionally focused
    C. Strategic
    D. Structural

(See answers next page.)

40. A) Enable the patient to see how they want their life to be different

The nurse practitioner has placed the patient in solution-focused therapy (SFT). SFT believes that the therapy process does not necessitate processing problems in order to resolve them. The therapy is solution-focused rather than problem-focused and is present and future oriented rather than past oriented. SFT seeks to empower the patient and is positive and non-pathologizing. The goal of SFT is to help the patient change by constructing solutions to problems rather than dwelling on them. The two key therapeutic goals are to determine (a) how the patient wants their life to be different, and (b) what it will take to make that happen. Helping patients move toward wholeness and self-actualization by helping them develop emotional awareness and adaptive emotional processing is a goal of emotion-focused therapy (EFT), not SFT. Another goal of EFT is to decrease the use of secondary and instrumental emotions so that patients are not encumbered by them.

41. D) Murray Bowen

Family systems theory, which operates on the belief that a person's problematic behavior may serve a purpose or function for the family, was originated by Murray Bowen. Salvador Minuchin originated structural family therapy, which emphasizes the manner in which family members relate to, understand, and change the family's structure. Virginia Satir pioneered experiential therapy, which emphasizes that behavior is determined by personal experience, not the external family. Jay Haley originated strategic therapy with a belief that symptoms are viewed as metaphors and reflect problems in the hierarchical structure of the family.

42. A) Conflict splits

A conflict split is marker for emotion-focused therapy where the goal is to develop the ability to access the important information that emotions provide and use that information to live a full, vital life. Self-concept and actualizing tendency are key concepts in person-centered therapy. Interruption is a key concept in gestalt therapy.

43. C) Directive

A directive, often used as an intervention in strategic family therapy, is a task given in expectation of a family member's compliance. Reframing is the act of relabeling problematic behaviors to have more positive meaning. A paradoxical intervention is a negative task given to family members who are resistant to change. An emotional cutoff is attempting to break contact with the family of origin.

44. C) Physical or psychological barriers that protect the integrity of family systems

Boundaries can be defined as physical or psychological barriers that protect the integrity of family systems. Assigning a negative task to a resistant family member demonstrates paradoxical intervention. Relabeling a problematic behavior to have a more positive meaning defines reframing. Dyads that decrease stress defines triangles, found in family systems theory.

45. B) Emotionally focused

Emotionally focused family therapy uses reflective statements and evocative questions. Family systems therapy uses interventions such as self-statements. Strategic family therapy uses directives and paradoxical interventions. Structural family therapy uses mapping.

46. According to Kurt Lewin's theory of change, the unfreezing stage is about:

    A. Getting ready to change
    B. Taking action toward change
    C. Solidifying a change
    D. Lacking the desire to change

47. When performing family therapy, the psychiatric-mental health nurse practitioner understands that the family system is a process that:

    A. Involves individuals of a family working on individual problems
    B. Involves family members working together
    C. Is not structured on family feedback
    D. Involves individuals in a family working in groups to achieve a common goal

48. The psychiatric-mental health nurse practitioner is working with a family and decides that the family could benefit from an approach using strategic family therapy. The nurse practitioner would:

    A. Examine how the family's dysfunctional patterns may be rooted in problematic behaviors that serve a purpose for the family
    B. Consider focusing directly on interventions around the problems identified within the family
    C. Work with an individual family member to perform psychotherapy
    D. Plan to rework in the present any solutions that have been beneficial for the family in the past

49. According to Kurt Lewin's theory of change, an older adult patient who decides that they are ready to quit smoking and sees the psychiatric-mental health nurse practitioner for interventions around smoking cessation demonstrates being in the stage of:

    A. Contemplation
    B. Precontemplation
    C. Freezing
    D. Action

50. The key concepts of structural family therapy are:

    A. Reframing and paradoxical interventions
    B. Family structure, subsystems, and boundaries
    C. Homeostasis and feedback loops
    D. Emotions and attachment styles

(See answers next page.)

46. A) Getting ready to change
According to Kurt Lewin's theory of change, the unfreezing stage is one of the most important stages of change, when the individual begins to prepare for change. Taking action toward change is indicative of the action or transition phase. Solidifying a change happens in the freezing phase of change. Lacking the desire to change does not indicate a phase of Lewin's theory.

47. B) Involves family members working together
A family system is a unit structured on feedback, including a process by which all family members work together. A family system is not promoted by working on individual problems or working in separate groups. A family system is structured on feedback.

48. B) Consider focusing directly on interventions around the problems identified within the family
Strategic family therapy is problem-focused, and interventions are geared to mitigate perpetuation of problems identified within the family. Examining how the family's dysfunctional patterns may be rooted in problematic behaviors that serve a purpose for the family is part of family systems theory. Working with an individual family member to perform psychotherapy would be done when performing individual psychotherapy. Planning to rework in the present any solutions that have been beneficial for the family in the past describes an approach for solution-focused therapy.

49. D) Action
According to Kurt Lewin's theory of change, the patient's readiness and action toward interventions demonstrates that the patient is in the transition, or action, phase. Contemplation and precontemplation are stages of the transtheoretical model of change, not Lewin's theory of change. Freezing would indicate that change has already occurred.

50. B) Family structure, subsystems, and boundaries
Family structure, subsystems, boundaries, and enmeshment are key concepts of structural family therapy. Reframing and paradoxical interventions are key interventions of strategic therapy. Homeostasis and feedback loops are key concepts of strategic family therapy. Emotions and attachment styles are discussed in emotionally focused family therapy.

51. The psychiatric-mental health nurse practitioner demonstrates family systems therapy when:

   A. Focusing on changing maladaptive behaviors by performing active behavioral techniques
   B. Focusing on emotional dysregulation, tolerance for distress, and individual self-management skills
   C. Placing emphasis on reflection of life and on self-confrontation
   D. Focusing on chronic anxiety within a family

52. Self-differentiation, which is an important concept of family systems theory, means the:

   A. Level achieved when one's self-worth is not dependent on external relationships
   B. Ability to differentiate problematic traits among family members
   C. Relabeling of problematic self-fulfilling behaviors to have more positive meaning
   D. Attempt to break contact between self and family members

(See answers next page.)

51. D) Focusing on chronic anxiety within a family

Family systems therapy focuses on chronic anxiety within families. Focusing on changing maladaptive behaviors by performing active behavioral techniques describes cognitive behavioral therapy, often used in individual psychotherapy. Focusing on emotional dysregulation, tolerance for distress, and self-management skills describes dialectical behavioral therapy, often used in individual psychotherapy, not family therapy. Placing emphasis on reflection of life and on self-confrontation describes an individual therapy technique with existential therapy.

52. A) Level achieved when one's self-worth is not dependent on external relationships

Self-differentiation is a key concept of family systems therapy and is the level achieved when one's self-worth is not dependent upon external relationships. Self-differentiation does not involve differentiating problematic traits; it is independent in nature. Relabeling of problematic self-fulfilling behaviors to have more positive meaning is an example of reframing. Attempting to break contact between self and family members is called cutting off, not self-differentiation.

Ethical and Legal Principles

1. An older adult patient comes into the office with concerns about changes in behavior. The psychiatric-mental health nurse practitioner demonstrates their role when:

   A. Collaborating with the patient's primary care provider
   B. Working independently from a supervising physician
   C. Giving no consideration to a referral to neurology
   D. Considering collaboration of care a responsibility of a psychiatrist

2. An older adult patient comes into the office of a psychiatric-mental health nurse practitioner for an initial visit. After assessment and evaluation, the nurse practitioner derives a diagnosis of major depressive disorder and recommends that the patient consider medication treatment to help alleviate the presenting symptoms. The patient explains that it is "against my religion" to take any medications for this reason. In an effort to promote cultural competence, the nurse practitioner:

   A. Advises the patient to take the medication in order to feel better
   B. Has a member of another religious background discuss the treatment plan with the patient
   C. Assumes that the patient is being resistant and is not listening
   D. Spends more time discussing the patient's religion and how it may impact decision-making

3. The psychiatric-mental health nurse practitioner's role in providing pharmacologic interventions includes:

   A. Only prescribing medications
   B. Prescribing medications and recommending pharmacologic agents
   C. Prescribing medications and ordering and interpreting diagnostic testing
   D. Only recommending medications

4. According to the American Nurses Association (ANA), an additional competency for the APRN for providing culturally congruent care:

   A. Leads interprofessional teams to identify the cultural and language needs of the consumer
   B. Identifies the stage of the consumer's acculturation and accompanying patterns of needs and engagement
   C. Communicates with appropriate language and behaviors, including the use of medical interpreters and translators in accordance with consumer preferences
   D. Advocates for policies that promote health and prevent harm among culturally diverse, underserved, or underrepresented consumers

1. A) Collaborating with the patient's primary care provider

Psychiatric-mental health nurse practitioners practice in primary care settings by collaboration and consultation with a primary care provider, providing behavioral healthcare in integrated settings, and/or unifying primary care and behavioral health within a mental health service site in what has been termed reverse co-location models. The nurse practitioner's role also includes collaboration with a supervising physician and consideration of referral to specialty care, such as neurology. Collaboration with a primary care physician is not solely the responsibility of a psychiatrist but is also that of a psychiatric-mental health nurse practitioner when providing care to patients.

2. D) Spends more time discussing the patient's religion and how it may impact decision-making

Cultural competence is demonstrated by the nurse practitioner's effort to seek a better understanding of the patient's religion and how it impacts their decision-making. Telling the patient that they have to take the medication to feel better or having a member of another religious background discuss the treatment plan with the patient does not demonstrate cultural competence or understanding. The nurse practitioner's assumption that the patient is being resistant does not demonstrate appropriate care.

3. C) Prescribing medications and ordering and interpreting diagnostic testing

Psychopharmacological interventions include prescribing or recommending pharmacologic agents and ordering and interpretation of diagnostic and laboratory testing. As a duty of the psychiatric nurse practitioner, prescribing medications only and/or recommending pharmacological agents is not the sole duty of the nurse practitioner. Providing pharmacological interventions such as prescribing medications is within the scope of practice of a psychiatric nurse practitioner.

4. A) Leads interprofessional teams to identify the cultural and language needs of the consumer

According to the ANA Practice Standards, the APRN competency regarding providing culturally congruent care is leading interprofessional teams to identify the cultural and language needs of the consumer. Competencies for the registered nurse in providing culturally competent care are identifying the stage of the consumer's acculturation and accompanying patterns of needs and engagement; communicating with appropriate language and behaviors, including the use of medical interpreters and translators in accordance with consumer preferences; advocating for policies that promote health and prevent harm among culturally diverse, underserved, or underrepresented consumers.

5. The competency that adheres to the American Nurses Association (ANA) Standards of Performance of the psychiatric-mental health nurse practitioner providing culturally congruent care is:

A. Assuming a leadership role in shaping or fashioning environments that promote healthy communication

B. Promoting shared decision-making solutions in planning, prescribing, and evaluating processes when the healthcare consumer's cultural preferences may create incompatibility with evidence-based practice

C. Providing leadership for establishing, improving, and sustaining collaborative relationships to achieve safe, quality care for healthcare consumers

D. Using the results of an evaluation to make or recommend process, policy, procedure, or protocol revisions when warranted

6. According to the Patient's Bill of Rights, the patient right that relates to protection of a patient's health information is the right to:

A. Have every consideration of privacy

B. Expect that all communication regarding care will be treated as confidential

C. Receive quality treatment

D. Know the identity of all healthcare staff involved in the patient's care

7. The psychiatric-mental health nurse practitioner role includes providing patient education. According to the Patient's Bill of Rights, this aspect of the nurse practitioner's role fulfills the patient's right to:

A. Know the identity of all involved in caring for a patient

B. Be informed of diagnosis, treatment, and prognosis

C. Be free from all forms of abuse or harassment

D. Receive care in a safe setting

8. According to the Patient's Bill of Rights, the psychiatric-mental health nurse practitioner is practicing according to patient rights when:

A. Providing patients a right to every consideration of privacy when time permits

B. Introducing the attending mental healthcare provider when treatment is handled by a resident

C. Furnishing the patient with informed consent documentation about their treatment

D. Arranging treatment after the patient expresses concern about the treatment

9. The psychiatric-mental health nurse practitioner is obtaining history from a patient's medical record for an upcoming appointment and finds that it will be helpful to obtain additional information by speaking with the patient's primary care provider. To ensure the patient's confidentiality, the nurse practitioner would:

A. Tell the primary care provider about the patient's history, including trauma and other details

B. Relay information to the primary care provider that pertains only to providing appropriate mental healthcare

C. Call the patient's family member to discuss information relayed from the primary care provider

D. Send all office notes to the primary care provider for review without discussing with the patient

(See answers next page.)

5. B) Promoting shared decision-making solutions in planning, prescribing, and evaluating processes when the healthcare consumer's cultural preferences may create incompatibility with evidence-based practice

According to the ANA Practice Standards, the APRN competency regarding providing culturally congruent care is promotion of shared decision-making solutions in planning, prescribing, and evaluating processes when the healthcare consumer's cultural preferences and norms may create incompatibility with evidence-based practice. A competency for communication is assuming a leadership role in shaping or fashioning environments that promote healthy communication. A competency for collaboration is providing leadership for establishing, improving, and sustaining collaborative relationships to achieve safe, quality care for healthcare consumers. A competency for evaluation is demonstrated by using the results of the evaluation to make or recommend process, policy, procedure, or protocol revisions when warranted.

6. B) Expect that all communication regarding care will be treated as confidential

The right to expect that all communication and records pertaining to a patient's care will be treated as confidential is specific to protection of a patient's health information. The right to every consideration of privacy, the right to quality treatment, and the right to know the identity of all healthcare staff involved in a patient's care are included in the Patient's Bill of Rights but do not pertain to protection of a patient's health information.

7. B) Be informed of diagnosis, treatment, and prognosis

According to the Patient's Bill of Rights, patients have a right to be informed of diagnosis, treatment, and prognosis, which is fulfilled by the nurse practitioner's role of providing patient education. The patient has a right to know the identity of those involved in their care, to be free from all forms of abuse/harassment, and to receive care in a safe setting, but these additional rights do not pertain to the nurse practitioner's role in patient education.

8. C) Furnishing the patient with informed consent documentation about their treatment

Patients have the right to receive informed consent about their treatment. According to the Patient's Bill of Rights, patients have a right to every consideration of privacy, not just when time permits. Patients have the right to know the identity of physicians, nurses, and all involved in their care, inclusive of students, residents, and trainees. Patients always have the right to refuse treatment or ask for more information regarding a treatment before the nurse practitioner arranges for the treatment.

9. B) Relay information to the primary care provider that pertains only to providing appropriate mental healthcare

Confidentiality is based on the duty to protect a patient's health information. Therefore, discussing only pertinent and necessary information with the primary care provider adheres to maintaining confidentiality. Discussing details with the primary care provider that are not relevant or necessary to provide appropriate care breaches confidentiality. Calling the patient's family member or sending office notes without the patient's consent is also a breach of patient confidentiality.

10. According to the APNA, the psychiatric-mental nurse practitioner role includes being "reliant on the overlapping skills and knowledge of each team member and discipline, resulting in synergistic effects where outcomes are enhanced and more comprehensive than the simple aggregation of the team members' individual efforts." The term for this description is:

    A. Interprofessional
    B. Nursing process
    C. Multidisciplinary
    D. Quality of care

11. A 16-year-old patient presents for a mental health evaluation because of parents' concerns about changes in the patient's mood with psychosis. After obtaining additional history from both the patient and the patient's parents, the psychiatric-mental health nurse practitioner suspects that the patient's current symptoms may have been exacerbated by recent marijuana use and orders a urine drug screen. To maintain the patient's confidentiality, the nurse practitioner:

    A. Immediately shares the results with the patient's parents without asking the patient
    B. Talks with the patient privately and then tells the patient's parents without the patient's consent
    C. Obtains the patient's consent to talk to the patient's parents about the results
    D. Does not share the results with the patient's parents even if the patient consents

12. The psychiatric-mental health nurse practitioner is consulted about an older adult patient in the emergency department. The patient has experienced behavioral changes and has made persistent threats to harm a neighbor. The nurse practitioner may notify the patient's neighbor about the threats due to a duty to disclose a threat of imminent physical harm. This action is called:

    A. Confidentiality
    B. Veracity
    C. Breach of confidentiality
    D. Nonmaleficence

13. According to the American Nurses Association (ANA), "the act or process of pleading for, supporting, recommending a cause or course of action" defines:

    A. Code of ethics
    B. Evaluation
    C. Assessment
    D. Advocacy

14. When the psychiatric-mental health nurse practitioner translates the consumer voice into policy and legislation that address such issues as control of healthcare access, regulation of healthcare, protection of the healthcare consumer, and environmental justice, this demonstrates advocacy at the level known as:

    A. Individual
    B. Policy
    C. Community
    D. Interpersonal

(See answers next page.)

10. A) Interprofessional
According to the APNA, the term interprofessional means being "reliant on the overlapping skills and knowledge of each team member and discipline, resulting in synergistic effects where outcomes are enhanced and more comprehensive than the simple aggregation of the team members' individual efforts." The APNA defines the nursing process as "a critical thinking model used by nurses that comprises the integration of the singular, concurrent actions of these six components: assessment, diagnosis, identification of outcomes, planning, implementation, and evaluation." The term multidisciplinary is defined as reliance on each team member or discipline contributing discipline-specific skills. Quality of care is defined as the degree to which health services increase the likelihood of desired outcomes and are consistent with current professional knowledge.

11. C) Obtains the patient's consent to talk to the patient's parents about the results
The patient's confidentiality is breached when the nurse practitioner does not obtain consent from the patient. To adhere to ethical practice guidelines, the nurse practitioner should not share any health information without the patient's consent. The nurse practitioner may speak with the patient's parents privately but may only do so upon the patient's consent. Due to the patient's age, consent is required from the patient to share health information, despite the patient living in the home with their parents.

12. C) Breach of confidentiality
Breach of confidentiality in this scenario is an authorized disclosure of patient information due to a threat of imminent physical harm to an identifiable person. Confidentiality refers to the duty to protect a patient's health information. Veracity refers to the duty to tell the truth. Nonmaleficence refers to the duty to do no harm.

13. D) Advocacy
According to the ANA, advocacy is "the act or process of pleading for, supporting, recommending a cause or course of action." A code of ethics is defined as a list of provisions that explain the primary goals, values, and obligations of the nursing profession. Evaluation is the process of determining the progress toward expected outcomes. Assessment is a systematic, dynamic process in which, through interaction with the patient, family, groups, communities, populations, and healthcare providers, nurse practitioners can collect and analyze data.

14. B) Policy
According to the APNA, the nurse practitioner translates the consumer voice into policy and legislation that address such issues as control of healthcare access, regulation of healthcare, protection of the healthcare consumer, and environmental justice at the policy level. Advocacy at the individual level includes the nurse engaging in informing healthcare consumers so they can consider actions, interventions, or choices in the light of their own personal beliefs, attitudes, and knowledge to achieve the desired outcome. At the community level, the nurse practitioner supports cultural transformation of organizations, communities, or populations. At the interpersonal level, the nurse practitioner empowers healthcare consumers by providing emotional support, attainment of resources, and necessary help through interactions with families and significant others in their social support network.

15. The three components of medical decision-making are:

    A. Diagnosis, documentation, and reviewing data

    B. Diagnosis, treatment, and reviewing data

    C. Treatment, documentation, and providing follow-up care

    D. Diagnosis, treatment, and providing follow-up care

16. A pediatric Spanish-speaking patient comes into the psychiatric-mental health nurse practitioner's office for an initial visit with parents who speak only Spanish. The nurse practitioner practices cultural competence by:

    A. Using a family member as an interpreter

    B. Using language services to provide an interpreter

    C. Moving forward with the patient without an interpreter

    D. Using a few known Spanish words to enhance the patient's understanding

17. Regarding elements of malpractice in clinical decision-making, *duty* refers to a:

    A. Patient relationship with ancillary staff in office

    B. Provider relationship with another provider

    C. Patient-provider relationship

    D. Patient relationship with another patient

18. The psychiatric-mental health nurse practitioner is caring for a 9-year-old patient who comes into the emergency department for psychiatric evaluation accompanied by parents. Upon discharge, the nurse practitioner provides emotional support to the patient and provides additional resources to the patient and family. This demonstrates patient advocacy at the:

    A. Individual level

    B. Organizational level

    C. Interpersonal level

    D. Policy level

19. The acronym LACE, a consensus model completed in 2008 by the APRN Consensus Work Group and the National Council of State Boards of Nursing APRN Advisory Committee, signifies:

    A. Litigation, accreditation, certification, and education

    B. Licensure, accreditation, certification, and education

    C. Litigation, access, certification, and education

    D. Licensure, application, certification, and education

20. A 14-year-old patient comes into the office accompanied by parents with a chief complaint of recent changes in mood. Upon evaluation, the psychiatric-mental health nurse practitioner finds that the patient had a recent concussion while playing soccer. The nurse practitioner best demonstrates clinical decision-making by:

    A. Further evaluating the patient's mood changes in relation to their being a teenager

    B. Employing evidence-based clinical practice guidelines about concussions to drive treatment

    C. Referring the patient to a sports medicine specialist for further evaluation

    D. Listening to the patient's parents to help determine diagnosis and treatment

(See answers next page.)

15. B) Diagnosis, treatment, and reviewing data

Medical decision-making has three components: (1) making a diagnosis, (2) choosing treatment options, and (3) reviewing data. While diagnosis and reviewing data are components of medical decision-making, documentation and providing follow-up care are not.

16. B) Using language services to provide an interpreter

Using an authorized Spanish interpreter demonstrates cultural competence, with an awareness of the need to enhance the patient's (and parents') understanding and communication with the provider to provide appropriate care. Family members should not be used as interpreters due to patient confidentiality and to ensure accurate information is being relayed to and from the patient. The nurse practitioner is not practicing cultural competence if continuing without an interpreter or attempting to communicate with the patient in a language without fluency.

17. C) Patient-provider relationship

A duty is established when there is a patient—provider relationship. A visit to the psychiatric-mental health nurse practitioner's office by a patient establishes the nurse practitioner's duty to that patient, and in any instance when a nurse practitioner gives professional advice or treatment in any setting, a duty may be established. Duty does not refer to a patient's relationship with office staff or another patient, nor does it refer to a provider's relationship with another provider.

18. C) Interpersonal level

According to the APNA, at the interpersonal level the nurse practitioner empowers healthcare consumers by providing emotional support, attainment of resources, and necessary help through interactions with families and significant others in their social support network. Advocacy at the individual level is engagement in informing healthcare consumers so they can consider actions, interventions, or choices in light of their own personal beliefs, attitudes, and knowledge to achieve the desired outcome. Advocacy at the organizational level is supporting cultural transformation of organizations, communities, or populations. Advocacy at the policy level is translating the consumer voice into policy and legislation that address issues such as control of healthcare access, regulation of healthcare, protection of the healthcare consumer, and environmental justice.

19. B) Licensure, accreditation, certification, and education

LACE is a consensus model that includes licensure, accreditation, certification, and education. Litigation, access, and application are not components of the LACE model.

20. A) Further evaluating the patient's mood changes in relation to their being a teenager

According to the APNA, the term interprofessional is being "reliant on the overlapping skills and knowledge of each team member and discipline, resulting in synergistic effects where outcomes are enhanced and more comprehensive than the simple aggregation of the team members' individual efforts." The APNA defines the nursing process as "a critical thinking model used by nurses that comprises the integration of the singular, concurrent actions of these six components: assessment, diagnosis, identification of outcomes, planning, implementation, and evaluation." The term multidisciplinary is defined as reliance on each team member or discipline contributing discipline-specific skills. Quality of care is defined as the degree to which health services increase the likelihood of desired outcomes and are consistent with current professional knowledge.

21. According to the American Nurses Association (ANA), the competency that concerns standards of professional performance regarding ethics is:

    A. Using current healthcare research findings and other evidence to support clinical knowledge
    B. Advocating for equitable healthcare consumer care
    C. Promoting a climate of research and clinical inquiry
    D. Disseminating research findings through activities such as publications

22. Medical decision-making refers to the:

    A. Process of focusing on the primary diagnosis
    B. Prescription of medications for therapeutic treatment
    C. Complex nature of diagnosing including appropriate treatment
    D. Establishment of a comprehensive treatment plan

23. According to the American Nurses Association (ANA), the integration of cultural expertise into practice when assessing, communicating with, and providing care for members of a racial, ethnic, or social group is known as:

    A. Cultural skills
    B. Cultural knowledge
    C. Continuity of care
    D. Competency

24. According to the American Nurses Association (ANA), codes of ethical practice:

    A. Educate professionals about sound ethical behavior and mandate a minimal standard of practice
    B. Do not apply to the practice of a psychiatric-mental health nurse practitioner
    C. Are used to guide the practice of a psychiatrist
    D. Are used when applicable to clinical practice

25. Prior to prescribing a medication to a patient, the psychiatric-mental health nurse practitioner must ensure that:

    A. The patient's family has agreed to the planned treatment
    B. They are prescribing the right medicine at the right time for the right indication for the right patient
    C. The patient has been treated with a similar medication in the past and has had no issues
    D. They have reviewed contraindications of the medication with the patient

26. A 19-year-old patient exhibiting self-destructive behavior has been recommended for seclusion. The psychiatric-mental health nurse practitioner will order the seclusion to be limited to:

    A. 1 hour
    B. 2 hours
    C. 3 hours
    D. 4 hours

(See answers next page.)

21. B) Advocating for equitable healthcare consumer care

According to the ANA, advocating for equitable healthcare consumer care is a competency of Standard 7: ethics. Using current healthcare research findings and other evidence to support clinical knowledge concerns a competency of education. Promoting a climate of research and clinical inquiry and disseminating research findings through activities such as publications are competencies of evidence-based practice and research.

22. C) Complex nature of diagnosing including appropriate treatment

Medical decision-making refers to the complexity of establishing a diagnosis and selecting a treatment management option. Medical decision-making is not solely establishing a diagnosis or treatment plan. It is also more inclusive than prescribing medications for therapeutic treatment.

23. A) Cultural skills

"Cultural skills" is defined as the integration of cultural knowledge and expertise into practice when assessing, communicating with, and providing care for members of a racial, ethnic, or social group. Cultural knowledge is defined as "the concepts and language of an ethnic or social group used to describe their health-related values, beliefs, and traditional practices, as well as the etiologies of their conditions, preferred treatments, and any contraindications for treatments or pharmacological interventions." Continuity of care is defined as "an interprofessional process that includes healthcare consumers, families, and other stakeholders in the development of a coordinated plan of care." Competency is defined as "an expected and measurable level of nursing performance that integrates knowledge, skills, abilities, and judgment, based on established scientific knowledge and expectations for nursing practice."

24. A) Educate professionals about sound ethical behavior and mandate a minimal standard of practice

According to the ANA, psychiatric-mental health nurse practitioners adhere to all aspects of Code of Ethics for Nurses with Interpretive Statements. Codes of ethical practice educate and inform professionals about sound ethical behavior while mandating a minimal standard of practice. Therefore, codes of ethical practice apply to the nurse practitioner and should always be adhered to by the psychiatric-mental health nurse practitioner.

25. B) They are prescribing the right medicine at the right time for the right indication for the right patient

Per standard of care, the nurse practitioner must ensure prescription of the right medicine at the right time for the right indication for the right patient. Ensuring that the patient's family agrees to treatment is not a mandatory standard of care when prescribing medications. While treatment with similar medications is an important part of the patient's history, it is not a necessary action to prescribe medications. The nurse practitioner should be cautious of contraindications when prescribing medications. Contraindications are not discussed with the patient.

26. D) 4 hours

Patients 18 and older are to be secluded due to self-destructive behavior for a maximum of 4 hours at a time. The nurse practitioner can have the order cover a period of up to 24 hours, but the length for each seclusion is 4 hours. Patients 9 to 17 are limited to 2 hours, and younger children are limited to 1 hour.

27. The psychiatric-mental health nurse practitioner is taking care of a newly pregnant patient with schizophrenia. The patient wants to continue the pregnancy, but her family insists that she should have an abortion. To promote the safety of the fetus, the patient's antipsychotic medication would need to be reduced, putting her at risk of exacerbating the psychiatric illness. Furthermore, the question has been raised as to whether the patient can safely care for the baby. Eventually, the patient decides to carry her pregnancy to term. The ethical principle that allows this decision is:

A. Autonomy

B. Beneficence

C. Fidelity

D. Veracity

28. The psychiatric-mental health nurse practitioner understands their role in practicing in a manner that is congruent with cultural diversity and inclusion principles by:

A. Practicing in a consistently ethical manner at all times

B. Advancing organizational policies and services that reflect respect, equity, and values

C. Communicating effectively in all areas of practice

D. Collaborating with healthcare consumers and other key stakeholders in the conduct of nursing practice

29. Refusing to discharge a voluntarily committed patient who is requesting to leave is an example of:

A. Negligence

B. Malpractice

C. Medical battery

D. Breach of duty

30. A patient with depression is admitted to the hospital in the first trimester of pregnancy. The spouse of the patient wants to continue the pregnancy; however, the patient feels that she might not be able to take care of the child. The spouse asks the psychiatric-mental health nurse practitioner to not inform the patient about the potential side effects of her antidepressants on fetal development. The nurse practitioner should:

A. Tell the patient about potential side effects only when the patient inquires

B. Listen to the spouse's request and not tell the patient about the effects of drugs

C. Ask the patient to undergo an abortion because the drugs might affect fetal development

D. Inform the patient about the side effects while prescribing the drugs

31. During evaluation, a patient with mental illness becomes agitated and begins to show aggressive behavior. To ensure the patient's right to a least restrictive environment is met, the psychiatric-mental health nurse practitioner will first:

A. Refer the patient to the psychiatrist for further evaluation

B. Attempt to deescalate the situation by removing stimulation

C. Ask a family member or guardian for permission to restrain the patient

D. Administer diazepam based on patient level of anxiety and aggression

(See answers next page.)

27. A) Autonomy

Autonomy is the ethical principle in which people respect the rights of others to make their own decisions. The patient has the right to decide whether to continue the pregnancy, so her situation falls under the autonomy principle. Beneficence can be defined as the duty to benefit or promote the health and well-being of others. The quality of being honest or truthful is veracity. Fidelity involves commitment and loyalty to a patient.

28. B) Advancing organizational policies and services that reflect respect, equity, and values

According to the ANA Standards of Professional Performance, practicing in a manner that is congruent with cultural diversity and inclusion principles adheres to Standard 8, culturally congruent practice, which concerns advancing organizational policies, programs, services, and practices that reflect respect, equity, and values. Practicing ethically is addressed in Standard 7 of the ANA Standards of Professional Performance. Communicating effectively in all areas of practice is addressed by Standard 9. Collaborating with the healthcare consumer and other key stakeholders in the conduct of nursing practice is addressed by Standard 10.

29. C) Medical battery

Medical battery is an intentionally harmful act that includes refusing to allow a patient to leave when requested, also known as false imprisonment. Negligence involves a breach of duty in providing reasonable care and results in harm to the patient. Malpractice, or "bad" practice, refers to failure to act in a reasonable manner according to skill and scope of practice. Breach of duty is a failure to practice based on standards of care for the profession.

30. D) Inform the patient about the side effects while prescribing the drugs

In the clinical setting, a practitioner often faces ethical dilemmas. However, the code of ethics indicates that the primary commitment of the nurse is toward the patient (Provision 2). The nurse should exercise the duty to inform the patient about necessary side effects so that the patient can make an informed decision. The patient should be informed about potential side effects even when the patient does not inquire; it is the patient's right to know. The nurse can listen to the spouse; however, the nurse should not hide anything from the patient regarding her medical treatment. It is the right of the patient to refuse treatment or to choose a certain available plan of treatment. Even when the nurse knows about the side effects, she should not ask the patient to abort because it is the patient's decision to make. In such situations, the practitioner should weigh the risks and benefits of a treatment and make a decision only after discussing it with the patient.

31. B) Attempt to de-escalate the situation by removing stimulation

The first step the nurse practitioner will take is to de-escalate the situation by removing stimuli, talking to the patient calmly and actively listening, and providing a diversion. Administering medication such as diazepam (Valium) would be a possible next step if these interventions are not successful. Referral to a psychiatrist may be needed, but all other attempts should be made to de-escalate the situation first. Asking the family for permission to restrain the patient is not needed legally but would be implemented if the patient is found to cause harm to self or others.

32. To promote a safe space for communication in group therapy, the psychiatric-mental health nurse practitioner should ask the members of the group to:

    A. Put their phones on silent mode during the session
    B. Switch their phones off during the session
    C. Not talk amongst each other after the therapy
    D. Not talk about their concerns outside the group

33. A 65-year-old patient visits the psychiatric-mental health nurse practitioner accompanied by two people. Before starting the interviewing process, to maintain the patient's confidentiality, the nurse practitioner should first:

    A. Avoid asking about the relationship between the two people and the patient
    B. Ask the two people accompanying the patient to wait outside the room
    C. Ask the permission of the patient to allow the two people to stay in the room
    D. Discuss the patient's issues in front of the two people

34. Advocating for healthcare that is sensitive to the needs of healthcare consumers with particular emphasis on the needs of diverse populations is a standard of nursing practice that reflects:

    A. Coordination of care
    B. Health teaching and promotion
    C. Consultation
    D. Implementation

35. A patient's right to confidentiality can be breached only:

    A. If communication is needed between law enforcement and the provider
    B. When information is needed to complete an insurance reimbursement
    C. If the patient has initiated conversation about treatment with family present
    D. When a patient has harmed another person or may injure someone

36. A patient being seen in the emergency department for delusions, hallucinations, and disorganized behavior requests to be discharged without further treatment. Prior to releasing the patient against medical advice, the psychiatric-mental health nurse practitioner will assess the:

    A. Available community resources to treat the patient as an outpatient
    B. History of family mental health illness and treatment provided
    C. Information provided to the patient regarding diagnosis and treatment options
    D. Patient's knowledge and understanding of mental illness and impact on daily life

(See answers next page.)

32. B) Switch their phones off during the session
Technology usage can be a challenge to confidentiality in group therapy. To avoid leakage of the information shared by members of the group, phones should be put in switched-off mode. Putting the phones on silent mode does not ensure confidentiality because the phones can still be used to take photos or record audio. Group members often share conversations beyond group sessions. Asking the members to not talk with each other outside the group can affect the purpose of the therapy.

33. C) Ask the permission of the patient to allow the two people to stay in the room
In order to maintain the confidentiality of the patient, the nurse practitioner should seek the patient's permission to allow the two people to stay. If the patient grants permission, the nurse practitioner should ask the visitors their names and what relationships they have with the patient before beginning any discussion with the patient. The nurse practitioner should not ask the visitors to leave the room before seeking the patient's permission.

34. D) Implementation
According to the American Nurses Association (ANA), advocating for healthcare that is sensitive to the needs of healthcare consumers reflects implementation of nursing practice. According to the ANA, coordination of care is demonstrated by providing leadership of coordination of interprofessional healthcare for integrated delivery of healthcare consumer services. Health teaching and promotion are demonstrated by conducting personalized health teaching and counseling. Consultation includes communicating consultation recommendations.

35. D) When a patient has harmed another person or may injure someone
The only time a patient's information can be shared is in the event the patient has harmed another person or will injure someone if not treated. This falls under a legal duty to warn in which all healthcare professionals are liable to report the patient's condition to authorities. Communication between law enforcement and the provider is not grounds for breaching confidentiality alone and must be based on the judgment that a patient has or will harm another. Only information needed to complete insurance claims is allowed to be released, which does not include specifics regarding patient conditions and protected information. The patient would have to sign a release to allow communication with the insurance company. Patients that initiate conversations about treatment are giving consent to speak in front of family; therefore, this does not constitute a breach of confidentiality. However, information is still protected, and the patient must be asked if they want certain information shared.

36. A) Available community resources to treat the patient as an outpatient
Patients have the right to refuse treatment and discontinue treatment at any time. Discharging a patient against medical advice, while not preferred, must be enforced. The nurse practitioner will, however, need to assess possible community resources that can offer the patient treatment as an outpatient. Family history and treatment, information provided to the patient, and the patient's knowledge and understanding are all important, but not what would be assessed for discharging a patient against medical advice.

37. The psychiatric-mental health nurse practitioner treats a patient who is at risk for suicide. The treatment sessions are conducted for a few months, and the patient responds positively. The nurse practitioner stays in touch with the patient and asks for feedback routinely to learn about the resolution of issues and how the patient is coping with life after therapy. Based on the standards of practice, the nurse practitioner is:

    A. Using appropriate resources
    B. Promoting futuristic thinking
    C. Improving leadership skills
    D. Ensuring environmentally safe practice

38. The condition necessary for voluntary admission involves:

    A. Written application by the patient to the faculty for admission
    B. Patient who has a proper understanding of treatment but does not consent
    C. Parent or guardian permission requirement if the patient is younger than 18
    D. Stipulation that the patient may discharged without reevaluation

39. Fidelity is:

    A. Providing information truthfully to the patient
    B. Maintaining loyalty and commitment to the patient
    C. Providing the same care regardless of personal attributes
    D. Acting to promote or benefit the good of the patient

40. A patient is admitted to the hospital and provided with basic information regarding risks, benefits, and treatment alternatives. The psychiatric-mental health nurse practitioner advises an experimental treatment, but the patient refuses to accept the recommendation. The patient is exercising the right:

    A. To treatment
    B. Regarding restraint and seclusion
    C. Regarding psychiatric advance directives
    D. To informed consent

(See answers next page.)

37. B) Promoting futuristic thinking

The nurse practitioner is promoting futuristic thinking. A skilled nurse practitioner attains knowledge and expertise that represents contemporary nursing practice and encourages forward thinking. It is an act of evidence-based practice and research and professional practice evaluation, and it enhances effective communication skills. The competencies of the standards of practice include resource utilization, which is not applicable in this patient's case. However, skilled nurse practitioners use appropriate resources to plan, provide, and maintain safe, effective, and cost-effective evidence-based nursing care. Another competency is leadership skills, which involves mentoring other healthcare professionals to promote safe and effective healthcare. In addition, nurse practitioners participate in professional organizations to contribute to the advancement of the profession and encourage health promotion. Another competency involves the nurse practitioner practicing in a safe environment and in a very healthy manner, which is important but not a concern for this patient.

38. A) Written application by the patient to the faculty for admission

For voluntary admission, the patient needs to submit a written application to the faculty. Also, the patient must have a proper understanding of the requirement of treatment and must give consent to it. Admission without consent or with a lack of willingness will not be a voluntary admission. The patient can independently seek admission if their age is between 16 and 18 years. However, if the age is below 16, then either a parent or a guardian has to seek the patient's admission. The patient possesses the right to be released or discharged on request. However, the patient can be released only after reevaluation because the psychiatric-mental health nurse practitioner may choose to facilitate an involuntary commitment if deemed necessary.

39. B) Maintaining loyalty and commitment to the patient

Fidelity is loyalty toward the patient. It is doing no wrong to the patient and maintaining expertise in nursing skills. Veracity is providing the information truthfully to the patient. The information should not be misleading or nontruthful. Justice involves providing the same or equitable distribution of resources or care. It does not base itself on any personal attributes or cultural or personal biases/stereotypes. Beneficence is the duty to act to promote the good of others.

40. D) To informed consent

Under the requirement for informed consent, the patient is provided with basic information regarding all aspects of the treatment. The patient must voluntarily accept the treatment. It is the responsibility of the practitioner to secure informed consent. Consent is secured for surgery, electroconvulsive treatment, or use of experimental drugs or procedures. Patients have the right to refuse participation in experimental treatments. One of the most fundamental rights of a patient admitted for psychiatric care is the right to quality care, which can be referred to as the right to treatment. Rights regarding restraint and seclusion are provided to ensure the safety of patients who are treated using restraints due to their violent nature. Rights regarding psychiatric advance directives allow patients who have experienced an episode of severe mental illness to have the opportunity to express their treatment preferences in a psychiatric advance directive.

41. The psychiatric-mental health nurse practitioner has been asked to strictly follow the 2003 Health Insurance Portability and Accountability Act (HIPAA) Privacy Rule regarding protecting the patient's confidentiality by the clinic. The nurse practitioner will share the patient's details with:

    A. No one without the patient's consent
    B. The patient's parents or spouse without the patient's consent
    C. The people involved in the patient's treatment plan without consent
    D. Any person who is at risk of being harmed by the patient without consent

42. "Least restrictive environment" in mental health treatment means:

    A. A patient cannot be restricted to a psychiatric facility when care can be successfully provided in the community
    B. Restraints can be used only when the patient is being evaluated and monitored in the emergency department
    C. Treatment settings must be in an outpatient clinic to promote patient autonomy and independence
    D. The patient has a right to interact with others in the same treatment facility without restriction

43. Metaethics studies the:

    A. Nature/meaning of moral reasoning
    B. Question of how to act as per ethics
    C. Morality in a particular situation
    D. Morality of a particular action

44. The psychiatric-mental health nurse practitioner intervention that follows ethical principles is:

    A. Administration of medicine without the consent of the patient
    B. Spending time with a patient having anxiety only during duty hours
    C. Giving equal attention to a patient who attempted suicide and a patient who had a brain aneurysm
    D. Not revealing the side effects of psychotropic drugs to the patient

(See answers next page.)

41. C) The people involved in the patient's treatment plan without consent
HIPAA deals with helping people to maintain the confidentiality of their medical records. The 2003 HIPAA Privacy Rule allows a psychiatric-mental health nurse practitioner to share information provided by the patient and also the medical record of the patient only to the people who are part of the patient's treatment without the patient's consent. The parents and spouse of the patient are not provided the information if they are not part of the patient's treatment plan. The nurse practitioner is strictly following the 2003 HIPAA Privacy Rule; hence, the nurse practitioner will not provide the details of the patient even to the person the patient can harm because it is against the rules.

42. A) A patient cannot be restricted to a psychiatric facility when care can be successfully provided in the community
Patients have the right to the least restrictive environment, which means they cannot be held or restricted to a psychiatric facility when treatment and care can be successful in the community setting. Restraint of patients is also an aspect of the least restrictive environment. However, restraint is not only used when patients are being evaluated and monitored in the emergency department; any emergency situation where the patient may harm themselves or others would warrant the use of restraints. Outpatient treatment settings are promoted when treatment can be successful in the community, but the goal to promote autonomy is not specific to outpatient clinics and is based on patient situations and diagnoses. Patient interaction with others in a facility is not an aspect of the least restrictive environment.

43. A) Nature/meaning of moral reasoning
Metaethics is a domain of ethics. It studies the nature of moral reasoning. It tries to understand the meaning of the terms used in ethics. The question of how to act comes under normative ethics, another domain of ethics. Studying or applying ethics in a particular situation or to an action comes under the third domain of ethics: applied ethics. It can apply to a single person, organization, or action of an individual entity.

44. C) Giving equal attention to a patient who attempted suicide and a patient who had a brain aneurysm
A nurse practitioner should provide equal attention to the patient who attempted suicide and the patient who just experienced a brain aneurysm. This falls under the ethical principle of justice, which dictates that the nurse practitioner should distribute care or health resources equally to the patients. The nurse practitioner should administer medicines only with the consent of patients because they have the right to refuse medication. This falls under the ethical principle of autonomy, which requires that the nurse practitioner respect and acknowledge others' rights of decision-making. Also, it is important for the nurse practitioner to spend extra time, not only in their work shift, if the patient is anxious. This act falls under the ethical principle of beneficence, which states that a nurse practitioner's duty is to promote the well-being of others. According to the ethical principle of veracity, while prescribing medicine, the nurse practitioner must inform the patient regarding the purpose of the drug prescription and also its adverse effects. This ethical principle involves the duty of nurse practitioners to communicate honestly.

45. While studying the history of a new patient, the psychiatric-mental health nurse practitioner discovers that the patient belongs to a different cultural background than the nurse practitioner. During the interview, the nurse practitioner notices that the patient suddenly seems uncomfortable and becomes reluctant to answer questions. The patient abruptly stands up and accuses the nurse practitioner of being harsh and disrespectful. Fearing unintentionally causing the patient pain, the nurse practitioner:

    A. Politely and directly asks the patient which behavior has offended the patient
    B. Offers reassurance to the patient and moves to the next question
    C. Asks another nurse practitioner to complete the interview
    D. Refrains from asking questions about the patient's culture and practices

46. The condition necessary for temporary admission is that the patient:

    A. May not be able to provide for their basic needs
    B. May be a danger to others
    C. Requires an emergency treatment
    D. Is diagnosed with a mental illness

47. The standard of practice involving a competent level of nursing care needed before executing a strategy is:

    A. Collaboration
    B. Education
    C. Leadership
    D. Planning

48. A patient visits a psychiatric-mental health nurse practitioner and reports anxiousness, restlessness, sweating, panting, and difficulty sleeping for a couple of weeks. The patient describes being separated from their spouse and facing a financial crisis because of a job layoff. According to the standards of practice, the first action by the nurse practitioner should be:

    A. Diagnosis
    B. Health promotion
    C. Planning
    D. Assessment

(See answers next page.)

45. A) Politely and directly asks the patient which behavior has offended the patient

Asking which kind of behavior has offended the patient helps to build rapport between the patient and the nurse practitioner and helps to regain the patient's trust. Offering reassurance to the patient may be warranted, but the nurse practitioner would determine the cause of offense before moving on to the next question. Asking culturally insensitive questions is a mistake that almost all nurse practitioners may make, but it does not mean that the nurse practitioner will stop the interview and turn the patient's care over to someone else. The nurse practitioner should ask the patient about the patient's culture because this will help the nurse practitioner to know more about the culture and to avoid causing the patient unintentional pain. It will also show the patient that the nurse practitioner has a desire to know more about the patient's culture.

46. C) Requires an emergency treatment

The criteria for temporary admission include that the patient experiences difficulty in making decisions by themselves or requires emergency treatment due to chronic illness or other conditions. Patients diagnosed with mental illness, those who are unable to provide for basic necessities, and those who may harm themselves or others are usually given assisted inpatient psychiatric treatment.

47. D) Planning

Among the components of standards of practice is planning. A competent level of nursing care includes proper planning. The psychiatric-mental health nurse practitioner should make proper planning and then execute the planned strategies to achieve the expected results. The standards of professional performance involve components like collaboration, education, and leadership. Collaboration with other healthcare professionals involved in the care of the patients is necessary to achieve desired results. Also, nurse practitioners must collaborate with stakeholders for executing treatment plans and other health practices. Attaining knowledge and competence beneficial in the execution of current or ongoing nursing practice and encouraging futuristic thinking are important as well. Leadership quality is also required in nurse practitioners. Within the professional practice context and the profession, the nurse practitioner must take the lead.

48. D) Assessment

Based on the standards of practice, the nurse practitioner should first collect the relevant data from the patient, which includes physical, emotional, occupational, transpersonal or spiritual, and age-related information. After the assessment, the nurse practitioner should make the diagnosis based on the assessment, technologies, and tools supporting the clinical decision. The symptoms of the patient signify the diagnosis of anxiety disorder. The next step involves making a treatment plan based on the diagnosis of the patient. Because the patient has an anxiety disorder, the nurse practitioner might make a treatment plan that involves psychological therapies and antidepressant therapy. Health promotion is the final step of the clinical process. It involves encouragement of a healthy lifestyle, which may include meditation, exercise, methods for managing stress, and healthy food habits.

49. The capacity of a psychiatric-mental health nurse practitioner to take effective action to demonstrate competency is known as:

A. Judgment

B. Skill

C. Ability

D. Knowledge

50. A tenet characteristic, central to nursing practice, that involves conscious judgment or deliberate decision exhibited in actions is:

A. Acknowledging individual's unique needs

B. Caring for individuals and populations

C. Establishing relationships for effective outcomes

D. Using the nursing process for planning and executing treatment plans

51. Informal admission is best suited for a patient who:

A. Is nonharmful

B. Has mental illness

C. Is self-harming

D. Has severe disability

52. The characteristic included in standards of professional performance is:

A. Assessment of patient's information

B. Implementation of the treatment plan

C. Utilization of resources for better outcomes

D. Evaluation of the outcomes

(See answers next page.)

49. C) Ability

Among the properties of competency are abilities. Ability is defined by the capacity to act in a timely and efficient manner. It necessitates listening, integrity, self-awareness, emotional intelligence, acknowledgment of one's talents and weaknesses, and receptivity to feedback. Aspects of judgment involve critical thinking skills, decision-making, ethical reasoning, and problem-solving skills. Another property of competency is skill. It involves diagnostic, psychomotor, communication, and interpersonal abilities. Thinking, comprehension of humanities and science, personal talents, practical experiences, professional practice standards, and leadership performance all fall under the purview of knowledge.

50. B) Caring for individuals and populations

Caring is defined as a conscious judgment or a deliberate decision that reveals itself in real interpersonal, verbal, and nonverbal behaviors. It is a tenet feature that is central to nursing practice. Nursing practice should be individualized. The psychiatric-mental health nurse practitioner must respect people of different communities and acknowledge the unique needs of individuals or situations. The nurse practitioner must cooperate with other healthcare professionals and family members of patients or their acquaintances for delivering quality and effective care. The nurse practitioner uses their evidence-based knowledge or the nursing process for assessment, diagnosis, and execution of the treatment plan. Every aspect of the nursing process, including problem solving and decision-making, is based on critical thinking.

51. A) Is nonharmful

Informal admission involves no formal application procedure. It is suited for a patient who is not prone to self-harm or is nonharmful. Such patients do not pose a threat to themselves or someone else. Patients with mental illness and self-harming patients are not suited for such admissions. A patient with severe disability who is not able to provide for basic necessities is not an appropriate candidate for informal admission. Such patients might be admitted without voluntary commitment.

52. C) Utilization of resources for better outcomes

The standards of professional performance define a competent degree of behavior in a professional capacity. Its components involve ethics, collaboration, culturally congruent practice, leadership, communication, education, environmental health, practice based on evidence, professional practice evaluation, and quality of practice. Apart from these, another important component is resource utilization. The psychiatric-mental health nurse practitioner should use appropriate resources to execute the treatment plan and for the sustenance of nursing services based on evidence. This is necessary to ensure effective, safe, and budget-conscious delivery of services and care. The critical thinking model is used to describe a competent level of nursing care in the standards of practice. This model includes assessment, implementation, and evaluation. Assessment of the healthcare consumer's data or health history should be done by the nurse practitioner. A good strategy should be made and implemented to achieve the effective and desired result. Progress should be evaluated for the achievement of the desired goal.

Part II
Practice Test and Answers With Rationales

Practice Exam 1

1. A patient presents to the psychiatric emergency department with a history of bipolar disorder. The patient reports occasional vomiting, abdominal pain, dry mouth, some dizziness, and weakness. The psychiatric-mental health nurse practitioner will expect a lithium level of:

   A. 0.8 mEq/L
   B. 1.8 mEq/L
   C. 2.5 mEq/L
   D. 3.0 mEq/L

2. The number of sessions typically needed for interpersonal therapy is:
   A. 0 to 5 sessions
   B. 5 to 10 sessions
   C. 12 to 20 sessions
   D. 20 to 30 sessions

3. The preoperational stage of cognitive development occurs at the age of:
   A. Birth to 2 years
   B. 2 to 7 years
   C. 7 to 11 years
   D. 11 years to adulthood

4. A patient presents to the psychiatric emergency department with a history of bipolar disorder and reports being well managed on a current medication regimen. However, the patient reports persistent nausea and vomiting, blurred vision, syncope, and hyperactive deep tendon reflexes. The nurse practitioner orders a laboratory test, expecting to see a lithium value of:

   A. 1.0 mEq/L
   B. 1.6 mEq/L
   C. 2.1 mEq/L
   D. 3.0 mEq/L

5. Urine testing to detect substance use must be performed within:

   A. 7 to 12 hours for alcohol
   B. 1 week for cocaine
   C. 3 months for marijuana
   D. 1 week for heroin

6. A patient who does not speak or understand English is admitted to the hospital. In such cases, the psychiatric-mental health nurse practitioner should ask:

   A. A relative of the patient who understands English to be an interpreter
   B. Another patient who understands the language of the patient to be an interpreter
   C. A trained medical interpreter to help with communication with the patient
   D. A fellow practitioner to help with the communication with the patient

7. A patient is taking olanzapine (Zyprexa) 10 mg each morning. This dosage works well in reducing the patient's psychotic symptoms of auditory hallucinations. The patient smokes between 10 and 20 cigarettes per day but is trying to quit cigarette smoking. If the patient successfully quits smoking, the nurse practitioner anticipates that the necessary change to the patient's olanzapine use will be:

   A. An increase in dosage
   B. A decrease in dosage
   C. Maintenance of the dosage
   D. Change to another medication

8. A patient with stimulant-related disorder experiences dysphoria and drug craving as a result of neurotoxic effects on neuron systems, causing:

   A. Positive reinforcement for stimulant use
   B. A state of intoxication
   C. A dopamine-deficient state
   D. Increased activation of dopamine (D1) receptors

9. The psychiatric-mental health nurse practitioner is reviewing autopsy results for a 70-year-old patient with Alzheimer's disease. The report notes that the brain has diffuse atrophy with flattened cortical sulci and enlarged ventricles. Microscopic examination of the brain most likely shows decreased:

   A. Dopamine
   B. Acetylcholine
   C. Serotonin
   D. Tryptophan

10. The psychiatric-mental health nurse practitioner is treating a patient with maladaptive anger management who now reports violent thoughts. The patient has not acted upon these feelings but is concerned that they could "snap at any time." Relaxation therapy introduced at the beginning of treatment has not provided any relief from symptoms. The nurse practitioner will now:

    A. Add cognitive behavior modification to the treatment plan
    B. Refer the patient to a psychiatrist for psychotherapy
    C. Perform a cultural assessment to recognize learned behavior
    D. Obtain blood work to rule out organic etiologies

11. A patient taking a selective serotonin reuptake inhibitor (SSRI) reports daytime somnolence that is affecting their job. The best action to take at this time is:

    A. Changing to a selective norepinephrine reuptake inhibitor (SNRI)
    B. Adjusting the time of administration of the SSRI
    C. Adding small doses of stimulants
    D. Prescribing a hypnotic for nighttime insomnia

12. A patient is brought to the mental health facility with court orders for involuntary commitment after attempting to murder their life partner, claiming voices were instructing them to rid the earth of their partner's "kind." When the patient becomes enraged and aggressive toward the staff, the psychiatric-mental health nurse practitioner will:

    A. Admit the patient for the appropriate state allowable days according to the law
    B. Contact law enforcement or security to have the patient restrained until evaluated
    C. Firmly instruct the patient to sit down so the intake process can be employed
    D. Administer olanzapine (Zyprexa) to calm the patient so intake evaluation can be performed

13. The initiation of signal transduction to its full effect is caused by the:

    A. Antagonist
    B. Inverse agonist
    C. Agonist
    D. Partial agonist

14. A patient reports to a psychiatric-mental health nurse practitioner that they avoid places that require standing in line or staying in an enclosed place due to feelings that they could get trapped. The patient also experiences panic whenever a situation becomes a bit difficult. The nurse practitioner diagnoses:

    A. Major depressive disorder
    B. Kleptomania
    C. Agoraphobia
    D. Hoarding disorder

15. A patient diagnosed with bipolar disorder is taking carbamazepine (Tegretol). The patient suddenly develops a fever, sore throat, and oral ulcerations. The patients' white blood cell count is 2,800 mm^3, and the absolute neutrophil count is 1,400 mm^3. The psychiatric-mental health nurse practitioner reviews the psychiatric medication history. The patient has not been prescribed other psychiatric medications in the past. The nurse practitioner discusses medication alternatives with the patient and agrees to discontinue the carbamazepine, understanding that the patient is currently experiencing:

    A. Neuroleptic malignant syndrome
    B. Serotonin syndrome
    C. Agranulocytosis
    D. Carbamazepine overdose

16. Rational-emotive therapy was developed by:

    A. John B. Watson
    B. Albert Ellis
    C. B. F. Skinner
    D. Ivan Pavlov

17. The first action to be taken when a patient becomes aggressive and starts shouting during a clinical interview is to:

    A. Ask the patient to stop shouting
    B. Move the patient to a different room
    C. Ask the patient to leave
    D. Alert security

18. A 70-year-old patient is being evaluated for cognitive impairment. The spouse reports that the impairment has gotten progressively worse over the past 2 years, with changes in object recognition and working memory. Genetic testing has revealed the presence of two apolipoprotein E4 genes, along with a mutation in the amyloid precursor protein (APP). Given this information, the psychiatric-mental health nurse practitioner further evaluates for:

    A. Down syndrome
    B. Alzheimer's disease
    C. Huntington's disease
    D. Prion disease

19. The area of the brain expected to be impacted with a diagnosis of posttraumatic stress disorder (PTSD) is the:

    A. Amygdala
    B. Brainstem
    C. Basal ganglia
    D. Cerebellum

20. During assessment, a child is noticed to be messy and defiant. The psychiatric-mental health nurse practitioner's assessment of the patient's psychosexual stage according to Freud is:

    A. Oral
    B. Anal
    C. Phallic
    D. Latency

21. A young adult patient is brought to the hospital by their parents in an unconscious state. The psychiatric-mental health nurse practitioner observes that the patient's body mass index (BMI) is 15.59. The parents inform the psychiatric-mental health nurse practitioner that the patient used to fear gaining weight and refused to eat most of the time. The parents explain that it started when the patient was bullied in high school for their weight. The nurse practitioner believes the most likely diagnosis is:

    A. Anorexia nervosa
    B. Bulimia nervosa
    C. Rumination disorder
    D. Factitious disorder

22. Patients who use antipsychotic medications and are poor metabolizers of CYP2D6 are at risk for:

    A. Inadequate dosing
    B. Antipsychotic-induced extrapyramidal symptoms
    C. Loss of efficacy
    D. Gene-drug interactions

23. The psychiatric-mental health nurse practitioner is part of the Assertive Case Management Team. The team visits a patient with chronic mental illness in a residential motel. The motel room is dirty and filled with garbage. The patient is oblivious to the conditions. The nurse practitioner decides to petition for involuntary hospital admission for a 72-hour mental health examination because the patient is at risk due to self-neglect. The nurse practitioner's actions:

    A. Violate the patient's rights of autonomy
    B. Violate the patient's privacy
    C. Are beyond the scope of practice
    D. Are an act of advocacy

24. While working with an interpreter during a clinical interview, a psychiatric-mental health nurse practitioner should:

    A. Keep questions detailed and explanatory
    B. Let the interpreter summarize
    C. Direct the interpreter to note important points
    D. Ask questions directed to the patient

25. A patient offers a cultural explanation of Hwa-byung that is indicative of depression. In an effort to provide culturally appropriate care, the psychiatric-mental health nurse practitioner:

    A. Asks the patient how their culture typically treats Hwa-byung
    B. Has the patient complete the Beck Depression Inventory
    C. Conducts a social and cultural assessment for depression
    D. Refers the patient to a practitioner of the same culture

26. When planning psychoeducational strategies with a patient, the psychiatric-mental health nurse practitioner will:

    A. Implement a token economy through behavior modification
    B. Counsel the patient on pyramidal effects of medications
    C. Assess the patient's current skills and readiness to learn
    D. Include rehabilitation therapy for the family and caregiver

27. A patient is admitted for emotional lability following a traumatic brain injury resulting from a car accident. The patient is from a different cultural practice than that of the nurse practitioner. In an effort to accurately develop a recovery-oriented treatment plan, the psychiatric-mental health nurse practitioner will first:

    A. Assess the uniqueness and experiences of the patient
    B. Determine the patient's willingness to receive treatment
    C. Evaluate the patient's hope and drive to recover
    D. Inquire as to healing modalities of the culture practiced

28. Teaching a patient with schizophrenia to recognize delusions and hallucinations related to the disorder is most effective:

    A. When diagnosis is made
    B. At discharge of patient to home
    C. When medication is prescribed
    D. At 2-week follow-up assessment

29. A 35-year-old patient with no medical history of seizures reports being unable to sit still and concentrate at a given task. The patient also informs the psychiatric-mental health nurse practitioner about frequent mood fluctuations. The nurse practitioner observes the patient talking very quickly and fidgeting constantly. The nurse practitioner suspects that the patient has symptoms related to:

    A. Attention deficit/hyperactivity disorder
    B. Personality disorder
    C. Mood disorder
    D. Cognitive disorder

30. A psychiatric-mental health nurse practitioner assesses a 6-year-old patient and observes that the patient does not focus on any particular thing and becomes distracted very easily. The patient's behavior is very impulsive. The nurse practitioner inquires about the patient's behavior and performance in school, to which the parents respond that the teacher always talks about incomplete homework submissions and careless mistakes. Based on the diagnostic criteria, the nurse practitioner determines the disorder known as:

    A. Attention deficit/hyperactivity
    B. Autism spectrum
    C. Specific learning
    D. Developmental coordination

31. During assessment of a patient diagnosed with depression, the patient reports drinking more alcohol lately, describing consumption of 6 to 8 beers at least 4 out of 7 days. To determine the severity of the drinking issue, the psychiatric-mental health nurse practitioner will choose the screening tool called:

    A. CAGE
    B. AUDIT
    C. T-ACE
    D. SBIRT

32. Parkinson's disease affects the area of the brain known as the:

    A. Cerebellum
    B. Brainstem
    C. Basal ganglia
    D. Hippocampus

33. The nurse practitioner has been given the duty to administer a drug to a patient. When the nurse enters the room, the patient shows anxiety. The nurse calms the patient, and only when the patient feels comfortable does the nurse administer the prescribed drug. This is an example of:

    A. Beneficence
    B. Justice
    C. Autonomy
    D. Veracity

34. Diazepam (Valium) is commonly prescribed to treat anxiety disorder and works by:

    A. Blocking voltage-sensitive sodium channels
    B. Blocking serotonin reuptake pumps
    C. Binding to the benzodiazepine receptors
    D. Blocking norepinephrine reuptake

35. A psychiatric-mental health nurse practitioner finds that a patient has experienced a hypomanic episode and two major depressive episodes. The patient has never experienced a manic episode. According to the given diagnostic criteria, the nurse practitioner infers that the patient has the disorder known as:

    A. Bipolar II
    B. Bipolar I
    C. Panic
    D. Cyclothymic

36. A 40-year-old patient reports a relationship breakup and passive suicidal thoughts. Mood is depressed, and the patient feels hopeless but denies feeling helpless for the last 2 weeks. The patient also reports angry outbursts and reduced need for sleep. Her speech is rapid and pressured. The patient has been receiving psychiatric services on and off since age 15. She reports a history of sexual abuse. She has a history of suicidal ideations and multiple hospitalizations and has been on "over a dozen medications." She has a history of cutting. Reality is intact, with no evidence of thought disorder. The patient has been married three times, with each relationship lasting 5 years or less. She has a history of marijuana and alcohol use but denies use in the last week. Differential diagnosis for this patient includes ruling out:

A. Borderline personality disorder and bipolar II disorder
B. Borderline personality disorder and other substance-related disorders
C. Obsessive–compulsive disorder and brief psychotic disorder
D. Borderline personality disorder and schizoaffective disorder

37. A patient reports nausea and difficulty in moving their shoulder. The patient is also feeling very sad and annoyed. The psychiatric-mental health nurse practitioner asks whether these conditions are accompanied by headaches. The patient replies affirmatively. The patient describes having a habit of drinking coffee every morning but states that they missed it today. The nurse practitioner suspects:

A. Caffeine intoxication
B. Caffeine withdrawal
C. Caffeine-induced anxiety disorder
D. Unspecified caffeine-related disorder

38. A patient with schizophrenia has severe hallucinations. The typical antipsychotic does not improve the condition of the patient. In such cases, the patient can be prescribed clozapine. The clozapine is chosen as the last resort in such cases because it:

A. Causes sedative side effects by blocking alpha 1 adrenergic receptors
B. Causes motor side effects by blocking dopamine 1 transporters
C. Reduces negative symptoms of schizophrenia by blocking dopamine 1 transporters
D. Reduces dopamine release in the brain as it blocks serotonin 2A receptors

39. In the theory of change outcome, the pathway involving the cessation of monitoring in a project that has no responsibility for outcomes, met or unmet, is:

A. Intervention
B. Rationale
C. Ceiling of accountability
D. Indicator

40. An example of a child's mesosystem is the:

A. Child's relationship with their family
B. Child's parents' relation with their school
C. Mass media's influence on the child's family
D. Impact of cultural belief on the teachings of the child's school

41. A patient with bipolar disorder visits the psychiatric-mental health nurse practitioner's clinic and reports severe stress along with anger issues. There has been a decline in appetite, sleep, and energy level of the patient since the last visit. Along with medications, the nurse practitioner would include the type of therapy known as:

    A. Family
    B. Behavioral
    C. Cognitive behavioral
    D. Interpersonal

42. A patient admitted from the emergency department for treatment of alcohol dependence syndrome suddenly becomes disoriented and demonstrates paranoid behaviors. When questioned, the patient states that "the voice" is telling them to set the bed on fire so they can get away and not have their "brain probed." After the psychiatric-mental health nurse practitioner administers lorazepam (Ativan), the next action is to:

    A. Admit the patient to observation with prn diazepam orders
    B. Provide the patient education on weaning from alcohol
    C. Administer naloxone stat followed by additional lorazepam 0.5 mg
    D. Collect blood specimen for thiamine level and start IV thiamine 200 mg

43. The psychiatric-mental health nurse practitioner is evaluating a 70-year-old patient. In the mental status exam, the nurse practitioner asks the patient to interpret proverbs. The patient's responses are literal. The nurse practitioner notes that the patient has a pattern of concrete interpretation. This indicates:

    A. Poor insight
    B. Poor judgment
    C. Delusional thought content
    D. Conceptualization deficit in cognitive thinking

44. After the psychiatric-mental health nurse practitioner assigns the "limited sick role" to a 13-year-old patient diagnosed with depression; the patient begins to show signs of improvement. During follow-up, the patient reports feelings of sadness and states that the parents are impatient and often angry with them. The current Children's Depression Inventory rating is 48, up five points from the last visit. The step the nurse practitioner takes first to ensure successful recovery is:

    A. Discussing positive reinforcement with the parents
    B. Conducting a "closeness circle" activity with the patient
    C. Referring the parents for cognitive behavior modification
    D. Explaining that the parents are upset with the illness, not with the patient

45. A 10-year-old patient is referred for evaluation of attention deficit disorder. After obtaining a thorough history and reviewing physical examination records, the psychiatric-mental health nurse practitioner determines that the child is healthy with no current medical issues or complaints and plans on prescribing methylphenidate (Concerta) 18 mg QD. The patient's parents are concerned about cardiac side effects because there is a family history of cardiac disease. Before initiating a stimulant to the child, the nurse practitioner orders a:

A. EEG

B. Single-photon emission computed tomography (SPECT)

C. PET

D. Consult to a pediatric cardiologist

46. People anticipate beginning to practice healthy habits in the foreseeable future (within the next 6 months) at the behavioral change stage of:

A. Preparation

B. Contemplation

C. Precontemplation

D. Action

47. Suffering within a cultural group is called:

A. Cultural explanation

B. Acculturation

C. Suffering of religiousness

D. Cultural idiom of distress

48. When determining an herbal supplement regimen for a patient, the psychiatric-mental health nurse practitioner would investigate specific ingredients based on the fact that:

A. Supplements include additional fillers that contribute to toxicity

B. A large percentage of poisonings is attributable to herbal supplements

C. DNA barcoding will provide needed information regarding supplement contents

D. Current regulatory requirements are not effective in management of supplements

49. A patient with schizophrenia believes the house manager of the group home is going to kill them. The patient is being discharged and shares that they plan to bomb the group home. The psychiatric-mental health nurse practitioner notifies the group home manager. The nurse practitioner:

A. Violated the patient's confidentiality

B. Violated the principle of justice

C. Should have the patient arrested

D. Demonstrated the duty to warn and protect

50. A patient makes everyday decisions only after receiving excessive advice and reassurances from different individuals. This patient's behavior is related to the personality disorder known as:

    A. Avoidant
    B. Dependent
    C. Narcissistic
    D. Histrionic

51. For more than 10 years, a psychiatric-mental health nurse practitioner has been counseling patients whose spouses have cancer. The nurse practitioner often asks the patients how the spouses' illness affects their mental and emotional life. To understand the coping mechanisms of these patients, a suitable study to conduct is a:

    A. Single randomized control study
    B. Descriptive study
    C. Opinion of practitioners
    D. Experimental study

52. A 32-year-old patient is brought to the emergency department with her two children by a neighbor, who reports witnessing a violent attack on the patient by her live-in partner. During the interview, the patient is reluctant to offer any specifics and simply states that her behavior triggers the partner's anger. When preparing psychoeducation materials and resources for this patient who wishes to return home, the psychiatric-mental health nurse practitioner will first:

    A. Provide information on battered women's shelters and other support in the community
    B. Help the patient develop an emergency plan for safety and possible escape
    C. Determine what would happen if the perpetrator found the educational material in the home
    D. Involve the children in the development of an escape plan and teach them how to call 911

53. A 29-year-old female patient is brought to the emergency department by a family member who reports that the patient has been "using again." The patient appears unkempt and disoriented and smells of alcohol. To determine which screening tool to use for substance use disorder, the psychiatric-mental health nurse practitioner needs to:

    A. Determine if the patient is pregnant
    B. Complete a review of patient records
    C. Collect a blood sample for toxicity
    D. Observe the patient's demeanor

54. The ideal goal in a therapeutic alliance developed by a psychiatric-mental health nurse practitioner is to:

    A. Assess the competency of the therapist
    B. Develop a basic level of trust
    C. Check medication side effects
    D. Understand technical interventions

55. The psychiatric-mental health nurse practitioner is evaluating a 12-year-old patient who falls frequently while running, is unable to kick an approaching ball, and is called "clumsy" by friends. With a previous diagnosis of attention deficit/hyperactivity disorder (ADHD) in second grade, the most likely diagnosis would be:

    A. Muscular dystrophy
    B. Developmental dyspraxia
    C. Stereotypic movement disorder
    D. Motor tic disorder

56. According to Mahler's stages of separation-individuation, a child recognizes separation from the caretaker in the phase called:

    A. Differentiation
    B. Practicing
    C. Rapprochement
    D. Consolidation

57. Critical incident stress debriefings, a part of the tertiary intervention, ensure confidentiality at the phase when the participants:

    A. Discuss the purpose of the meeting and introduce themselves
    B. Discuss their first thoughts about the incident
    C. Discuss the worst or most painful part of the incident
    D. Review the material discussed and bring closure

58. A patient reports temper outbursts for a year. The anger is expressed verbally and is recurrent (3–4 times a week). The psychiatric-mental health nurse practitioner diagnoses the disorder called:

    A. Disruptive mood dysregulation
    B. Persistent depressive
    C. Oppositional defiant
    D. Intermittent explosive

59. A patient with a history of alcohol use disorder (AUD) and generalized anxiety disorder (GAD) presents to the emergency department with palpitations, nausea, vomiting, headache, and flushing. The patient has been prescribed sertraline, thiamine, naltrexone, and disulfiram. The patient admits to drinking several glasses of champagne earlier in the evening. The nurse practitioner knows that the agent related to the symptoms is:

    A. Disulfiram
    B. Naltrexone
    C. Thiamine
    D. Sertraline

60. The period when the psychiatric-mental health nurse practitioner initiates therapeutic alliance is:

    A. During the first visit
    B. During the second visit
    C. After 1 month of therapy
    D. At the end of therapy

61. A 70-year-old patient in therapy is noticed to have extreme alienation. According to Erikson's psychosocial stages, the patient's stage-specific conflict is:

    A. Ego integrity versus despair
    B. Intimacy versus isolation
    C. Initiative versus guilt
    D. Identity versus role confusion

62. A 5-year-old patient is brought to the clinic with the report of feces passage on the floor and clothing. The patient's parents inform the psychiatric-mental health nurse practitioner that their child had been continent until the last 4 months. Various diagnostic tests have been done, which have showed no major diagnosis except for constipation. The patient has no other medical conditions and has not taken laxatives. The nurse practitioner infers that the patient has the disorder called:

    A. Encopresis
    B. Enuresis
    C. Bulimia
    D. Hoarding

63. The repeated passage of urine either intentionally or involuntarily, occurring twice a week for at least 3 months, that is not consistent with the patient's developmental age is the diagnostic criterion of:

    A. Enuresis
    B. Bulimia
    C. Encopresis
    D. Hoarding

64. The process of self-reappraisal to assess the effect of a particular unhealthy behavior on others is:

    A. Self–reevaluation
    B. Environmental reevaluation
    C. Counter-conditioning
    D. Consciousness-raising

65. In an effort to gain accurate information and conduct a meaningful assessment of a patient of a differing culture, it is most important for the psychiatric-mental health nurse practitioner to:

    A. Educate all patients about mental illness regardless of culture
    B. Tailor the intervention and treatment to the individual
    C. Conduct a thorough social and cultural interview
    D. Establish a trusting and collaborative relationship

66. The first step of a clinical interview is:

    A. Establishing rapport
    B. Identifying emotional clues
    C. Taking notes
    D. Generating a diagnostic hypothesis

67. A 54-year-old patient is being seen for tremors and shuffling gait that began approximately 1 week ago. He has had several falls during this time frame. The patient is being treated for bipolar disorder and was switched to risperidone (Risperdal) 3 months ago. Upon assessment, the psychiatric-mental health nurse practitioner finds the patient to have orthostatic hypotension and slight neurocognitive dysfunction. A Mini-Cog exam is given, with a result of three. To further evaluate this patient to determine accurate diagnosis, the nurse practitioner would first:

   A. Evaluate medication dosage and efficacy
   B. Send the patient for an MRI of the brain
   C. Admit the patient for 72 hours for observation
   D. Schedule physical therapy to reduce risk of falls

68. The process in which an electrical impulse is converted into a chemical impulse at the synapse is:

   A. Synaptogenesis
   B. Signal transduction cascade
   C. Excitation-secretion coupling
   D. Volume neurotransmission

69. A 7-year-old child visits the clinic with a parent. The patient has anger management issues that began several months ago. The parent informs the psychiatric-mental health nurse practitioner that the child does not fear punishment and has to be promised rewards for staying calm. During the clinical interview, the patient denies being mischievous and blames problems on others. To make an accurate diagnosis, the nurse practitioner asks the parent if the child has:

   A. Demonstrated consistent behavior for at least 3 months
   B. Exhibited spiteful or vindictive behaviors at least twice in the past 6 months
   C. Ever apologized or demonstrated feelings of guilt
   D. Aggressive tendencies shown by behaviors such as setting things on fire or harming animals

70. Becoming sexually aroused from the exposure of one's genitals to another person because of urges and fantasies is a diagnostic criterion of the disorder called:

   A. Exhibitionist
   B. Frotteuristic
   C. Pedophilic
   D. Fetishistic

71. A diagnostic criterion of nightmare disorder is that the patient:

   A. Experiences frightening dreams during rapid-eye-movement sleep
   B. Does not remember the details of dreams after waking up
   C. Always wakes up from sleep directly after having dreams
   D. Feels bewildered regarding the patient's location upon waking

72. The concept of emotional triangles is part of the theory known as:

    A. Family systems
    B. Functionalism
    C. Conflict
    D. Symbolic interactionism

73. A 54-year-old patient comes into the office for an initial visit accompanied by their spouse, with concerns of speech problems, trouble finding words and understanding written communication, and inappropriate, abrupt behavioral changes. These changes have been slowly worsening. After further testing, the psychiatric-mental health nurse practitioner orders an MRI. The nurse practitioner expects to see atrophy in the:

    A. Cerebellum
    B. Frontal and temporal lobes
    C. Brainstem
    D. Parietal lobe

74. The lobe of the brain responsible for executive functioning is:

    A. Parietal
    B. Occipital
    C. Frontal
    D. Temporal

75. An example of a macro theory is:

    A. Family systems
    B. Social exchange
    C. Functionalism
    D. Symbolic interactionism

76. A 21-year-old male patient has reported using alcohol to self-medicate for depression after losing a friend to drug overdose. The patient completes the AUDIT screening for risk for alcohol use disorder (AUD) and scores an 8. Based on this score, the psychiatric-mental health nurse practitioner will:

    A. Refer the patient for outpatient rehabilitation
    B. Provide education on the risks for alcohol dependency
    C. Further assess for alcohol use disorder
    D. Admit the patient for inpatient treatment for alcohol use disorder

77. The neurotransmitter that is responsible for the inhibition of wakefulness is:

    A. Gamma-aminobutyric acid (GABA)
    B. Histamine
    C. Serotonin
    D. Dopamine

78. The psychiatric-mental health nurse practitioner is treating a 65-year-old patient who wants to take only "natural medicine." The patient is showing difficulty with memory and cognitive performance. The nurse practitioner recommends a trial of:

    A. Valerian 450 mg per day
    B. Melatonin 3 mg per day
    C. Ginkgo biloba 120 mg per day
    D. Omega-3 fatty acids 1 g per day

79. The excitatory neurotransmitter involved in kindling, seizure disorders, and possible bipolar disorder is:

    A. Glutamate
    B. Gamma-aminobutyric acid (GABA)
    C. Acetylcholine
    D. Glycine

80. The psychiatric-mental health nurse practitioner is dealing with a family that reports dysfunctional communication with each other. While interviewing the family members to determine if they manipulate each other, the nurse practitioner should ask if they:

    A. Grant each other's requests only after keeping some strings attached
    B. Introduce irrelevant issues when one family member is discussing any problem
    C. Accuse each other of responsibility for the issues occurring in the family
    D. Pretend to be well-meaning to maintain peace within the family

81. A 22-year-old patient is brought to the emergency department by law enforcement after an explosive outburst at a local bar, where the patient physically assaulted a customer causing injuries to the customer as well as property damage. The officers report that witnesses say the patient was laughing and having fun when she suddenly became enraged and attacked the other person. The patient is now combative, screaming obscenities, and threatening both officers and health professionals. The action the psychiatric-mental health nurse practitioner would take first to address the emergency is:

    A. Ensure that the officers contain the patient in a holding area until they can be seen
    B. Have security assist officers in holding the patient's limbs while administering lorazepam
    C. Restrain the patient to the hospital bed until they can be evaluated by the nurse practitioner
    D. Contact a family member or significant other to determine any medications the patient is on

82. The act that protects the right of psychiatric patients to have medical records kept confidential is the:

    A. Community Mental Health Centers Act
    B. Patient Protection and Affordable Care Act
    C. Health Insurance Portability and Accountability Act
    D. Oregon Death with Dignity Act

83. A 50-year-old teacher, treated for a 3-year history of major depression that has recently worsened, is seen via telemedicine session. During the session, the psychiatric-mental health nurse practitioner notices that the room the patient is speaking from is filled floor to ceiling with stacks of clothing, books, educational toys, and arts and crafts. Upon further inquiry, the patient shares that every room in their apartment is filled with things they "cannot let go of" and that the patient has had panic attacks when friends and family have tried to help clean the apartment. The patient reports significant functional impairment, as friends and family no longer visit and the patient feels gravely ashamed and distressed. The most likely DSM-5 diagnosis is:

A. Hoarding disorder and dysthymia

B. Obsessive-compulsive disorder and persistent depressive disorder

C. Mixed obsessive-compulsive disorder and hoarding disorder

D. Hoarding disorder and major depression

84. A parent receives a phone call that their son has had a major accident while playing football and is asked to go to the hospital where their son has been transported. The parent suddenly feels anxious and stressed and has a panic attack. This response involves:

A. Inhibition of cortisol secretion

B. Increased production of gamma-aminobutyric acid (GABA)

C. Hyperactivation of the amygdala

D. Deactivation of the sympathetic nervous system

85. The disorder with diagnostic criteria of excessive sleeping every week for 3 months is called:

A. Hypersomnolence

B. Narcolepsy

C. Insomnia

D. Excoriation

86. The patient has been diagnosed with narcolepsy. The psychiatric-mental health nurse practitioner knows that:

A. Cerebrospinal fluid (CSF) orexin-c level is high

B. Hypnagogic hallucinations are common

C. Polysomnography shows absence of rapid eye movement (REM) sleep

D. Presence of catalepsy is one of the defining characteristics

87. Carol Gilligan's concept supported Kohlberg's:

A. Method of developing the theory of moral development based on a sample of boys and men

B. Favor for males' methods of reasoning

C. Justice view of morality in the theory of moral development

D. Idea that the progression of moral development occurs in three major divisions

88. An older patient is diagnosed with sarcoma, and the prognosis states that the patient has approximately 3 months to live. The patient prefers other remedial methods to the suggestions for treatment provided in the hospital. The psychiatric-mental health nurse practitioner should first:

    A. Identify the cultural values of the patient
    B. Speak with the family about the patient's decision
    C. Identify advanced medical solutions for the patient
    D. Instruct the patient to not leave the hospital

89. A patient has stopped taking aripiprazole (Abilify) suddenly and has been brought to the emergency department reporting suicidal ideations with anger and irritability. When conducting a recovery-oriented assessment to address the immediate danger, the psychiatric-mental health nurse practitioner will:

    A. Identify new or additional risk factors for the patient
    B. Determine the level of self-esteem of the patient
    C. Involve the parents in creating a recovery plan
    D. Measure the current stress level and depression score

90. Developmental coordination disorder may be considered in an 11-year-old patient when physical coordination is substantially below the expectation for the patient's age and the patient demonstrates:

    A. Hyperextensible joints
    B. Lack of motor competence due to distractibility or impulsiveness
    C. Lack of interest in participating in tasks requiring complex coordination skills
    D. Inaccurate performance of motor skills such as catching a ball or riding a bicycle.
       (D) Impairment of skills requiring motor coordination that interferes with daily activities is a cornerstone of developmental coordination disorder. Joint hypermobility syndrome causes hyperextensible joints. Attention deficit/hyperactivity disorder may cause a lack of motor competence due to distractibility and impulsiveness. Patients with autism spectrum disorder may be uninterested in participating in tasks requiring complex coordination skills

91. A 17-year-old patient being treated for bipolar disorder has a history of relapse and has been admitted for monitoring and intervention. Upon admission interview, the patient reports feelings of irritability, being increasingly hungry, and vacillating between events of extreme energy and wanting to sleep. Based on this patient's self-observation, the nurse will:

    A. Enhance social and occupational functioning
    B. Implement sleep/light manipulation in therapy
    C. Include an emergency plan in psychoeducation
    D. Provide the patient with information on support groups

92. The FDA mandated boxed warnings for atypical antipsychotic use in older adults for the treatment of psychosis due to:

    A. Increased mortality risk when used to treat behavioral disturbances of dementia
    B. Higher susceptibility for adverse cardiac effects in that population
    C. Slower metabolism and excretion rates of all drugs in that population
    D. Questionable reduced capacity for giving informed consent

93. According to Erikson's eight stages of development, egocentricity can come as an unsuccessful resolution of the psychosocial crisis called:

    A. Identity versus role confusion
    B. Intimacy versus isolation
    C. Generativity versus self-absorption
    D. Integrity versus despair

94. The psychiatric-mental health nurse practitioner should maintain confidentiality when the patient:

    A. Is suicidal and can self-harm
    B. Reports domestic violence.
    C. Is nonharmful to self and others
    D. Expresses intent to harm a known person

95. The scientist who noted a discernible pattern in the difference in cognitive processing between young children and older children while scoring Binet Intelligence Tests is:

    A. Jean Piaget
    B. Erik Erikson
    C. Carol Gilligan
    D. Lawrence Kohlberg

96. The patient is admitted for treatment for alcoholism after a driving under the influence citation. The patient was involved in a motor vehicle crash, and another driver was physically hurt. The patient shares the details in a group session on the unit. Afterward, the patient feels that patients and staff on the unit are judging them negatively. The patient states that other patients have more privileges and that staff seem to be avoiding them. The psychiatric-mental health nurse practitioner agrees to look into the problem. The ethical principle guiding the nurse practitioner's action is the patient's right to:

    A. Justice
    B. Beneficence
    C. Nonmaleficence
    D. Fidelity

97. The disorder that involves failure to control the impulse to steal objects not needed for use or monetary value is called:

    A. Kleptomania
    B. Pyromania
    C. Cognitive dissonance
    D. Conduct disorder

98. The nurse practitioner is working in the psychiatric emergency department when a patient with a history of bipolar disorder who takes valproate (Depakote) comes in with a red maculopapular rash. The patient reports being started on a new medication. The medication the nurse practitioner suspects to be the cause for these symptoms is:

    A. Lithium carbonate (Lithobid)
    B. Lurasidone (Latuda)
    C. Cariprazine (Vraylar)
    D. Lamotrigine (Lamictal)

99. The patient reports consistent sadness, lack of interest in activities usually enjoyed, grief, and self-doubt. The patient states that they feel "worthless." The patient has lost weight, cannot sleep through the night, and feels like "giving up." The patient denies any physical complaints and reports having begun to use marijuana to sleep. The differential diagnosis the psychiatric-mental health nurse practitioner considers is:

    A. Malingering and factitious disorder
    B. Substance abuse
    C. Persistent complex bereavement disorder
    D. Major depression

100. A patient consults the psychiatric-mental health nurse practitioner and reports a lack of interest in activities. The patient shares that they experienced the death of a family member more than a year ago. The patient does not feel like eating, has made three suicide attempts, and has had difficulty getting a full night's sleep for a year. The patient recently lost their job and has no hope of finding another. All the diagnostic reports of the patient are normal. The nurse practitioner suspects:

     A. Unspecified depressive disorder
     B. Depressive disorder as a result of other medical reasons
     C. Substance or drug-induced depressive disorder
     D. Major depressive disorder

101. Overactivation of the hypothalamic-pituitary-adrenal (HPA) axis resulting in glucocorticoid cortisol elevation is one consideration in the treatment of:

     A. Major depressive disorder
     B. Anxiety
     C. Substance use disorders
     D. Personality disorders

102. A 65-year-old patient reports difficulty with memory. The patient finds it harder to learn new things and frequently becomes disorganized. There is no change in level of independence and no reported difficulty with ability to manage day-to-day responsibilities. The patient reports an increased need for lists and reminders to compensate for memory problems. There are no signs of delirium. The patient has no history of psychiatric illnesses. The most likely diagnosis is:

     A. Mild neurocognitive disorder without behavioral disturbances
     B. Mild neurocognitive disorder
     C. Dementia
     D. Mild neurocognitive disorder due to Alzheimer's disease

103. When providing teaching to a patient with schizoaffective disorder who is newly admitted to a group home, the immediate psychoeducational support that the psychiatric-mental health nurse practitioner will include is:

    A. Milieu therapy
    B. Recovery strategies
    C. Wellness strategies
    D. Cognitive behavior modification

104. A patient presenting with severe hyperthermia, muscle rigidity, diaphoresis, and ocular clonus reports having taken an overdose of a prescribed psychiatric medication approximately 12-hours-ago. The nurse practitioner suspects an overdose of:

    A. Benzodiazepine
    B. Serotonin norepinephrine reuptake inhibitor anticholinergics
    C. Monoamine oxidase inhibitor (MAOI)
    D. Tricyclic antidepressant (TCA)

105. A patient presents to the emergency department reporting extreme fatigue, subjective feeling of overall weakness, and uncharacteristically sad mood lasting for 10 days. The patient states, "I am not acting like myself," and denies suicidal/homicidal thoughts. Immunoglobulin M (IgM) and immunoglobulin G (IgG) antibodies are elevated. White blood cell count (WBC) is elevated. Liver enzymes (ALT and AST) and bilirubin also are elevated. There is no previous psychiatric history or recent trauma. The psychiatric-mental health nurse practitioner orders Epstein-Barr virus (EBV)-specific antibody and antigen and suspects a diagnosis of:

    A. Major depression
    B. Mononucleosis
    C. Chronic fatigue syndrome
    D. Malingering

106. The cognitive screening tool that can be used to assess for dementia is the:

    A. Montreal Cognitive Assessment
    B. Modified Ashworth scale
    C. Tardieu scale
    D. Glasgow Coma Scale

107. A patient is brought to the emergency department after experiencing a seizure at home. Upon evaluation, the patient is found to have heart palpitations, hypertension, dyspnea, and tremors. The patient scores a 14 on the Clinical Institute Withdrawal Assessment Alcohol Scale, revised (CIWA-Ar scale). Based on this information, the initial approach the psychiatric-mental health nurse practitioner will take is:

    A. Pharmacotherapy
    B. Psychoeducation
    C. Peer-centered care
    D. Motivational interviewing

108. The interviewing process:

    A. Is a written or spoken framework for arranging a patient's information
    B. Necessitates acute awareness of the patient's emotions and behavioral cues
    C. Standardizes communication with other healthcare professionals engaged in the patient's care
    D. Is a clinician-centered and closed-ended "yes-no" method of questioning

109. Disorders involving changes in brain structure and function that result in impaired learning, orientation, and judgment can be classified as:

    A. Alcohol-related
    B. Substance-related
    C. Personality
    D. Neurocognitive

110. A 19-year-old patient has lifelong symptoms of awkward social skills, including being overtalkative, inattentive, and hyperactive. The patient is of average intelligence and has difficulty following instructions and staying employed. History is significant for delayed developmental milestones and congenital heart defects. The patient has short stature, ocular hypertelorism, and low-set ears. The differential diagnosis includes:

    A. Attention deficit/hyperactivity disorder (ADHD)
    B. Autism spectrum disorder (ASD)
    C. Noonan syndrome (NS)
    D. Turner syndrome

111. When teaching a family how to handle stressors of mental illness, an area of focus will be:

    A. Normalization
    B. Bibliotherapy
    C. Group experiences
    D. Social skills training

112. It is appropriate for the psychiatric-mental health nurse practitioner to breach a patient's confidentiality and share private health information when:

    A. Treating older adult patients
    B. Observing evidence of abuse of an older adult patient
    C. Caring for an older adult patient whose adult child wants information because they live together
    D. Obtaining family members' health information

113. A patient who has suffered a cerebral vascular accident with vision loss likely has damage to the:

    A. Parietal lobe
    B. Occipital lobe
    C. Medulla oblongata
    D. Temporal lobe

114. A 50-year old patient with a history of bipolar disorder and type 2 diabetes reports 25-lb weight gain, especially in the abdominal area. Their HbA1c is 10.6%, and the lipid profile indicates total cholesterol 240 mg/dL and low-density lipoprotein (LDL) 200 mg/dL. The patient reports they started a new medication 6 months ago. The most likely medication is:

    A. Citalopram (Celexa)
    B. Olanzapine (Zyprexa)
    C. Dextro-amphetamine (Adderall)
    D. Sertraline (Zoloft)

115. Parents bring their 10-year-old child to a mental health clinic. The parents tell the psychiatric-mental health nurse practitioner that the child has been damaging furniture at school, behaving badly with classmates, and not paying attention to teachers. There are daily complaints about the patient's school-related issues. The nurse practitioner interacts with the child and determines that the best medication for the patient is:

    A. Olanzapine (Zyprexa)
    B. Sertraline (Zoloft)
    C. Ondansetron (Zofran)
    D. Fluoxetine (Prozac)

116. The questions asked during a clinical interview should be:
    A. In a series, all at once
    B. Open-ended to focused
    C. Leading
    D. Answerable with yes or no

117. A patient is discharged after being treated for substance use disorder. The patient's employer and a friend are present to drive the patient to the supportive housing unit where the patient will reside for the next 90 days. In addition to referral for supportive housing placement, as part of the recovery-oriented treatment plan the psychiatric-mental health nurse practitioner will include:

    A. Support employment
    B. E-mental health
    C. Outpatient substance use treatment
    D. Family and caregiver support

118. A patient feels sudden trembling, sweating, and increased heart rate, accompanied by intense fear. The psychiatric-mental health nurse practitioner correlates these diagnostic criteria to the disorder called:

    A. Panic
    B. Bipolar
    C. Hoarding
    D. Excoriation

119. The personality disorder involving distrust and suspiciousness as its diagnostic criteria is:

    A. Schizotypal
    B. Borderline
    C. Paranoid
    D. Antisocial

120. A patient presents with a unilateral hand tremor and states that it is interfering with activities of daily living. The presence of the tremor is not consistent throughout the examination; it is less present with voluntary movement. The tremors occur at rest and during walking. The patient is prescribed lithium and has levels within the normal range. The psychiatric-mental health nurse practitioner suspects the tremor is:

    A. Cerebellar
    B. Tardive dyskinesia
    C. Parkinson's disease
    D. Physiological

121. The psychiatric-mental health nurse practitioner demonstrates a clear understanding of the ethical scope and standard of practice by:

    A. Participating on a hospital committee to ensure that patients with substance use disorders have equal access to care
    B. Informing a voluntarily hospitalized patient that they do not have the right to request to be discharged against medical advice
    C. Deciding not to notify someone a patient has stated they wish to harm because the potential victim lives out of state
    D. Failing to report illegal actions taken toward a patient in a mental health clinic because of fear of retribution

122. Home visits by nurses improve postpartum depression in patients. However, a patient experiencing postpartum depression refuses such visits when the nurse calls the patient. The dominant element of the clinical decision-making model of evidence-based practice affecting the treatment here is:

    A. Internal evidence
    B. Patient preferences
    C. Research evidence
    D. Healthcare resources

123. The psychiatric-mental health nurse practitioner overhears a staff member tell a 12-year-old patient, "If you don't behave, you're going to the restraint room." The nurse practitioner intervenes by meeting with the staff member and providing education on laws and clinical aspects related to seclusion and restraint. The nurse practitioner's intervention is an example of:

    A. Quality assurance
    B. Plan-do-study-act
    C. Evidence-based practice
    D. Patient advocacy

124. The psychiatric-mental health nurse practitioner observes a patient as flat and constricted. In the mental status exam, the nurse practitioner documents this as:

    A. Patient affect
    B. Patient mood
    C. Thought content
    D. Thought process

125. The explanation that best describes how self-determination impacts treatment of mental health patients is:

    A. Self-determination allows patients to understand their rights while obtaining mental health treatment
    B. Promoting self-determination in a patient with mental illness can result in irrational decision making with poor outcomes
    C. Patients who feel autonomous and independent are more receptive to treatment and have more successful outcomes
    D. When patients feel their rights are being upheld and they can choose care options, they most often will make informed decisions

126. The stages of the transtheoretical model of change include:

    A. Contemplation, freezing, unfreezing, and action
    B. Precontemplation, contemplation, preparation, action, and maintenance
    C. Plan, do, study, act, and maintain
    D. Freezing, transition, action, unfreezing, and maintenance

127. Self-liberation is a process found in the behavioral change stage of:

    A. Precontemplation
    B. Contemplation
    C. Preparation
    D. Action

128. According to Erikson's eight stages of development, the psychosocial crisis of initiative versus guilt arrives in:

    A. Infancy
    B. Preschool
    C. Adolescence
    D. Early adulthood

129. A patient reports dizziness, insomnia, nervousness, dry mouth, sweating, anorexia, somnolence, and sensory disturbances after beginning to taper off venlafaxine (Effexor) according to the treatment plan. The psychiatric-mental health nurse practitioner will:

    A. Admit the patient to the hospital for observation
    B. Prescribe several doses of fluoxetine (Prozac)
    C. Resume the previous dosage of venlafaxine immediately
    D. Immediately discontinue venlafaxine completely

130. A 10-year-old patient was referred by a school nurse for a psychiatric evaluation after the patient was found to be talking to the bulletin board every day during recess. The psychiatric-mental health nurse practitioner observes that the patient becomes very agitated and has cuts all over their arms and legs. When asked about the cuts, the patient becomes angry, breaks a glass, and tries to hit the nurse practitioner. The nurse practitioner decides the patient should take an antipsychotic. The nurse practitioner makes this decision using:

   A. Prescriptive authority
   B. Milieu therapy
   C. Counseling
   D. Cultural assessment

131. After initial emergency treatment for aggressive and violent behavior, a committed patient has shown improvement over the past 24 hours. When told social privileges cannot be reinstated until after an additional 24-hour monitoring, the patient begins to bang on the table, raises their voice, and becomes aggressive toward the psychiatric-mental health nurse practitioner. After de-escalating the situation, the nurse practitioner determines that therapy needs to be added to the treatment plan. The therapy that will be most effective for this patient is:

   A. Prevention strategies
   B. Cognitive behavior modification
   C. Reducing stimulation
   D. Providing choices and options

132. Psychiatric-mental health nurse practitioners can function as advocates for policy change by:

   A. Protecting patients from harm
   B. Providing expert testimony to help inform policy decisions
   C. Communicating patient preferences
   D. Providing essential information to inform decision making

133. A patient comes to the psychiatric-mental health nurse practitioner's office and discusses problems with the nurse practitioner. The patient has been experiencing insomnia and feels tired. The nurse discovers that the patient has been having these problems for the past 7 months. The nurse identifies additional symptoms of major depression. The immediate intervention should be:

   A. Electroconvulsive therapy
   B. Immediate hospitalization
   C. Psychotherapy
   D. Dialectal behavior therapy

134. A diagnostic feature of trichotillomania is:

   A. An excessive urge to set something on fire
   B. Pulling one's own hair recurrently
   C. Picking one's own skin recurrently
   D. A tendency to purposeless repetitive movement

135. A patient with impaired resilience expresses a willingness to learn skills to improve their functioning in this area. To accurately add goals for recovery, the updated diagnosis the psychiatric-mental health nurse practitioner determines is appropriate for this patient is:

    A. Increased readiness to learn
    B. Improved readiness for teaching
    C. Readiness for enhanced resilience
    D. Enhanced awareness of disorder

136. The psychiatric-mental health nurse practitioner recognizes the resilience in a pediatric patient being evaluated for abuse and understands this resilience has protected the patient by:

    A. Giving strength during times of abuse so they can retreat to safety
    B. Regulating their emotions to not fall victim to self-defeating thoughts
    C. Allowing heightened awareness during fight-or-flight responses
    D. Repressing fear during times of heightened physiological response

137. When performing family psychotherapy, the psychiatric-mental health nurse practitioner begins to use a strategic family therapy approach by helping the family to reframe their belief systems. This is demonstrated when the nurse practitioner:

    A. Creates family triangles to decrease stress
    B. Maps relationships using symbols
    C. Relabels control to caring
    D. Gives family a task in expectation of their compliance

138. The process in which an impulse travels from the postsynaptic neuron to the presynaptic neuron is the neurotransmission called:

    A. Volume
    B. Classic
    C. Retrograde
    D. Nonsynaptic diffusion

139. Parents bring their preschool-aged daughter for evaluation. The patient has begun to show disinterest in playing, loss of eye contact, and persistent hand-wringing. The patient has had normal growth patterns and reached early developmental milestones on target. Medical record review confirms that at approximately 12 months old, the patient's head circumference growth began to slow down. The psychiatric-mental health nurse practitioner suspects the syndrome called:

    A. Heller's
    B. Rett
    C. Fragile X
    D. Fetal alcohol

140. An adult patient is diagnosed with bipolar disorder. The patient wants to stop medications due to side effects that impact their quality of life. The patient, once physically very active, now has gained weight and feels lethargic. The patient has a history of multiple inpatient admissions due to severe decompensation and psychosis. The psychiatric-mental health nurse practitioner believes that discontinuation of medication may exacerbate the patient's chronic mental illness. At this time, the patient shows no signs of impaired thought process. The best course of action for the nurse practitioner is to provide information regarding the risks, benefits, and treatment alternatives, and to:

    A. Begin proceedings for court-ordered medication
    B. Contact the patient's family and inform them of the patient's decision
    C. Revise the treatment plan to taper medication with supervision
    D. Discharge the patient for noncompliance

141. When providing pharmacological interventions, the psychiatric-mental health nurse practitioner accurately demonstrates their role by:

    A. Collaborating with patients' primary care providers with each medication adjustment
    B. Prescribing microdoses of psychotropic medications, anticipating common side effects
    C. Safeguarding against adverse drug interactions
    D. Spacing new medications a month apart to safely monitor for unintended responses

142. The psychiatric-mental health nurse practitioner discusses psychogenetic testing with a patient. The nurse practitioner explains that the FDA:

    A. Says that identifying a patient's genotype may aid in determining therapeutic strategy and appropriate dosages
    B. Does not support the scientific evidence of pharmacogenetic associations of certain drugs with altered drug metabolism or other effects
    C. Advocates using pharmacogenetic testing before prescribing any medications
    D. Is neutral on the subject of psychogenetic testing

143. While working with a new patient admitted for bipolar disorder, the psychiatric-mental health nurse practitioner smells alcohol and notices that the patient's appearance is somewhat disheveled. The nurse practitioner proceeds with the initial interview and includes an assessment with:

    A. CAGE
    B. AUDIT
    C. T-ACE
    D. SBIRT

144. In the rapprochement phase of Mahler's stages of separation-individuation, the task a child is observed to complete is to:

    A. Fulfill basic needs for survival and comfort
    B. Recognize separateness from the caretaker
    C. Seek emotional refueling from the caretaker
    D. Establish a sense of separateness

145. The psychiatric-mental health nurse practitioner wishes to prescribe a medication and has choices of both generic and brand-name agents. The nurse practitioner demonstrates patient advocacy by:

    A. Contacting the patient's primary care provider
    B. Seeking prior authorization from the insurance company
    C. Prescribing a generic brand due to cost
    D. Encouraging the patient to find coupons for medication discounts

146. The nurse practitioner is working in the psychiatric emergency department when a 65-year-old patient with a history of major depression and Parkinson's disease reports fever, uncontrollable shivering, diarrhea, restlessness, and hyperreflexia. The patient reports taking paroxetine (Paxil) and just starting on a new medication for Parkinson's disease. The medication the nurse practitioner suspects was recently started is:

    A. Selegiline (Eldepryl)
    B. Levodopa/carbidopa (Sinemet)
    C. Cyproheptadine (Periactin)
    D. Loratadine (Claritin)

147. The psychiatric-mental health nurse practitioner would expect a patient who presents with signs and symptoms of depression to have low:

    A. Acetylcholine
    B. Glucose
    C. Glutamate
    D. Serotonin

148. When speaking with a talkative patient in a clinical interview, the psychiatric-mental health nurse practitioner should:

    A. Interrupt the patient
    B. Show interest by interrogating further
    C. Ask the patient to stop talking
    D. Give cues by showing impatience

149. The psychiatric-mental health nurse practitioner has a follow-up visit with a 16-year-old patient. Upon evaluation, the patient states that they were using marijuana occasionally to cope with anxiety but now use it daily to get through the day. Indication that the patient remains in the precontemplation phase of change is noted when the patient:

    A. States that they want to change over the next month
    B. States that their marijuana use is not a big deal
    C. Agrees to reduce marijuana use before the next visit
    D. States that their marijuana use is a problem and they want to do something about it

150. The psychiatric-mental health nurse practitioner is evaluating a 28-year-old male patient brought in after experiencing a psychotic episode at home. The patient appears calm and oriented to people, place, and time. Suddenly the patient becomes agitated, is talking to himself, and begins pacing back and forth, moving closer and closer to the nurse practitioner. The nurse practitioner, feeling unsafe, will:

   A. Calmly speak to the patient in a slow manner, asking what has happened to upset them

   B. Softly ask the patient to have a seat and engage them in conversation on how they are feeling

   C. Remove themselves from the room for safety and have another provider continue evaluation

   D. Step away from the patient and call for security to be present for the remainder of the assessment

151. A patient visits the psychiatric-mental health nurse practitioner for further evaluation of major depression and attention deficit disorder. The patient is currently prescribed tranylcypromine 30 mg. The patient's depression has minimally improved. The patient is having increased difficulty managing attention and concentration, which is affecting work function. The nurse practitioner suggests amphetamine (Adderall), and the plan of care is updated to:

   A. Start amphetamine with tranylcypromine immediately

   B. Taper tranylcypromine over 14 days before starting amphetamine

   C. Stop tranylcypromine and wait 30 days before starting amphetamine

   D. Stop tranylcypromine and wait 14 days before starting amphetamine

152. A 25-year-old patient with marked functional decline for the past 10 months has been diagnosed with schizophrenia and prescribed aripiprazole (Abilify). The patient has elevated hemoglobin A1c, hyperlipidemia, and weight gain. The patient presents with active auditory hallucinations (command type) and persecutory delusions. The priority of the assessment should be:

   A. Medication compliance

   B. Side effects of aripiprazole

   C. Focus on reality testing

   D. Suicidal behavior

153. A patient is admitted from a rural mental health clinic for substance use disorder. Outpatient treatment has not been successful, and the patient now reports losing their job due to missing work. After stabilizing the patient and developing an immediate treatment plan, the psychiatric-mental health nurse practitioner adds to the recovery-oriented plan with a focus on:

   A. E-mental health

   B. Supported employment

   C. Technology-based care

   D. Alternative housing arrangements

154. The action that defines implied consent is:

    A. The patient is informed about the health condition
    B. The patient is told about the risks of the treatment
    C. A preferred physician and a therapist are designated
    D. The patient shows willingness to receive the medication

155. The psychiatric-mental health nurse practitioner caring for patients knows that patient self-determination is a right based on:

    A. The right to choose one's health-related options and behaviors
    B. Cognition and competence to make informed decisions
    C. Legal protection from forced commitment for treatment
    D. The right to appoint a healthcare proxy to make decisions in emergencies

156. A 15-year-old patient is undergoing treatment for substance use disorder and intermittent explosive disorder. The parents are going through a hostile divorce, which resulted in the mother and children relocating to an apartment in a new school district. These changes have resulted in crisis that has affected the patient's recovery. The patient reports that the patient's mother imposes punitive measures for infractions, so the psychiatric-mental health nurse practitioner determines at this time that:

    A. The patient and family can benefit from functional family therapy
    B. Treatment will be compromised further without group therapy
    C. Drugs and alcohol have become a crutch for the patient
    D. The patient would benefit from placement in a less hostile environment

157. When preparing for a psychiatric evaluation of a school-aged child, the psychiatric-mental health nurse practitioner understands that:

    A. The child should be able to sit quietly in a chair during the evaluation
    B. They should avoid looking directly at the child to decrease anxiety
    C. A parent or guardian should remain in the room with the child
    D. The manner of conducting the interview varies with age and developmental status

158. Under the Health Insurance Portability and Accountability Act of 1996 (HIPAA), the psychiatric-mental health nurse practitioner understands that:

    A. The patient may ask for a copy of medical records
    B. The patient should not authorize release of information
    C. Patient privacy rights should not be shared with the patient
    D. Patient information can be shared with those who call the facility to speak with the patient

159. An older adult patient begins to recognize patterns of familial dysfunction with poor communication and convinces their family to commit to family therapy. Upon evaluation, the psychiatric-mental health nurse practitioner decides to use interventions with an approach in strategic family therapy. In doing so, the nurse practitioner must focus on:

    A. Family structure to effectively manage problems
    B. The problem and the sequence of interactions that maintain the problem
    C. Self-confrontation of each family member
    D. Self-differentiation of each family member

160. The psychiatric-mental health nurse practitioner is assessing a patient who reports low mood, lethargy, weight gain, cold intolerance, and "brain fog." Before starting this patient on an antidepressant, the nurse practitioner would first assess laboratory values for:

    A. Vitamin B1
    B. Vitamin D
    C. Thyroid panel
    D. Complete blood count

161. The psychiatric-mental health nurse practitioner is conducting a psychiatric evaluation on a patient who states, "I'm so anxious. I feel like my heart is racing." The patient has a tremor and some pressure to speech. The patient also reports increase in sweating and weight loss. Before initiating treatment, the nurse practitioner should first assess the laboratory results for:

    A. Thyroid panel
    B. Complete blood count
    C. Vitamin B12
    D. Liver function test

162. A patient with substance use disorder has to ingest more substance than previously needed to maintain their "high." This behavior demonstrates:

    A. Tolerance
    B. Confabulation
    C. Withdrawal
    D. Addiction

163. A patient with recent emotional and social behavior changes presents for an office visit. The patient has concerns about the changes, particularly outbursts of inappropriate anger, having a significant impact on functional ability in social settings. The psychiatric-mental health nurse practitioner would screen the patient for:

    A. Traumatic brain injury
    B. Huntington's disease
    C. Cyclothymic disorder
    D. Pick's disease

164. A patient describes their habit of picking their own hair. They wish to resist this habit, because it is causing embarrassment in society and difficulty in their work concentration. It has been a year since this issue began, and while it seemed normal to the patient at first, it has gradually led to hair loss. The psychiatric-mental health nurse practitioner inquires as to whether this habit is due to any dermatological reason, which the patient denies. Based on the diagnostic criteria, the nurse practitioner diagnoses the disorder known as:

A. Trichotillomania
B. Excoriation
C. Hoarding
D. Body dysmorphia

165. One way to protect a patient's medical records and maintain confidentiality is by:

A. Resaving the records after edits
B. Deleting records after use
C. Using password-protected records
D. Using records on paper only

166. The psychiatric-mental health nurse practitioner can avoid misdiagnosis of a patient from a differing culture by:

A. Conducting a thorough physical and diagnostic assessment
B. Using culturally appropriate assessment tools
C. Interviewing family members for past medical history
D. Ordering a wide variety of laboratory and diagnostic tests

167. The corneal reflex is controlled by the cranial nerve:

A. II optic
B. III oculomotor
C. IV trochlear
D. V trigeminal

168. Techniques for empowering a patient involve:

A. Conveying an interest in only the problem of the patient
B. Validating the emotions of the patient
C. Obscuring the clinical explanation for the patient
D. Concealing the nurse practitioner's knowledge

169. An older patient visits the psychiatric-mental health nurse practitioner with his adult daughter. The daughter states that the patient frequently becomes confused and is not able to make proper decisions when dealing with problems. The patient also suffers from urinary incontinence. The daughter says that the patient forgets things, but that this issue is quite mild and not troubling to the patient or anyone else. That daughter also says that the patient has never behaved as if he is having hallucinations. The nurse practitioner orders an MRI (magnetic resonance imaging) to confirm a diagnosis of:

A. Vascular dementia
B. Dementia with Lewy bodies
C. Alzheimer's disease
D. Huntington's disease

170. The psychiatric-mental nurse practitioner promises to share community resources with a patient by a certain date. The nurse practitioner forgets to prepare and send the information on time. The nurse practitioner calls the patient and lets them know the information is not yet available. This is an example of:

A. Fidelity
B. Nonmaleficence
C. Veracity
D. Beneficence

171. A 22-year-old patient is admitted to a hospital for treatment for schizophrenia and is prescribed the antipsychotic clozapine. Within the first week of treatment, the patient shows signs of spasms, muscle stiffness, dry mouth, and cramping. This is immediately reported and treated with an anticholinergic drug. The nurse practitioner suspects that the patient:

A. Had an overdose of antipsychotics
B. Was experiencing extrapyramidal symptoms
C. Has developed myocarditis
D. Needs to change the medication

172. An adolescent patient has been taking fluoxetine (Prozac) 60 mg per day for 2 months with little improvement in obsessive–compulsive disorder (OCD). When planning to discontinue this medication, the most important issue for the psychiatric-mental health nurse practitioner is:

A. Assessing for rebound compulsions
B. Ensuring the maximum therapeutic dose has been achieved
C. Weaning off the medication while continuously assessing for increased suicidal ideation
D. Prescribing a different selective serotonin reuptake inhibitor immediately

173. A patient is admitted for detoxification with the last alcoholic drink approximately 13 hours ago. The patient seems confused and has trouble maintaining balance when walking. When the patient reports blurry vision, the diagnosis the psychiatric-mental health nurse practitioner will evaluate for is:

    A. Detoxification
    B. Delirium tremens
    C. Wernicke encephalopathy
    D. Korsakoff's amnestic syndrome

174. The psychiatric-mental health nurse practitioner is creating a treatment plan for a patient diagnosed with posttraumatic stress disorder who wishes to employ alternative therapies. The spirit-mind-body therapy the nurse practitioner will include in the treatment plan is:

    A. Yoga and guided imagery
    B. Sertraline and reiki
    C. Exercise and qigong
    D. Omega-3 fatty acids and music

175. Cultivating a spirit of inquiry is the:

    A. Zero step of evidence-based practice
    B. First step of evidence-based practice
    C. Second step of evidence-based practice
    D. Third step of evidence-based practice

Practice Exam 1 Answers

1. B) 1.8 mEq/L

The patient is exhibiting mild to moderate intoxication of lithium, which presents with symptoms of vomiting, abdominal pain, dry mouth, ataxia, dizziness, slurred speech, nystagmus, lethargy or excitement, and muscle weakness. Mild to moderate lithium toxicity can be seen at lithium levels between 1.5 and 2.0 mEq/L. A level of 0.8 mEq/L is a therapeutic level for bipolar maintenance. Levels between 2.0 and 2.5 mEq/L indicate moderate to severe lithium intoxication, and greater than 2.5 mEq/L indicates severe lithium toxicity.

2. C) 12 to 20 sessions

Interpersonal therapy is generally short-term therapy and takes about 12 to 20 sessions to complete. Behavioral therapy generally takes fewer than 10 sessions; it varies with the patient's condition. Psychodynamic therapy generally takes more than 20 sessions. Cognitive behavioral therapy takes about 5 to 20 sessions to complete. It is also known as a short-term therapy session.

3. B) 2 to 7 years

The child is in the preoperational stage at age 2 to 7 years. The sensorimotor stage begins at birth and lasts through age 2 years. The concrete operational stage begins at age 7 years and lasts until age 11 years. The formal operational stage begins at age 11 years and continues until adulthood.

4. C) 2.1 mEq/L

This patient is exhibiting signs and symptoms of moderate to severe lithium toxicity as illustrated with lithium levels of 2.0 to 2.5 mEq/L. A level of 1.0 mEq/L is considered a therapeutic level for bipolar maintenance. Levels between 1.5 and 2.0 mEq/L indicate mild to moderate lithium intoxication, and greater than 2.5 mEq/L indicates severe lithium toxicity.

5. A) 7 to 12 hours for alcohol

Unless there is a contributing medical history (e.g., liver disease), alcohol is detected in urine toxicology testing for 7 to 12 hours. Cocaine is detected for 6 to 8 hours, marijuana for 3 days to 4 weeks, and heroin for 36 to 72 hours.

6. C) A trained medical interpreter to help with communication with the patient

The nurse practitioner should call a trained medical interpreter to communicate with the patient because effective communication is essential to provide quality care. The nurse practitioner should not ask a family member, another patient, or another practitioner to help with communication because that would be a breach of confidentiality. Even though the family member can be permitted by the patient to interpret, it is not an ideal practice.

7. B) A decrease in dosage

When taking a medication that involves metabolism by CYP-450 1A2, the patient who smokes cigarettes requires a higher dose of medication than the patient who does not smoke. If the patient stops smoking, the dose should be decreased. Cigarette smoking causes the induction of CYP-450 1A2, which causes more of this enzyme to be synthesized. Maximum enzyme induction occurs with 7 to 12 cigarettes per day for some medications, such as clozapine (Clozaril) and olanzapine. This leads to a 40% to 50% reduction in serum level. If a patient smokes half of a pack or more, a higher dose of medication is needed. Maintenance of the dosage would not be appropriate if the patient quits smoking. Change to another medication would not be necessary.

8. C) A dopamine-deficient state

A pattern of sustained stimulant use through avoidance of the aversive withdrawal/abstinence state (negative reinforcement) is mediated through dopamine downregulation and neurotoxic effects on neuron systems, resulting in a dopamine-deficient state. Stimulant use disorders include operant conditioning, which is a positive reinforcement mechanism wherein a given behavior is controlled by consequences. Stimulant intoxication results in changes in mood, social interactions, or judgment and may include physical symptoms such as changes in blood pressure, heart rate, motor changes, and neurological problems. Mood is not dysphoric; it is euphoric with stimulant use.

9. B) Acetylcholine

Acetylcholine is associated with attention and memory and is decreased in Alzheimer's disease. The treatments used to help manage Alzheimer's disease are acetylcholinesterase inhibitors, which help to reduce the breakdown of acetylcholine. Dopamine is also involved with thinking but is implicated in Parkinson's disease, where dopamine is decreased. Serotonin is associated with regulation of sleep and mood; it is most implicated as being decreased in depression and anxiety. Tryptophan is not a neurotransmitter, but an amino acid and precursor to serotonin.

10. A) Add cognitive behavior modification to the treatment plan

The patient has provided clues that they recognize the issue and are not ready to implement intervention techniques. Therefore, cognitive behavior modification would be added to the plan so the patient can learn how to avoid stimuli and self-monitor for cues of anger arousal. The patient has not escalated to a point that referral to a psychiatrist is needed, and a cultural assessment has not been determined to be needed at this point. Likewise, obtaining blood work may be warranted, but not at this time based on the patient's report.

11. B) Adjusting the time of administration of the SSRI

Adjustment of the timing of administration of the SSRI may resolve unwanted daytime sleepiness and should be the first step to manage this side effect. Difficulty with sleep is a common symptom for patients with mood disorders. Medications that also promote sleep because of sedating side effects should be taken in the evening. Changing the medication to a SNRI (a different class) may be considered only after assessing the impact of evening administration of the SSRI. Adding a small dose of stimulants may be effective; however, polypharmacy is to be avoided whenever possible. If the patient is experiencing nighttime insomnia, other non-narcotic approaches would be considered first.

12. A) Admit the patient for the appropriate state allowable days according to the law

The patient is exhibiting behavior that supports emergency commitment. The appropriate step would be to follow through with the admission so the patient can be further evaluated and treated. Having law enforcement or security restrain the patient is not recommended unless it is a last option. Firmly speaking to the patient may be needed, but most often speaking in a calm voice has better results. Administering olanzapine will not immediately calm the patient because it is a mood stabilizer that must be administered on a titrated regimen over the course of hours to days.

13. C) Agonist

An agonist causes a conformational change in the G-protein-linked receptor, thereby turning on the synthesis of the second messenger and initiating the signal transduction to its full extent. Antagonists fully block the action of a neurotransmitter. The inverse agonist causes a functional reduction in signal transduction. The partial agonist neither fully inhibits the transduction nor fully initiates it.

14. C) Agoraphobia

The tendency to avoid staying in an enclosed place or boarding public transport for fear of getting trapped is a diagnostic feature of agoraphobia. This disorder also makes one feel panicked in an adverse situation. In major depressive disorder, patients may avoid public transport or leaving the home because they feel a loss of energy and low self-esteem, but fear is not the reason. Kleptomania is an uncontrollable urge to steal. It brings tension before committing the theft but does not bring panic. Feeling challenged to throw away possessions even if they do not have value is a sign of hoarding disorder; it is not related to panic.

15. C) Agranulocytosis

Bipolar disorder can be successfully treated with a variety of psychotropic agents. A medication that has been effective but is now causing significant side effects may be discontinued. The patient has not experienced previous treatment failure with other psychiatric drugs. This factor supports the decision to discontinue carbamazepine and explore alternatives. Carbamazepine is an anticonvulsant agent often used as an off-label treatment for bipolar disorder. Among the adverse reactions to carbamazepine are blood dyscrasias such as agranulocytosis and aplastic anemia. Symptoms of agranulocytosis include sore throat, fever, and oral and perianal ulcerations. Neuroleptic malignant syndrome is associated with use of antipsychotics. Serotonin syndrome is caused by use of antidepressants and other medications concurrently that increase levels of serotonin. Anticonvulsant intoxication or an overdose of carbamazepine would present with delirium or psychosis.

16. B) Albert Ellis

Albert Ellis developed rational-emotive therapy in the year 1955. John B. Watson developed the concept of behaviorism in 1919. B. F. Skinner researched operant conditioning theory. Ivan Pavlov invented the classic conditioned theory.

17. D) Alert security
The first action that should be taken by a psychiatric-mental health nurse practitioner when faced with an aggressive patient who starts shouting is to alert security. Ensuring a safe environment is the foremost thing to do. Asking the patient to stop shouting or to lower their voice right away may only make matters worse. Once a safe environment is ensured, the nurse practitioner should try to calm the patient. After the matter is under control and rapport has been established, the nurse practitioner can then ask the patient to move to a different location as appropriate. Asking the patient to leave as a first resort does not follow correct decorum. Once the patient has calmed down, the nurse practitioner should continue with the interview or reschedule it for a different date.

18. B) Alzheimer's disease
Alzheimer's disease is a form of progressive dementia seen commonly in older adults with impairments in several memory tasks. Mutations of the APP gene are highly indicated in Alzheimer's, leading to amyloid plaques, which are the hallmark of this disease. Also, patients with multiple copies of E4 genes have been shown to have an eight times greater risk of Alzheimer's than those with no E4 gene. Those with only one copy of E4 are three times as likely to develop Alzheimer's. Down syndrome is caused by an extra copy of chromosome 21. Huntington's disease is caused by a defective gene on chromosome 4. The genetic form of prion disease (Creutzfeldt–Jakob disease) is a single gene mutation on the prion protein gene.

19. A) Amygdala
Adults with PTSD have been found to have an overactive amygdala and decreased hippocampal volume. Brainstem involvement may occur with conditions such as pseudobulbar affect, commonly associated with strokes with injury to the brainstem. Parkinsonism is a disease of the basal ganglia, also commonly associated with dementia and depression. Cerebellar involvement is implicated in other psychiatric disorders such as anxiety disorders, attention deficit/hyperactivity disorder, depressive disorder, bipolar disorder, and schizophrenia.

20. B) Anal
The problematic traits seen in the anal stage of Freud's psychosexual stages are messiness, defiance, and rage. Traits in the oral stage include excessive dependency, envy, and jealousy. Phallic stage characteristics include sexual identity issues. The latency stage includes traits of excessive inner control.

21. A) Anorexia nervosa
The patient's BMI signifies that the patient is underweight. The diagnostic criteria of fear of weight gain, being underweight, and refusing to eat suggest that the patient has anorexia nervosa. A patient with bulimia nervosa eats food in large quantities and then, due to fear of weight gain, purges with laxatives or by vomiting. The patient experiencing rumination disorder spits out food, re-chews, and re-swallows it. Factitious disorder is related to the mental condition in which a patient behaves as an ill person in front of others.

22. B) Antipsychotic-induced extrapyramidal symptoms

Poor metabolizers of CYP2D6 may develop higher levels of antipsychotic drugs, resulting in adverse effects such as extrapyramidal symptoms (EPS) and hyperprolactinemia. Multiple studies have shown a relationship between dysfunctional CYP2D6 variants and antipsychotic-induced EPS, especially tardive dyskinesia. Inadequate dosing is a risk for patients who are ultrarapid metabolizers. They require higher doses; without alteration in dose, ultrarapid metabolizers may experience decrease or loss in efficacy. Poor metabolizers are not at risk for gene–drug interactions.

23. D) Are an act of advocacy

The nurse practitioner's actions are those of an advocate when acting to protect patients who cannot protect themselves due to mental status. The patient does have the right to autonomy; however, that right is superseded by the need for patient safety. The fear of being accused of violation of rights should not prevent the nurse practitioner from providing legally sound, ethical psychiatric care in the best interests of the patient. The patient's privacy rights are not violated because the nurse practitioner acts in the role of medical provider. Scope of practice is legislated by the state boards of nursing. Most states acknowledge advanced psychiatric nurse practitioners as professionals who may execute a certificate stating that they have evaluated the patient within the last 48 hours and the patient appears to meet the criteria for involuntary evaluation.

24. D) Ask questions directed to the patient

While working with an interpreter during a clinical interview, the nurse practitioner should direct questions to the patient and not the interpreter. This helps to establish rapport and connection with the patient. The nurse practitioner should keep the questions as simple and short as possible. This ensures that the questions are translated properly and that words are not misinterpreted. The nurse practitioner should ask the interpreter to translate everything, not just summarize. This leaves no scope for confusion. The nurse practitioner should make notes and list points for review, not ask the interpreter to do so.

25. A) Asks the patient how their culture typically treats Hwa-byung

The nurse practitioner will conduct an interview with the patient and inquire as to how their culture typically treats depression. This will allow the nurse practitioner to provide culturally appropriate care. Completing a depression inventory or a cultural assessment for depression should not be done until the nurse practitioner determines how these actions fit into the patient's cultural practices. It is not necessary to immediately refer the patient to another practitioner.

26. C) Assess the patient's current skills and readiness to learn

When planning psychoeducational strategies to address patient needs and skills that are altered due to mental illness, the nurse practitioner will assess current skill set and readiness to learn. This will allow the plan to be focused on individualized teaching to improve and build on current experiences. Token economy is a tool used to apply behavior modification techniques to several different behaviors. Teaching the patient about pyramidal effects of medication would be included in medication therapy teaching. Rehabilitative therapy for family and caregivers is a separate treatment on its own.

27. A) Assess the uniqueness and experiences of the patient

Recovery-oriented treatment is based on the uniqueness of the individual and the experiences they have had in life. The progress of the patient is based on this information, so recovery is not a step-by-step process; recovery plans would be individualized toward the experiences, attitudes, and health of the patient. Determining the patient's willingness to receive treatment, performing cultural inquiry, and evaluating the patient's hope and drive for recovery are steps that would follow the assessment.

28. D) At 2-week follow-up assessment

Psychoeducational teaching is best received and implemented once the patient has had time for medication to begin working effectively. Typically, this is after 2 weeks. This will allow the patient to recognize that they have a mental illness that causes hallucinations and delusions, which need to be recognized and compared with reality. At diagnosis and when medication is prescribed are both too soon for this teaching because the medication has not had time to take effect. At discharge to home is not an appropriate time for this teaching unless the patient had been admitted for longer than 2 weeks.

29. A) Attention deficit/hyperactivity disorder

The patient is experiencing attention deficit/hyperactivity disorder. The disorder is characterized by difficulty in concentrating on particular tasks, impulsive behavior, mood fluctuations, and constant fidgeting as the diagnostic symptoms. Personality disorders are marked by episodic changes in the behavior of an individual with aggression as a diagnostic symptom. Mood disorders are a group of disorders that affect the mood of an individual, ranging from mania to depression. Cognitive disorders are characterized by changes in the thinking ability of an individual.

30. A) Attention deficit/hyperactivity

Lack of attention and impulsive nature are the diagnostic criteria for attention deficit/ hyperactivity disorder. Careless nature in school activities signifies this as well. Autism spectrum disorder is related to difficulty in interacting with people. Specific learning disorder correlates to difficulty in understanding or learning the meaning of different words and their application. Developmental coordination disorder causes difficulty in carrying out coordinated motor skills.

31. B) AUDIT

The Alcohol Use Disorders Identification Test (AUDIT tool) is a widely used tool to determine the severity of alcohol use and is especially beneficial when patients self-identify there may be a problem. The tool can be administered by either the practitioner or the patient and is an early identifier of risk for alcohol use disorder (AUD). The CAGE assessment tool is an excellent initial tool if the practitioner suspects alcohol use may be an issue, but it is brief and used to identify a patient's alcohol use that the patient may not report. The T-ACE screening tool is specific to patients who are pregnant, and screening, brief intervention, referral to treatment (SBIRT) is a screening and intervention approach used to determine and treat high-risk behaviors that may lead to AUD. This approach integrates screen, assessment, and intervention and is a tool that can be used alone or with other tools.

32. C) Basal ganglia

Parkinson's disease is a disease of the basal ganglia, also commonly associated with dementia and depression. Parkinson's disease affects the dopaminergic neurons of the substantia nigra. The cerebellum, brainstem, and hippocampus are regions of the brain that are not specific for Parkinson's disease; disorders of these areas of the brain affect various bodily functions that are not consistent with Parkinson's disease.

33. A) Beneficence

The nurse helping the patient feel calm before administering the drug shows beneficence. It is promoting the good of the patient. The nurse must administer the drug but also act to benefit the patient. Justice involves providing an equitable distribution of resources or care without any prejudices or differentiation. Autonomy allows the patient to refuse a treatment or to prefer a certain treatment plan. The patient is not refusing the drug or requesting a different one. Veracity is the truthful communication of relevant information related to the drug or treatment to the patient.

34. C) Binding to the benzodiazepine receptors

Diazepam works by binding to the benzodiazepine receptors at the gamma-aminobutyric acid-A (GABA-A) ligand-gated chloride channel complex, thereby enhancing the inhibitory effects of GABA, which further inhibits neuronal activity and helps in treating anxiety. Valproate is an antiepileptic that works by blocking voltage-sensitive sodium channels. This further results in an increase in GABA concentration in the brain. Fluoxetine (Prozac) works by blocking the serotonin reuptake pump, thereby increasing serotonin concentration and helping alleviate depression. Protriptyline (Vivactil) works by blocking norepinephrine reuptake, thereby increasing noradrenergic neurotransmission; it is used to treat depression.

35. A) Bipolar II

The diagnostic criteria for bipolar II disorder include at least one hypomanic episode and at least one major depressive episode. Therefore, the nurse practitioner diagnoses bipolar II disorder. The diagnostic criteria for bipolar I disorder include these episodes along with one or more manic episodes. Panic disorder is a subset of anxiety disorder. Its diagnostic criteria involve palpitations, dizziness, chest pain, choking, and fear of dying. The criteria for cyclothymic disorder include hypomanic episodes and major depressive episodes, but these do not abide by the diagnostic criteria of major depressive episodes.

36. A) Borderline personality disorder and bipolar II disorder

The patient's presentation shows evidence of borderline personality disorder (i.e., with a pattern of unstable relationships, recurrent suicidal threats, self-mutilating behavior, and inappropriate anger). The patient also shows evidence of bipolar II disorder, with decreased need for sleep and pressured speech with a major depressive episode. A diagnosis of other substance-related disorders requires a problematic pattern of using intoxicating substances not classified elsewhere; the patient's use of marijuana and alcohol shows no evidence of problematic use. The diagnosis of obsessive-compulsive disorder requires "obsessions or compulsions that cause distress, are time-consuming (more than 1 hour per day), and substantially interfere with normal functioning." The patient does not meet the criteria for schizoaffective disorder because she has no delusions, hallucinations, disorganized behavior, or negative symptoms.

37. B) Caffeine withdrawal

If a person consumes caffeine daily and suddenly withdraws it, symptoms such as headache, dysphoric mood, agitation, symptoms of flu, and muscle pain are often experienced. The patient is experiencing caffeine withdrawal. People experience excitability, nervousness, twitching of muscles, difficulty sleeping, diuresis, and gastrointestinal distress due to caffeine intoxication. People experiencing caffeine-induced anxiety disorder have symptoms of anxiety disorder like restlessness, anxiousness, insomnia, and muscle pain due to excessive consumption of caffeine. People with unspecified caffeine-related disorder show symptoms similar to caffeine-related disorders, resulting in great distress in public and workplaces, but they also do not completely exhibit the diagnostic criteria of caffeine-related disorder.

38. A) Causes sedative side effects by blocking alpha 1 adrenergic receptors

Clozapine can cause hypotension, tachycardia, and sedation by blocking alpha 1 adrenergic receptors. Clozapine is a second-generation antipsychotic or atypical antipsychotic. It is prescribed when the standard course of antipsychotic therapy has failed. Clozapine is prescribed to balance serotonin and dopamine. Rare motor side effects are caused due to blocking of dopamine 2 transporters by this drug. Clozapine is used to reduce the positive symptoms by blocking dopamine 2 transporters. The dopamine release is increased in some parts of the brain due to clozapine, and it blocks serotonin 2A receptors.

39. C) Ceiling of accountability

The ceiling of accountability is the level at which monitoring is ceased. It is irrespective of the attainment of intermediate results. Intervention is also known as strategy. Rationales are the basic ideas behind one intermediate outcome being a prerequisite for the next. Indicators are the measurable things that are visible when a person is about to or has already reached an intermediate result.

40. B) Child's parents' relation with their school

How the child's parents interact with their school has an indirect impact on the child–parent relationship. It is an example of a mesosystem because both the child's parents and their school are related to it. The child's interaction with their family is their microsystem. The effect of mass media on their family is the exosystem, and the effect of cultural beliefs on their school is the macrosystem.

41. C) Cognitive behavioral

Cognitive behavioral therapy (CBT) acts along with medications to treat depression. Due to the seriousness of the patient's issues, the proper active and challenging therapy is necessary. Family therapy helps the patient and the patient's family to recover from distressing situations. In general, behavioral therapy can treat behavior or anger management problems, but for depression, CBT incorporates additional attention. Behavioral therapy can help the patient to open up, but it is not sufficient for severe depression. Interpersonal therapy is focused on improving the relationships or conflicts in the social or personal life of a patient; it is suited for interpersonal conflicts.

42. D) Collect blood specimen for thiamine level and start IV thiamine 200 mg
Thiamine and niacin levels are low in patients with alcohol use disorders due to poor eating habits and malabsorption of minerals. Severe thiamine deficiency can cause delirium, confusion, and hallucinations and should be treated with IV thiamine. Admitting the patient for observation will not address the patient's current needs. Providing education on proper weaning and administering naloxone are not appropriate actions at this stage. There is no need to give the patient additional lorazepam because the initial dose should be adequate.

43. D) Conceptualization deficit in cognitive thinking
Abstraction requires higher cognitive or intellectual functioning. Abstract reasoning is the ability to shift back and forth between general concepts and specific examples. The inability to think abstractly indicates concrete or literal thinking. This may be seen in an older adult as a sign of early dementia. Insight refers to the patient's understanding of how they feel. Judgment refers to the patient's capacity to make good decisions and act on them. Delusional thought content refers to false beliefs not shared by others.

44. B) Conducting a "closeness circle" activity with the patient
The nurse practitioner would first conduct a "closeness circle" to determine the people in the patient's life that contribute to the depression and those the patient feels safe with. This will allow the nurse practitioner to develop a plan for recovery that will include the people the patient can trust and feel safe with so recovery will be successful. Positive reinforcement and cognitive behavior modification will need to be addressed with the parents but would be conducted after the closeness circle activity. The patient may need to be told again that the diagnosis of depression is the same as any other illness and that the parents are upset with the illness, not the patient, but this would have been covered during the initial assignment of the limited sick role.

45. D) Consult to a pediatric cardiologist
Before initiating therapy with a stimulant, an evaluation by a cardiologist should be done if there are any significant findings on physical examination, ECG, or patient or family history. Unless there is a strong history of medical comorbidities, neurological studies (i.e., EEG, SPECT, PET) are not indicated, and practice guidelines advise against children's exposure to radioactive substances.

46. B) Contemplation
In the contemplation stage, people become increasingly conscious of the possible advantages of making a change, but the disadvantages tend to stand out more. This contradiction causes a significant sense of apprehension when it comes to change. Because of this ambiguity, the period of change contemplation might continue for months. In the preparation stage, people are ready to act within the next 30 days. People begin to modify their behavior in modest increments, believing that changing their conduct will lead to a healthier existence. In the precontemplation stage, people do not intend to take action within the next 6 months. People at this stage frequently undervalue the benefits of altering their behavior and place much more focus on the disadvantages. In the action stage, people have recently modified their behavior (within the previous 6 months) and aim to continue with that behavior modification. Behavior modifications include changing troublesome habits and learning new healthy ones.

47. D) Cultural idiom of distress
Cultural idiom of distress is the term used to refer to the suffering within a cultural group. Cultural explanation refers to perceived causes of symptoms. Acculturation is the process of socialization of a minority group that learns and adapts to the culture of the dominant group. Religiousness is the participation of a group in a community who gather to worship in a common way. Suffering within this group would be suffering of religiousness.

48. D) Current regulatory requirements are not effective in management of supplements
Lack of an effective management process is a main concern for practitioners wanting to practice complementary and alternative medicine. Fillers are often tainted or not included on the label. These fillers do not contribute to toxicity; however, and the highest percentage of poisonings come from prescribed medications. DNA barcoding is not currently available, but it would reduce the risk of tainted products through product ingredient identification.

49. D) Demonstrated the duty to warn and protect
The landmark Tarasoff case (*Tarasoff v. Regents of the University of California 1976*) defined the duty to protect third parties when there is an imminent danger. By notifying the group manager, the nurse practitioner has demonstrated the duty to warn and protect. The nurse practitioner did not violate the patient's confidentiality because confidentiality does not apply when there is a risk to the life of another person. The principle of justice was not violated because this decision is consistent with the standard of care and applies to all patients. Different states have various versions and clinical interventions; all state courts have upheld that the need to safeguard the public overrides confidentiality, so the duty to protect is a national standard of practice. The nurse practitioner does not function in law enforcement and cannot have the patient arrested.

50. B) Dependent
The patient with dependent personality disorder faces difficulty in making everyday decisions on their own. The patient seeks the help of others and makes decisions based on their advice and reassurances. Individuals with avoidant personality disorder have a constant fear of rejection, criticism, and disapproval. The diagnostic criteria for narcissistic personality disorder involve lack of empathy, need for admiration from others, and self-importance. The need to be the center of attention is an important aspect of histrionic personality disorder.

51. B) Descriptive study
To understand the patient's coping mechanisms, a descriptive study should be conducted. This study will provide multiple sources of evidence and will dive into the complex nature of the question. These studies look at the participants in nature where variables cannot be controlled. Coping mechanisms can be diverse. A single randomized control study is not suited for such studies because it requires two interventions to be compared to conduct the trial; the focus here is to understand or observe only. Opinions are not considered a good source of evidence and are not based on objective studies. Experimental studies are suitable where interventions have been made to see how one variable will affect another variable; in these, variables can be manipulated.

52. C) Determine what would happen if the perpetrator found the educational material in the home

Before providing the patient with any written material or information on resources, emergency plans, or documented telephone numbers for the children, the nurse practitioner will determine what would happen if the live-in partner found the material. Would this discovery trigger a violent reaction toward the patient and the children? This must be established first so any information on resources can be safeguarded for the patient's use. Once this issue is addressed, the patient can be provided with specific information on support, emergency plans, and escape mapping, and the children can be included in the teaching for their safety.

53. A) Determine if the patient is pregnant

When a female patient is within the childbearing age group, determining pregnancy status is the first step in selecting a tool that can be used to identify risk for alcohol use disorder. The screening tool to use if the patient is pregnant is the Substance Use Risk Profile-Pregnant scale. Completing a review of patient records and observing the patient's demeanor are both part of the overall assessment and would not be specific to choosing a screening tool. Collecting a blood sample for toxicity would be needed only if the patient was unresponsive.

54. B) Develop a basic level of trust

The ideal goal in a therapeutic alliance is to develop a basic level of trust and a shared agenda between the patient and the nurse practitioner. This also includes the collaborative goals of therapy. The ideal goal is not to assess the competency of the therapist, to check medication side effects, or to develop an understanding of technical interventions.

55. B) Developmental dyspraxia

Gross motor symptoms of developmental dyspraxia include poor timing and impaired balance that interfere with daily activities. Developmental dyspraxia is a form of developmental coordination disorder. Its symptoms are often comorbid with ADHD. Muscular dystrophy is a group of diseases that cause progressive weakness and loss of muscle mass. Frequent falls, difficulty rising from a lying or sitting position, trouble running and jumping, waddling gait, walking on the toes, and delayed growth are some of the presenting symptoms. It is not associated with ADHD. Stereotypic movement disorder is a condition that is typified by a variety of repetitive and uncontrolled movements, such as body rocking, head banging, nail-biting, tics, self-mutilating actions such as self-hitting or skin picking, and hand waving or wringing. A motor tic disorder is a chronic condition that involves quick, uncontrollable movements, not coordination deficits.

56. A) Differentiation

According to Mahler's stages of separation-individuation, a child recognizes separation from the caretaker at 5 to 10 months in the differentiation phase. In the practicing phase, the child experiences increased independence and separateness of self. In the rapprochement phase, the child seeks emotional refueling from the caretaker, and in the consolidation phase, the sense of separateness is established.

57. A) Discuss the purpose of the meeting and introduce themselves

The introductory phase of a group meeting for critical incident stress debriefing involves setting the goals of the meeting. Confidentiality is ensured at this phase. During later phases, the discussion is conducted. During the thought phase, the participants of the group share their thoughts about the particular incident that caused the crisis. During the reaction phase, the participants share the worst memory or the most painful part of the incident. During the re-entry phase, reviewing is done to bring closure to the briefing.

58. A) Disruptive mood dysregulation

The diagnostic criteria for disruptive mood dysregulation disorder involves a problem in dealing with anger management. The anger is expressed verbally or physically. The duration of the condition should be 12 months or more. In persistent depressive disorder, the patient experiences symptoms of chronic depression for 2 years or more. People with oppositional defiant disorder often indulge in arguments with others and are easily agitated, frequently blaming their mistakes on other people. The duration for diagnosis of this condition should be at least 6 months. People with intermittent explosive disorder find difficulty in controlling their anger, leading to property destruction or physical assault. The diagnosis for this disorder is made if the patient experiences at least three anger outbursts resulting in harm or destruction over a duration of 12 months.

59. A) Disulfiram

Disulfiram (Antabuse) for AUD is prescribed as a deterrent; it produces unpleasant side effects and sensitivity to alcohol. Thiamine is used to treat alcohol misuse but is not associated with palpitations, nausea, vomiting, headache, and flushing. Naltrexone (Revia) works to reduce cravings associated with alcohol use, and sertraline (Zoloft) is used for generalized GAD; neither is associated with palpitations, nausea, vomiting, headache, and flushing with ingestion of alcohol.

60. A) During the first visit

During the first visit or contact with the patient, the nurse practitioner initiates the therapeutic alliance. The first several sessions play a crucial role in laying the foundation for the therapist's connection with the patient. The therapeutic alliance enables the patient to continue and benefit from treatment. It continues throughout therapy.

61. A) Ego integrity versus despair

According to Erikson's psychosocial stages, extreme alienation is seen in older age (65 years to death), and the stage-specific conflict is ego integrity versus despair. Intimacy versus isolation is seen in young adulthood, where schizoid personality is a pathological outcome. Initiative versus guilt is the conflict in late childhood where phobias are seen, and identity versus role confusion is seen in adolescence with a possible pathological outcome of delinquency.

62. A) Encopresis

The repeated passage of feces in inappropriate places occurs in encopresis disorder. The patient should face this issue for at least 3 months in order to be diagnosed with encopresis. Enuresis disorder is related to the involuntary repeated passage of urine by the patient in inappropriate places. The patient faces episodes of binge eating and purging in bulimia disorder. Hoarding disorder occurs when an individual faces problems in parting with their belongings.

63. A) Enuresis

The intentional or unintentional voiding of urine, occurring twice a week for at least 3 months, that is not consistent with the patient's developmental age is the diagnostic criterion for enuresis disorder. Binge eating and then vomiting or misusing laxatives are signs of bulimia disorder. Encopresis is a type of elimination disorder in which feces are eliminated in inappropriate places. A patient who cannot bear the feeling of separation from their possessions may be diagnosed with hoarding disorder.

64. B) Environmental re-evaluation

Environmental re-evaluation involves self-reappraisal to assess the effect of an unhealthy behavior on others or on the physical environment. Self–re-evaluation involves evaluation of the effect of healthy behavior and how it affects the thinking of that person. Counter-conditioning involves the substitution of a healthy behavior with an unhealthy behavior upon development of a problem. Consciousness-raising involves creating awareness among people regarding healthy behavior.

65. D) Establish a trusting and collaborative relationship

Establishing a trusting and open relationship that is collaborative builds a therapeutic relationship in which the nurse practitioner can gain accurate information from the patient. While educating all patients on mental illness regardless of culture, as well as tailoring interventions, is important, building a trusting relationship is the first priority. Conducting a thorough social and cultural interview can take place only if the trusting relationship has been established first.

66. A) Establishing rapport

The first step of a clinical interview is to establish rapport and connection with the patient. This is important before taking the process further. Identification of emotional clues is a very important step but not the first one. The second step of a clinical interview is to take thorough notes, which helps in maintaining records. Generation of a diagnostic hypothesis is the last step before concluding an interview.

67. A) Evaluate medication dosage and efficacy

The patient's symptoms and signs indicate the possibility of dementia with Lewy bodies or Parkinson's disease; however, the patient has recently been started on a new medication that attributes to the depletion of dopamine, resulting in the shuffling gait and tremors. The first step would be to evaluate the dosage of medication and adjust accordingly. If additional interventions are needed, then the patient would be sent for an MRI and/or observation. Physical therapy would be scheduled as needed if falls and gait are determined to be an ongoing issue.

68. C) Excitation-secretion coupling

Excitation-secretion coupling is the process in which an electrical impulse is converted to a chemical impulse at the synapse. Synaptogenesis is the process of the formation of synapses. Signal transduction cascade is the series of events that occurs after postsynaptic receptor stimulation. Volume neurotransmission is a process that does not involve a synapse.

69. B) Exhibited spiteful or vindictive behaviors at least twice in the past 6 months

Oppositional defiant disorder (ODD) in a child older than 5 years is exhibited by anger and the tendency to blame others for their own mischief. Patients do not care about punishment but can be controlled by the promise of larger rewards. Asking the parent questions regarding how long the behavior has occurred and whether spiteful or vindicative behavior has been exhibited is key to diagnosis of ODD. Behaviors must be consistent, at least once per week, for 6 months with a minimum of two spiteful and/or vindictive behaviors during this time. Apologizing and feeling guilty, as well as showing aggressive tendencies through behaviors such as setting fires or harming animals, are not in the diagnostic criteria for ODD.

70. A) Exhibitionist

The patient who becomes sexually aroused when exposing their genitals to another person shows signs of exhibitionist disorder. Frotteuristic disorder involves sexual arousal from rubbing genitals against a person without consent. The individual with pedophilic disorder has fantasies or sexual desires related to prepubescent children. Fetishistic disorder is sexual excitement toward nonliving things or nongenital body parts.

71. A) Experiences frightening dreams during rapid-eye-movement sleep

A person experiences nightmares during rapid-eye-movement sleep. The person clearly recalls and can describe what they have seen in the dreams after waking up. People with sleep terror disorder forget about the details of their dreams after waking up. The person with nightmare disorder does not always wake up immediately after dreams, but whenever the person wakes up, the dream will still be in the person's mind and the person will feel completely alert and oriented to place.

72. A) Family systems

One of the five key concepts of the family systems theory is the concept of emotional triangles. In general, two sides of the triangle depict harmony, while the other side denotes conflict. The emotional triangle concept is not related to functionalism theory, conflict theory, or symbolic interactionism theory.

73. B) Frontal and temporal lobes

The patient's concerns suggest Pick's disease. In patients with Pick's disease, imaging studies show atrophy to both the frontal and the temporal lobes, referred to as frontotemporal dementia. Pick's disease MRI results show atrophy that will increase and spread to the temporal areas. The cerebellum, brainstem, and parietal lobe are not consistently involved with Pick's disease. The cerebellum is responsible for the body's coordination, balance, and posture. The brainstem plays an important role in the body's core functions of awareness, consciousness, and movement. The parietal lobe is the area of the brain that is responsible for sensation and processing of stimuli from outside the body.

74. C) Frontal

The frontal lobe is responsible for executive functions such as emotional regulation, planning, and reasoning. The parietal lobe is responsible for language processing. The occipital lobe plays an important role in vision processing. The temporal lobe plays an important role in listening and communication.

75. C) Functionalism

Functionalism theory is a macro theory or a large-scale theory. Family systems theory, social exchange theory, and symbolic interactionism theory are examples of micro theories.

76. C) Further assess for alcohol use disorder

A score of 8 for men on AUDIT screening provides insight that there could be a possible risk for alcohol dependency and AUD. Therefore, the nurse practitioner will further assess the patient for AUD using a variety of tools and assessment methods. The needs for referral for outpatient rehabilitation, for admission, or for providing education have not yet been established.

77. A) Gamma-aminobutyric acid (GABA)

GABA is the neurotransmitter that is responsible for the regulation of the sleep–wake cycle and is released in the tuberomammillary nucleus to inhibit wakefulness. Histamine is the neurotransmitter that is responsible for the regulation of wakefulness. Serotonin is associated with mood-stabilizing functions. Dopamine is associated with reward pathways.

78. C) Ginkgo biloba 120 mg per day

Ginkgo biloba has been used to treat impaired cognition with convincing results, improving cognitive function, neuropsychiatric symptoms with age-related cognitive decline, mild cognitive impairment, and mild to moderate dementia. Valerian (Valeriana officinalis) treats anxiety and insomnia. Melatonin is used for the regulation of sleep. Intake of omega-3 fatty acids is thought to lower the risk of developing major depression, prenatal depression, and bipolar depression.

79. A) Glutamate

Glutamate is the universal excitatory neurotransmitter. It is involved with kindling, seizure disorders, and possibly bipolar disorder. The universal inhibitory neurotransmitter is GABA. Acetylcholine is cholinergic and not associated with kindling, seizure disorders, or bipolar disorder. Glycine is also an inhibitory neurotransmitter.

80. A) Grant each other's requests only after keeping some strings attached

Granting a request while keeping strings attached is a type of manipulation. An example of distraction is talking about irrelevant things when family problems are being discussed. Accusing each other is known as blaming, not manipulating. Acting well-meaning in front of other family members is an example of placating.

81. B) Have security assist officers in holding the patient's limbs while administering lorazepam

The patient is exhibiting behavior indicative of intermittent explosive disorder. The nurse practitioner would ask security and other aides to hold each limb or ask security to help the officers to temporarily restrain the patient's limbs while administering an initial dose of lorazepam to calm the patient. Holding the patient in another area may be needed, but is not the first option, nor is restraining the patient to the bed. The family may need to be contacted, but this would occur after the patient has been calmed.

82. C) Health Insurance Portability and Accountability Act

The Health Insurance Portability and Accountability Act of 1996 provided for patient record confidentiality. The Community Mental Health Centers Act (1963) promoted the deinstitutionalization of patients with mental illness. The Affordable Care Act (earlier known as the Patient Protection and Affordable Care Act) of 2010 expanded Medicaid funding eligibility. Oregon's Death with Dignity Act (1997) allows Oregonians who are terminally ill to end their lives through the voluntary self-administration of lethal medications.

83. D) Hoarding disorder and major depression

Hoarding disorder reflects "persistent difficulty discarding or parting with possessions due to a perceived need to save the items and distress associated with discarding them." DSM-5 has changed the diagnosis of chronic forms of depression. Dysthymia now falls under the category of persistent depressive disorder, which now includes both chronic major depressive disorder and the previous dysthymic disorder.

84. C) Hyperactivation of the amygdala

The brain images of patients with panic attacks reveal that their amygdalae are hyperactive. The amygdala is associated with emotions and is called the "fear center" of the brain. A fear response called the hypothalamic-pituitary-adrenal axis is also triggered in situations of stress or fear; this response ends with the secretion of the cortisol hormone. GABA is usually decreased in anxiety disorders or panic attacks. GABA is a neurotransmitter that has a calming effect and helps with anxiety. The sympathetic nervous system is activated in response to signals received from the hypothalamus. This manifests in increased heartbeat rate and breathing rate.

85. A) Hypersomnolence

Hypersomnolence disorder is diagnosed by self-reported excessive sleeping every week for at least 3 months. Narcolepsy disorder is related to episodes of napping by the patient multiple times within a day. A person with insomnia disorder is unable to achieve healthy and sound sleep. Excoriation disorder is a type of compulsive disorder in which the patient repeatedly picks the skin, resulting in the formation of skin lesions.

86. B) Hypnagogic hallucinations are common

The diagnosis of narcolepsy requires the symptoms of daytime sleepiness and one of the following: cataplexy (episodic loss of muscle function triggered by emotional responses); hypnagogic hallucinations (dreamlike experiences while falling asleep, dozing, or awakening); sleep paralysis (inability to move on awakening); or decreased orexin in the CSF. Polysomonographs of patients with narcolepsy show REM sleep that is disturbed, not absent. Catalepsy is seen in catatonic schizophrenia; the patient maintains the body position they are placed in without moving.

87. D) Idea that the progression of moral development occurs in three major divisions

Both Kohlberg and Gilligan had similar ideas regarding the stages of moral development, which are preconventional, conventional, and postconventional. Gilligan criticized Kohlberg's sampling method and believed that Kohlberg favored the method of reasoning of the male samples over the female samples. Gilligan also suggested the replacement of Kohlberg's justice view of morality with the morality of care.

88. A) Identify the cultural values of the patient

The nurse practitioner faces an ethical dilemma. The nurse practitioner cannot take away the patient's autonomy, but it is their duty to promote the safety of the patient. The patient has the right to refuse treatment. The nurse practitioner in such cases should identify why the patient may not have faith in the treatment provided at the hospital. The nurse needs to first understand the cultural values, personal beliefs, and values of the patient. This can help the nurse practitioner to provide culturally competent care. Speaking with family, with the patient's consent, is an option; however, the family may not be able to supply any insight into the patient's beliefs. Identifying new medical solutions can help the patient only if they are willing to be treated. The nurse practitioner should respect of the autonomy of the patient and should not instruct them not to leave the hospital.

89. A) Identify new or additional risk factors for the patient

Risk factors that have not been properly addressed could hinder the recovery process, so it is critical for the nurse practitioner to identify new and/or additional risk factors that could impede the patient's progress. Determining self-esteem and conducting a depression inventory are needed but are not the priority to address the immediate need. Involving the patient's parents in the recovery plan would need to be addressed with the patient first.

90. D) Inaccurate performance of motor skills such as catching a ball or riding a bicycle

Impairment of skills requiring motor coordination that interferes with daily activities is a cornerstone of developmental coordination disorder. Joint hypermobility syndrome causes hyperextensible joints. Attention deficit/hyperactivity disorder may cause a lack of motor competence due to distractibility and impulsiveness. Patients with autism spectrum disorder may be uninterested in participating in tasks requiring complex coordination skills.

91. C) Include an emergency plan in psychoeducation

Including an emergency plan for relapse is critical in helping the patient recognize signs of relapse and how to manage them. Enhancing social and occupational functioning and sleep/light manipulation are psychotherapies that may or may not be needed but have no correlation to what has been discovered or reported in self-observation. Information on support groups would be provided at a later time, such as in a therapy session or upon discharge.

92. A) Increased mortality risk when used to treat behavioral disturbances of dementia

FDA boxed warnings regarding atypical agents in this patient population are due to increased risk of cerebrovascular adverse events, including stroke, in older adults with dementia. These drugs are not approved for the treatment of patients with dementia-related psychosis. Potential serious consequences can occur with any medication; on its own, this would not justify a boxed warning. It is a recommended practice to use lower starting doses in older adults due to possible age-related changes in renal clearance and hepatic metabolism. Ethical dilemmas may be present with medically ill older adults or those with dementia, making obtaining informed consent difficult, but these dilemmas do not relate to FDA boxed warnings.

93. B) Intimacy versus isolation
Egocentricity comes in early adulthood when the psychosocial crisis of intimacy versus isolation remains unresolved. Confusion about oneself comes when identity versus role confusion remains unresolved. Obstacles in the path come when generativity versus self-absorption remains unresolved. Life dissatisfaction comes when integrity versus despair remains unresolved.

94. C) Is nonharmful to self and others
There are exceptional cases in which the nurse practitioner can share the information revealed during a therapy session with someone outside the therapy. When the patient does not show any sign of harm to self or others, the nurse practitioner should maintain confidentiality. However, when the patient is suicidal, for protection of the patient, the nurse practitioner should connect with concerned persons or authorities. When the nurse practitioner notices abuse like domestic violence or child abuse, the nurse practitioner must report that to a third party. When the nurse practitioner learns that the patient may harm a known person, the nurse practitioner should inform that person and other concerned authorities.

95. A) Jean Piaget
While helping with scoring some Binet Intelligence Tests, Jean Piaget found that the cognitive processing of young children is dissimilar to that of older children and adults. Erik Erikson, Carol Gilligan, and Lawrence Kohlberg did not make a similar finding.

96. A) Justice
The nurse practitioner will look into violations of the justice principle, which is demonstrated by actions to provide similar medical and nursing care for patients with similar characteristics and needs. Beneficence is providing/promoting the well-being of the patient. Nonmaleficence is doing no harm. Fidelity is honoring commitments made and being truthful.

97. A) Kleptomania
Kleptomania is associated with the inability of the patient to control the impulse to steal objects. The patient with pyromania disorder lights fires anywhere on impulse. Cognitive dissonance involves inconsistent thoughts, beliefs, or attitudes; it is not a disorder. Conduct disorder leads to disturbed behavior and disrupts the normal cognitive functioning of the patient.

98. D) Lamotrigine (Lamictal)
Stevens–Johnson syndrome is life-threatening epidermal necrolysis that can occur in patients taking lamotrigine. The risk of Stevens–Johnson syndrome is increased with concomitant use of valproate. Concurrent use of lamotrigine and valproate should be avoided if at all possible; however, if coadministration is deemed warranted, then the dose of lamotrigine must be decreased by half and tapered slowly to avoid Stevens–Johnson syndrome. Lithium carbonate, lurasidone, and cariprazine are used in the treatment of bipolar depression; however, risk of Stevens–Johnson syndrome is not a concern with these medications.

99. D) Major depression

The patient shows symptoms of grief, including sadness and withdrawal from usual activities. Their mood is consistently sad. In grief, patients usually maintain their feelings of self-worth. The patient reports feeling worthless and having vague suicidal ideation. Insomnia and loss of appetite as evidenced by weight loss suggest major depression. There are no signs of malingering or factious disorder. Lack of medical complaints and recent marijuana use reportedly not in excess rule out substance abuse. There are no significant reported losses that would be needed for complex bereavement.

100. D) Major depressive disorder

Being hopeless, along with a loss of interest in everyday activities, signifies that the patient is depressed. These diagnostic criteria are accompanied by insomnia, thoughts of suicide, and loss of appetite, which suggest that the patient is experiencing major depressive disorder. People showing symptoms of depression due to or associated with other medical conditions like brain injury or Parkinson's disease fall under the category of depressive disorder as a result of other medical conditions. Because all the diagnostic reports of the patient are normal, they cannot be diagnosed with depressive disorder due to other medical conditions. People developing symptoms of depression due to substance use or withdrawal fall under the category of substance or drug-induced depressive disorder. Because the patient does not claim to be using any substance and the depressive symptoms seem related to the loss of a loved one, the patient cannot be diagnosed with substance or drug-induced depressive disorder. People with unspecified depressive disorder show symptoms similar to depressive disorder but do not completely fall under the diagnostic criteria of depressive disorders. The patient's symptoms completely meet all the diagnostic criteria of major depressive disorder.

101. A) Major depressive disorder

The HPA axis is implicated in major depressive disorder and other stress-related conditions. In depression, research suggests evidence of overactivation of the HPA axis, which is seen as elevated levels of cortisol and adrenal hyperplasia. The pathophysiological basis for anxiety is the response of the amygdala to anxiety-producing stimuli. Substance use disorder development stems from neurophysiologic reinforcement (reward). Usually abnormalities in the frontal, temporal, and parietal lobes are the pathophysiological basis of personality disorders.

102. A) Mild neurocognitive disorder without behavioral disturbances

Mild neurocognitive disorder without behavioral disturbances is a new DSM-5 diagnosis that describes clinical symptoms showing a noticeable decline in cognitive functioning that goes beyond normal changes seen in aging. The four criteria refer to cognitive changes, functional activities, delirium exclusion, and competing mental disorders. The patient does not report any behavioral disturbances or meet the criteria for dementia or Alzheimer's disease.

103. A) Milieu therapy

When introducing a patient with mental health illness to new surroundings with new faces and personalities, it is important to include milieu therapy to teach the patient how to live harmoniously with others as well as how to perform self-care. Recovery and wellness strategies, as well as cognitive behavior modification, are support therapies and strategies that may be included in the treatment plan, but only after a full evaluation has occurred.

104. C) Monoamine oxidase inhibitor (MAOI)

Signs and symptoms of MAOI overdose range from mild to severe. Severe symptoms include severe hyperthermia, seizures, central nervous system depression, muscle rigidity, and myoclonus. Clinical features of acute intoxication with a benzodiazepine include slurred speech, incoordination, unsteady gait, and impaired attention or memory; physical signs include nystagmus and decreased reflexes. Anticholinergic syndrome presents with flushing, dry mucous membranes and skin, fever, and altered mental status. TCAs are common agents used in cases of fatal overdose, with signs and symptoms that include fever, drowsiness, confusion, and cardiac arrest.

105. B) Mononucleosis

EBV produces infectious mononucleosis. Mononucleosis is associated with weakness, depression, and personality changes. Testing for this condition include tests for EBV-specific antibody and antigen. IgM and IgG antibodies are usually elevated during the acute phase. With EBV infection, WBC, liver enzymes (ALT and AST), and bilirubin are elevated during acute illness. Major depression and malingering do not cause similar lab abnormalities. Chronic fatigue syndrome involves extreme fatigue that lasts for 6 months or more.

106. A) Montreal Cognitive Assessment

The Montreal Cognitive Assessment allows for assessment of several cognitive domains. It may be used for dementia, parkinsonism, Huntington's disease, and other neurological diseases to test cognitive function. The modified Ashworth scale is a clinical tool used to measure increase in muscle tone. Tardieu is a scale for measuring spasticity that takes into account resistance to passive movement at both slow and fast speeds. The Glasgow Coma Scale provides a practical method for assessing impairment of consciousness in response to defined stimuli.

107. D) Motivational interviewing

Motivational interviewing will help guide the patient through the process of change by using a person-centered approach to strengthen motivation. Pharmacotherapy and psychoeducation may be needed, but the motivational interview will be conducted first. Peer-centered care is part of the self-discovery and self-reporting phase of the initial evaluation.

108. B) Necessitates acute awareness of the patient's emotions and behavioral cues

To respond successfully to patient signals, sentiments, and worries, the interviewing process is flexible and depends on a variety of relationship abilities. It involves active listening, empathetic responses, affirmation without speaking, reassurance, and validation. The health history format is a structure helpful in organizing the information of patients in either written or verbal format. This makes communication with other healthcare professionals involved in the patient's care concise and effective. The interviewing process should be a patient-centered conversation rather than clinician-centered, and questioning should be open-ended to make the patient comfortable enough to share their feelings.

109. D) Neurocognitive

Neurocognitive disorders involve changes in brain structure and function, resulting in intellectual and memory impairments and impaired learning, orientation, and judgment. Substance-related disorders are disorders related to substance use or misuse and include alcohol-related disorders. Personality disorders are described as lifelong maladaptive patterns of behavior that are typically recognized at adolescence.

110. C) Noonan syndrome (NS)

NS is a genetically heterogeneous developmental disorder with classic facial and/or cardiac features. Patients often have mental, emotional, and behavioral issues that are similar in presentation to ADHD and ASD. In this case, social skill difficulty could suggest ASD, and being overtalkative, inattentive, and hyperactive suggest ADHD; however, neither condition has hallmark physical characteristics. Turner syndrome is also a disorder caused by chromosomal abnormalities and shares some clinical features of Noonan syndrome (i.e., short stature), but the psychiatric symptoms are not similar.

111.A) Normalization

When teaching family how to deal with the stressors of having a family member with mental illness, the focus will be on normalization, which teaches normal behaviors and what the expected responses should be. Teaching typical developmental processes and how to react to these when they are altered reduces stress in the family. Bibliotherapy is providing personal education through reading and supplemental material, which the family and patient can do on their own time. Social skills training and group experiences help teach children how to interact with peers and adults more effectively.

112. B) Observing evidence of abuse of an older adult patient

There are few instances when breach of confidentiality is necessary for the provider, including when there is evidence of abuse of a minor or an older adult. General treatment of older adult patients, without suspected abuse, is not an appropriate or necessary reason to breach a patient's confidentiality. Breach of confidentiality and discussion of health information with family members is only appropriate for adult patients with patient consent.

113. B) Occipital lobe

The occipital lobe is primarily responsible for vision processing. Damage to the occipital lobe may result in vision loss. The parietal lobe is responsible for language processing. The temporal lobe plays an important role in listening and communication. The medulla oblongata is a lower part of the brainstem and has the same functions as the brainstem.

114. B) Olanzapine (Zyprexa)

Olanzapine (Zyprexa) is an atypical antipsychotic. Atypical antipsychotics are known to increase risk factors for metabolic syndrome. The patient's elevated HbA1c, lipid profile, weight gain, and increase in abdominal girth are signs of metabolic syndrome. Citalopram (Celexa) is an selective serotonin reuptake inhibitor (SSRI) and not known to contribute to metabolic syndrome. Dextroamphetamine (Adderall) is a stimulant; weight loss would be more likely with this medication. Sertraline (Zoloft) is an SSRI with no association with metabolic syndrome.

115. A) Olanzapine (Zyprexa)

The nurse practitioner diagnoses the child with conduct disorder. Olanzapine is an antipsychotic drug used to treat behavioral disturbances in children and should help with the conduct disorder of the patient. Sertraline is an antidepressant drug that will not be effective in treating conduct disorder. Ondansetron is an antiemetic that is used in the treatment of cancer. Fluoxetine is used to treat depression.

116. B) Open-ended to focused

Questions asked in a clinical interview should follow the sequence of open-ended to focused questions. This helps the interview to proceed in a general to a more specific manner that will not overwhelm the patient. If asked in a series, questions should not be directed all at once, because this might result in the patient responding in a greatly generalized manner instead of answering questions separately and specifically. Leading questions in a clinical interview are discouraged because such questions might lead to curtailed answers. Questions that are answered with a "yes" or "no" should be avoided because they might lead to curtailed interpretation. Instead, questions should be asked that result in a more graded response.

117. C) Outpatient substance use treatment

Supportive housing does not guarantee that substance use treatment will be provided to patients in recovery. Therefore, it is imperative to include this in the recovery-oriented plan to reduce the risk of relapse. At this time, the patient is not in need of support employment. Family and caregiver support may be needed just prior to the patient leaving the supportive house but are not needed upon admission to supportive housing.

118. A) Panic

Trembling, sweating, and increased heart rate are some of the diagnostic criteria of panic disorder. The diagnostic criteria of bipolar disorder include hypomanic, manic, and major depressive episodes. Patients with hoarding disorder face difficulty in parting from their possessions and fear the distress that parting with them may induce. Excoriation disorder includes diagnostic criteria such as the presence of skin lesions and repeated acts of skin picking.

119. C) Paranoid

Individuals with paranoid personality disorder do not trust anyone easily and remain suspicious that others may try to hurt them. Schizotypal personality disorder leads to difficulty in having close relationships and in performing at full potential in social situations. Individuals with borderline personality disorder have abandonment issues and find difficulty in developing good interpersonal relationships. People with antisocial personality disorder become manipulative and deceitful for their own needs. Disregard for responsibilities, tendency to take risks, and impulsive behavior are diagnostic features for this disorder.

120. C) Parkinson's disease

Tremor is an involuntary, repetitive movement that is common in clinical practice and more prevalent with the use of psychotropic medications. Distinguishing causation involves assessment of its presence at rest or in action, whether it is positional, when it is active or not active, and its frequency and body distribution (e.g., bilateral). Causes can be medication related or part of a neurological syndrome such as multiple sclerosis, Parkinson's tremors, cerebellar tremors, or neuropathy. Parkinson's tremors are asymmetric at onset and while walking. Tremors occurring at rest is a diagnostic criterion for Parkinson's disease. Cerebellar tremors are present with voluntary motion but not at rest; multiple sclerosis is a common cause of cerebellar tremor. Tardive tremors are persistent and do not diminish during the course examination and voluntary movement; the patient must be on a dopaminergic-blocking medication for this diagnosis. Physiological tremor is seen in all people when muscles are activated. It is a common side effect of many drugs as well as a result of stress, fatigue, and caffeine intake. Physiological tremors rarely interfere with activities of daily living.

121. A) Participating on a hospital committee to ensure that patients with substance use disorders have equal access to care

According to the American Psychiatric Nurses Association (APNA), a core competency for ethical practice includes advocating for access and parity of services for mental health problems, psychiatric disorders, and substance use disorder services. Participation in interprofessional teams to discuss risks, benefits, and outcomes adheres to APRN ethical practice standards. Scope of practice involves informing the patient of all aspects of their care, including their right to be discharged against medical advice when their hospitalization is voluntary. According to the APNA, ethical competency also includes reporting illegal, incompetent, or impaired practices. The patient's confidentiality can be breached without the patient's permission is when the patient has revealed a determined intention to injure or kill a specific person.

122. B) Patient preferences

The clinical decision-making model has four components: internal evidence, patient preferences, research evidence, and healthcare resources. When a patient is denying a visit, the patient is expressing their preference. Internal evidence includes the clinical status and circumstances of the patient; circumstances include accessibility and location of the patient's home. Research evidence comes from the research done in related fields; that home visits improve depression is one such piece of evidence. The healthcare resource component is not dominant because whether the nurse visiting the patient has the expertise to deliver the same results or not is not known.

123. D) Patient advocacy

According to the American Nurses Association Code of Ethics for Nurses, the nurse promotes, advocates for, and strives to protect the health, safety, and rights of the patient. Patient advocacy principles center on the respect of human dignity and protection of the rights of patients. The use of seclusion and restraint to punish patients violates the patient's rights. Quality assurance is the process of evaluating the efficacy of nursing interventions and making recommendations for future improvements. Plan-do-study-act is a quality assurance method. It is a four-step process for implementing change, solving problems, and continuously improving processes. Evidence-based practice incorporates research findings in practice to improve treatment efficacy using a scholarly and systematic problem-solving approach.

124. A) Patient affect

Affect is the expression of mood that is reflected in the patient's appearance and in what the nurse practitioner observes. Terms used to describe the quality of a patient's affect include dysphoric, happy, euthymic, irritable, angry, agitated, tearful, sobbing, and flat. Quantity of affect should also be noted using terms such mild, moderate, or severe. The nurse practitioner should also document the appropriateness of the expressed mood: Is it congruent with what the patient has told the nurse practitioner, or is it incongruent? Mood differs from affect in that it is defined as the patient's internal and sustained emotional state; it is a subjective report of what the patient states about how they feel, rather than what is observed. Thought content is what the patient is thinking and whether there are abnormalities such as delusional, obsessive, suicidal, or homicidal ideas. Thought process differs from thought content because it describes how thoughts are formulated rather than what the person is thinking.

125. C) Patients who feel autonomous and independent are more receptive to treatment and have more successful outcomes

Autonomy and independence are integral components of self-determination, and patients who feel empowered by these characteristics will be more receptive to treatment and thus will have more successful outcomes. While self-determination allows patients to competently make decisions based on understanding their rights, this is based on competence. Likewise, promoting self-determination is an ethically sound practice; however, irrational decision making is not always the result, and patients can often make rational, sound decisions. Patients feel more empowered when they feel their rights are being protected and supported, but self-determination is not related only to patient rights.

126. B) Precontemplation, contemplation, preparation, action, and maintenance

The transtheoretical model of change includes the stages of precontemplation, contemplation, preparation, action, and maintenance. Freezing, unfreezing, and action are components of Kurt Lewin's change theory, which does not include contemplation, transition, or maintenance. Plan, do, study, and act are stages of the plan do study act model, but maintain is not a stage in this model, and it is unrelated to the transtheoretical model of change.

127. C) Preparation

Self-liberation is the stage at which an individual is intending to take action. Self-liberation is found in the preparation stage. The process of consciousness-raising, dramatic belief, and re-evaluation is found in precontemplation. The process of self–re-evaluation is found in contemplation. The process of counter-conditioning, stimulus control, and helping relationship is found in the action stage.

128. B) Preschool

The psychological crisis of initiative versus guilt occurs in the preschool stage (36 years). Trust versus mistrust occurs in the infancy stage (0–1.5 years). Identity versus role confusion occurs in the adolescent stage (12–20 years). Intimacy versus isolation occurs in the early adulthood stage (20–35 years).

129. B) Prescribe several doses of fluoxetine (Prozac)

Tapering off the medication is part of the treatment plan, and the patient is experiencing symptoms of discontinuation syndrome that can be helped by adding a few doses of fluoxetine, which is has a long half-life to help bridge the transition. Hospitalization, resuming the previous dosage, or discontinuing the medication entirely are not necessary given that administration of fluoxetine will help alleviate the symptoms of discontinuation syndrome.

130. A) Prescriptive authority

Prescribing drugs is a part of evidence-based practice. The nurse practitioner prescribes medications under prescriptive authority. It is an advanced role. Milieu therapy focuses on providing a secure environment to the patient for their recovery. It is usually used for inpatients. Counseling helps the nurse practitioner understand the problems faced by the patient. Cultural assessment is done before initiating treatment or therapy.

131. A) Prevention strategies
Prevention strategies that are developed with the patient's input are the most effective way to address aggression and violent tendencies when the patient has demonstrated the ability to practice restraint. Cognitive behavior modification and providing choices/options would be included once the prevention strategies have been determined. Reducing stimulation would be added to the treatment plan upon first admission to the unit.

132. B) Providing expert testimony to help inform policy decisions
The Public Health Policy Advocacy Guide Book and Tool Kit published by the Association of Public Health Nurses (APHN) recommends providing testimony to help inform policy decisions. The APHN points out that nurses make up the largest single group of health professionals (3.4 million), which translates to significant potential influence at all levels of government. APHN's resource also includes other examples of ways nurses can be effective advocates for policy change, including learning about the legislative process, participating in listservs and legislative action alerts, participating in coalitions, and contacting and meeting with elected officials. Examples of how the nurse can be a personal advocate for patients include protecting patients from harm, communicating patient preferences, fostering collaboration, and providing essential information to inform decision making.

133. C) Psychotherapy
The patient is experiencing the continuation phase of depression. In this phase, the patient needs proper depression-specific psychotherapy, pharmacotherapy, and education. Electroconvulsive therapy is used when pharmacological and psychotherapeutic interventions have failed to achieve the desired effect on the patient. The patient is usually admitted to the hospital when the patient can cause harm to self or others. Dialectal behavior therapy is more suited to when the patient is suicidal or has other disorders like borderline personality disorder.

134. B) Pulling one's own hair recurrently
Recurrent pulling of one's own hair, causing hair loss, is a diagnostic feature of the disease called trichotillomania. Excessive and unusual urges to set things on fire or to watch fires are the diagnostic features of pyromania. In an excoriation or skin-picking disorder, one has a tendency to constantly pick their own skin. Skin rubbing and biting are also diagnostic features of this disorder, but hair pulling is not. Skin picking may be seen in body dysmorphic disorder as well. The tendency toward purposeless repetitive movement is seen in stereotypic movement disorder and tic disorders.

135. C) Readiness for enhanced resilience
The patient has demonstrated a readiness to learn new interventions for building, or enhancing, resilience skills and would therefore have a new nursing diagnosis: readiness for enhanced resilience. Increased readiness to learn, improved readiness for teaching, and enhanced awareness of disorder do not accurately represent the patient's desire to learn new skills related to the specific current diagnosis.

136. B) Regulating their emotions to not fall victim to self-defeating thoughts
Resilience is a quality found in many children who are victims of abuse, and it allows them
to find the resources needed to protect their well-being and survive. By regulating emotions, children will not fall victim to the negative and often self-destructive thoughts that
come with the trauma of abuse. Resilience does not give strength for retreating to safety; it
provides the cognitive ability to overcome trauma. Heightened awareness and repression
of fear during times of fight or flight is not due to resilience but to a physiological response
of the body. Resilience is a psychological response.

137. C) Relabels control to caring
Reframing, an intervention used in strategic family therapy, is relabeling a problematic
behavior to have a more positive meaning. Creating family triangles to decrease stress is an
intervention in family systems theory. Mapping relationships using symbols, also known as
structural mapping, is an intervention used in structural family therapy. While giving family members a task in expectation of their compliance is an intervention used in strategic
family therapy, it is considered a directive, not reframing.

138. C) Retrograde
Retrograde neurotransmission is the transmission of the impulse from the postsynaptic to
the presynaptic neuron. Volume neurotransmission is a process that does not involve a synapse. Classic neurotransmission is the process in which the impulse is transmitted from the
presynaptic neuron to the postsynaptic neuron. Nonsynaptic diffusion neurotransmission
is another name for volume neurotransmission, which requires no synapse.

139. B) Rett
Rett syndrome is a neurodevelopmental disorder that affects girls almost exclusively. It is
characterized by normal early growth and development, followed by a slowing of development, loss of purposeful use of the hands, distinctive hand movements (characteristi-
cally hand-wringing), slowed brain and head growth, problems with walking, seizures,
and intellectual disability. Heller's syndrome is also known as childhood disintegrative
disorder. Affected children have often achieved normal developmental milestones before
the regression of skills. The age of onset is variable but is typically seen after 3 years of
reaching normal milestones. Fragile X patients have moderate intellectual disability. They
have a particular facial appearance, characterized by large head size, a long face, prominent
forehead and chin, and protruding ears. Behavioral problems are often present, such as
hyperactivity, hand flapping, hand biting, and temper tantrums. Fetal alcohol syndrome
patients have distinctive physical features such as short stature, midface hypoplasia, and
mild to moderate mental retardation. Behavioral problems are common, particularly hyperactivity and inattention.

140. C) Revise the treatment plan to taper medication with supervision
The patient is given the opportunity to consent to the change in treatment plan, which
acknowledges the patient's decision and gives the opportunity to educate the patient as to
the risks of no treatment. It also allows for a medication taper, which provides the opportunity for continued medical evaluation. The patient is not a risk to themselves or others
at this point; court-ordered medication efforts will further alienate the patient. Due process
protections must be complied with before forcing the patient to take medications in a non-
emergency situation. Contacting the patient's family without consent is a violation of the
patient's right to confidentiality. Discharging the patient from care could potentially harm
the patient because the lack of provider availability affects continuity and access to care.

141. C) Safeguarding against adverse drug interactions

According to the APNA, the nurse practitioner safeguards against adverse drug interactions. Collaboration with patients' primary care providers is generally appropriate; however, collaboration only with major changes to the treatment plan is recommended. The nurse practitioner seeks specific therapeutic responses, anticipates common side effects, and monitors for unintended or toxic responses. Microdosing is not necessary and may lengthen the patients' severity of symptoms. One month's delay between initiations of most psychotropic medications is unnecessary.

142. A) Says that identifying a patient's genotype may aid in determining therapeutic strategy and appropriate dosages

The FDA acknowledges that identification of a patient's genotype may be used to aid in determining a therapeutic strategy, determining an appropriate dosage, or assessing the likelihood of benefit or toxicity. The FDA has evaluated pharmacogenetic associations of certain drugs and supports the belief that there is sufficient scientific evidence to suggest that subgroups of patients with certain genetic variants, or genetic variant-inferred phenotypes, are likely to have altered drug metabolism, and, in certain cases, differential therapeutic effects, including differences in risks of adverse events. The FDA does not support the use of pharmacogenetic testing before prescribing any medications. The FDA has compiled a table of pharmacogenetic associations for which the data support therapeutic management recommendations. The FDA recommends testing before prescribing certain drugs to identify patients for which the drug is contraindicated.

143. D) SBIRT

SBIRT is a screening and intervention approach used to determine and treat high-risk behaviors that may lead to AUD. This approach integrates screen, assessment, and intervention and is a tool that can be used alone or with other tools to determine the severity of AUD. It is an initial screening for patients who have not self-reported alcohol use. The AUDIT tool is a widely used tool to determine the severity of alcohol use and is especially beneficial when patients self-identify that there may be a problem. The tool can be administered by either the nurse practitioner or the patient and is an early identifier of risk for AUD. The CAGE assessment tool is an excellent initial tool if the practitioner suspects alcohol use may be an issue. The assessment is brief and used to identify a patient's alcohol use that the patient may not report. The T-ACE screening tool is specific to patients who are pregnant.

144. C) Seek emotional refueling from the caretaker

According to Mahler's stages of separation-individuation, in the rapprochement phase the child seeks emotional refueling from the caretaker. Fulfillment of basic needs for survival and comfort is observed in the normal autism phase; a child recognizes separation from the caretaker at 5 to 10 months in the differentiation phase; and in the consolidation phase, the sense of separateness is established.

145. B) Seeking prior authorization from the insurance company

The American Nurses Association Code of Ethics states, "The nurse promotes, advocates for, and protects the rights, health, and safety of the patient." The nurse practitioner should prescribe based on the best pharmaceutical option for the patient's condition. Brand-name medications are often denied or are a higher cost due to insurance company tiers. Should the preferred choice be a brand-name medication, the nurse practitioner can advocate for the patient by providing the medical information needed to obtain a prior authorization. This is time consuming and unreimbursable. However, if the medication choice can be justified, the nurse practitioner should proceed. Contacting the patient's primary care provider is evidence of collaborating with other providers, but it does not address the problem of ensuring the best medication choice for the patient. Prescribing a generic medication because it is less time consuming for the nurse practitioner and cheaper for the patient is unethical. Providing patients with resources is a positive intervention; however, finding coupons for pharmaceutical company discounts is an administrative burden that should not be delegated to the patient.

146. A) Selegiline (Eldepryl)

The patient is prescribed paroxetine (Paxil), which is an selective serotonin reuptake inhibitor (SSRI). Serotonin syndrome is a psychiatric emergency that occurs when an SSRI dosage is increased or when it is combined with a medication that can raise plasma levels of serotonin to toxic concentrations. Mild cases are resolved by stopping either the SSRI or the additional medication that is causing the drug–drug interaction. Severe serotonin syndrome can be life-threatening. Symptoms rising to the level of an emergency include fever, seizures, cardiac arrhythmias, and an altered level of consciousness. Offending medications include monoamine oxidase inhibitors (MAOIs), lithium, L-tryptophan, and others. Selegiline (Eldepryl), which is often used to treat Parkinson's disease, is an MAOI. Levodopa/carbidopa, used to treat Parkinson's, is not associated with serotonin syndrome. Cyproheptadine is an antihistamine agent that decreases serotonin levels and is often used in the treatment of serotonin syndrome. Loratadine is an antihistamine that is not associated with serotonin syndrome.

147. D) Serotonin

The following six neurotransmitters are found in the brain: serotonin, norepinephrine, dopamine, acetylcholine, glutamate, and gamma-aminobutyric acid (GABA). A patient with depression has low serotonin. Glucose is not a neurotransmitter. Acetylcholine is expected to be low in a patient with Huntington's disease and high in a patient with Alzheimer's dementia. Glutamate plays an essential role in normal brain function, including nerve cell function and nerve communication.

148. B) Show interest by interrogating further

When dealing with a talkative patient, the nurse practitioner should show interest by interrogating further. This might help exclude unimportant topics and lead the interview forward with relevant topics. Interrupting should be avoided because it is impolite to do so. Asking the patient to stop talking is rude and should be avoided. The nurse practitioner should not show impatience because it might break the connection and rapport with the patient.

149. B) States that their marijuana use is not a big deal
During the precontemplation phase, the individual does not identify problematic behavior and does not demonstrate readiness for change. The patient stating that they want to change within the next month and acknowledging that marijuana use is a problem with a desire to take action show that the patient is ready to change and is planning interventions for change in the near future. This indicates that the patient is in the contemplation phase of change. The patient's agreement to reduce marijuana use before the next visit demonstrates action that the patient is willing to take by setting goals to reduce problematic behavior.

150. D) Step away from the patient and call for security to be present for the remainder of the assessment
The most appropriate action would be to step away from the patient, go to the door or phone, and call for assistance. The nurse practitioner would not leave the patient alone because they may injure themselves or possibly leave. Speaking calmly and softly is an appropriate way to communicate with the patient, but if feeling unsafe, the nurse practitioner should trust their instincts and not engage the patient because they may become aggressive.

151. D) Stop tranylcypromine and wait 14 days before starting amphetamine
The patient was taking tranylcypromine 30 mg, which is a monoamine oxidase inhibitor (MAOI). MAOIs interact with many drugs, especially stimulants. Adverse reactions include elevated blood pressure, headache, and arrhythmias. Concurrent use with stimulants that are sympathomimetic could result in death. Stimulants should not be started until 14 days after stopping the MAOI. Tapering is not necessary. Waiting 30 days is not required and may contribute to worsening function.

152. D) Suicidal behavior
Suicide is the leading cause of death in schizophrenic patients. A command hallucination is a false perception of instructions or orders the patient may feel obligated to obey or is unable to resist. The content of the command auditory hallucinations may include messages to self-harm. Command hallucinations and persecutory hallucinations are associated with a high risk for suicidal behavior. The assessment of the risk for self-harm is the priority. Monitoring medication compliance is important because nonadherence may be contributing to current mental status, but it is not the main priority. Aripiprazole is a second-generation atypical psychotic with well-documented risks for metabolic syndrome. Monitoring for all side effects is an important component of care to assess the overall health of the patient; it does not present an imminent risk for loss of life. Refocusing the patient on reality is a therapeutic intervention and should be included in the plan of care. However, the priority is the suicidal assessment.

153. B) Supported employment
The patient would benefit most from a supported employment program, which provides the stability and self-esteem needed for ultimate recovery results. E-mental health and technology-based care would be alternatives once the patient is established in recovery. At this point, there is no indication that the patient needs alternative housing arrangements, but they should be monitored for this need.

154. D) The patient shows willingness to receive the medication
When a caregiver approaches the patient with medications in hand and the patient shows a willingness to take the medication, it is considered implied consent. The patient is informed about the health condition to avoid risks. Patients are told about the risks of treatment because of their right to informed consent. In the case of rights regarding psychiatric directives, designation of preferred physician and therapist is mentioned to the patient.

155. A) The right to choose one's health-related options and behaviors
Self-determination is based on patient autonomy to make sound healthcare decisions. The Self-Determination Act states that self-determination is a right patients have to make these decisions based on options, behaviors, and informed practice. Cognition and competence are important components of assessing for a patient's ability to make informed decisions, but they are not rights regarding self-determination. Legal protection from forced commitment and the right to appoint a healthcare proxy are patient rights but are not related specifically to self-determination.

156. A) The patient and family can benefit from functional family therapy
In a situation where there is conflict in the family unit, the best treatment plan for optimal recovery is to treat the family as a whole with functional family therapy. Conflict in the family has been determined to be a cause of relapse and failure to recover in patients with substance use disorder. Treatment may or may not be compromised without group therapy because working within a group is not the challenge for this patient. Drugs and alcohol are a crutch for this patient, as is evidenced by the treatment plan, so this would not be a new determination or discovery. While the patient may benefit from being placed in another home that is a hostility-free environment, that is a determination that would be made after further evaluation.

157. D) The manner of conducting the interview varies with age and developmental status
To conduct a useful interview of a child of any age, the nurse practitioner should be familiar with normal child development and approach the evaluation with appropriate techniques according to the child's developmental status. Depending on the condition, a child may find it difficult to sit still during the entire evaluation. Some children are at ease with adults, while others experience anxiety or oppositional behaviors. Research has shown that eye contact is important for child development. It is preferable for the child's parent or guardian to be present when a child is being evaluated; however, there may be times when the child is seen alone, as in cases of suspected child abuse or neglect.

158. A) The patient may ask for a copy of medical records
Under HIPAA, patients may ask for a copy of their medical records. Patients can authorize and release information and receive a copy of privacy rights. No patient information should be given to those who call the facility unless patient consent is given.

159. B) The problem and the sequence of interactions that maintain the problem
Strategic family therapy is problem focused, and techniques include those that focus on changing the sequence of interactions that is causing the problem. Focusing on family structure to effectively manage problems is important when using structural family therapy. Focusing on self-confrontation of each family member is important in an individual therapy approach with existential therapy. Self-differentiation is a key concept in family systems theory.

160. C) Thyroid panel

Hypothyroidism often mimics the signs and symptoms of depression. Common signs of hypothyroidism include apathy, weight gain, thin and dry hair, cold intolerance, facial puffiness, and slowed thinking. Although assessment of vitamin B1 and vitamin D and a complete blood count would be helpful to rule out medical causes for depressive symptoms, the patient is exhibiting signs of hypothyroidism, and therefore assessing the thyroid panel is the priority.

161. A) Thyroid panel

Hyperthyroidism is characterized by increased pulse, fine tremor, heat intolerance with excessive sweating, weight loss, menstrual irregularities, muscle weakness, and exophthalmos. Some symptoms of hyperthyroidism mimic anxiety and manic symptoms, such as nervousness, exaggerated startle response, and hyperverbal speech. In its severe form, patients may even experience delusions or hallucinations. Therefore, checking a thyroid panel for this patient is a priority. Assessment of complete blood count, vitamin B12 level, and liver function test should also be included in the initial workup; however, because the patient is exhibiting signs and symptoms of hyperthyroidism, the first priority is to assess the thyroid panel.

162. A) Tolerance

Tolerance occurs when a person has to ingest more and more of a substance over a period of time to feel any effect, such as a "high." The build-up of the substance leads to a tolerance level, and subsequently the substance must be ingested in increasingly higher amounts to have an effect on the body. Confabulation is "honest lying," where a patient makes inaccurate statements but truly believes they are telling the truth. It is common in advanced alcoholism. Withdrawal involves reduced substance ingestion, and addiction involves compulsive physiological need for the substance and continued use regardless of the adverse effects.

163. A) Traumatic brain injury

Damage to the brain, particularly the frontal lobe, could impact behavioral and emotional responses. Anger, irritability, or aggressive outbursts occur in up to one third of patients after a traumatic brain injury. Therefore, it would be important to obtain a thorough patient history as well as imaging studies to rule out possible sources of the patient's presenting symptoms. Huntington's disease is characterized by involuntary jerking movements and social withdrawal. Cyclothymic disorders present with mood shifts that are not usually extreme. Symptoms of Pick's disease often include difficulty in social settings such as disinhibition, restlessness, and personality changes. It has a slow progression and would not present as a recent change.

164. A) Trichotillomania

Picking of one's own hair that results in alopecia and does not involve any dermatological conditions is due to trichotillomania disorder. Difficulty in the ability to resist this condition, causing great distress in work and in public, signifies trichotillomania as well. Excoriation disorder involves the habit of recurrent picking of the skin, resulting in lesions where the picking occurs. This may cause difficulty in social involvement. The condition involving difficulty in discarding one's possessions, resulting in excessive accumulation, is called hoarding disorder; this disorder should not be associated with other mental disorders or medical conditions. In the case of body dysmorphic disorder, the patient spends much of their time occupied with thoughts of perceived flaws in their physical appearance. They are primarily engaged in grooming, asking for reassurances, and making comparisons with others' appearances.

165. C) Using password-protected records

Protecting a patient's confidentiality is crucial. It can be done by maintaining password-protected records. Resaving records after edits is important for the accuracy and currency of the records, but it does not help maintain confidentiality. Deleting records is a negative approach because keeping records is important for credibility and future directions. Paper records are important, but electronic medical records are the need of the hour. Breach of confidentiality is possible with both. It is important to be mindful that paper records are kept safely from the reach of any person who should not have access to them.

166. B) Using culturally appropriate assessment tools

Using culturally appropriate assessment tools such as cultural explanation and appropriate social and cultural interviewing will guide the nurse practitioner in choosing additional diagnostic tests that are culturally appropriate. Conducting a thorough physical and diagnostic assessment may be seen as invasive and inappropriate in some cultures. Reviewing medical records would be an appropriate step for all patients, but interviewing the family for this information is not always appropriate. Ordering excessive testing is not needed and may not be seen as appropriate.

167. D) V trigeminal

Testing for a corneal reflex by touching the cornea with a fine wisp of cotton is an assessment of cranial nerve V, trigeminal. Cranial nerves II and III are assessed when testing pupillary reactions, and cranial nerves III and IV are assessed by checking for extraocular movements.

168. B) Validating the emotions of the patient

One of the methods for empowering the patient includes validating the patient's emotions. This helps the patient feel like their emotions are understandable and legitimate. Another method for empowering the patient involves showing interest in both the patient and the problem. Therefore, just showing interest in the problem and not the patient or vice versa is not a technique of skilled interviewing. The skilled psychiatric-mental health nurse practitioner keeps their clinical reasoning transparent with patients. This helps in understanding the cause of the concerns and the effectiveness of treatment and also makes the connection stronger. The limits of the nurse practitioner's knowledge should not be concealed; in fact, nurse practitioners should share their knowledge because it offers the patient a better understanding of the cause of the patient's problem and the potential therapies.

169. A) Vascular dementia
A patient with vascular dementia generally faces issues like confusion, problems in decision making, and urinary incontinence. It can be detected using MRI because a blockage or damage present in the blood vessels of the brain can cause this disease. Dementia with Lewy bodies cannot be confirmed using MRI, and it has a high likelihood of hallucinations as a symptom. Alzheimer's disease can also be detected by MRI, but its most common symptom is memory-related issues that disrupt the patient's daily life. Huntington's disease cannot be confirmed through MRI; genetic testing is needed.

170. C) Veracity
Veracity is the obligation to tell the truth. The nurse practitioner is truthful with the patient about the failure to provide information as promised. Fidelity is faithfulness to one's duties. Nonmaleficence means that a medical practitioner has a duty to do no harm or allow harm to be caused to a patient through neglect. Beneficence means that all medical practitioners have a moral duty to promote the course of action that they believe is in the best interests of the patient.

171. B) Was experiencing extrapyramidal symptoms
The patient experienced extrapyramidal symptoms due to use of an antipsychotic drug. This usually occurs young adults and is treated with anticholinergic drugs to increase the transmission of dopamine blocked by the antipsychotic. An overdose of antipsychotics causes an altered state of consciousness, excess salivation, and respiratory depression. Myocarditis should be suspected only if troponin levels are elevated and other related features are observed. Clozapine should be stopped in cases such as when C-reactive protein level is higher than 100 mg/L.

172. C) Weaning off the medication while continuously assessing for increased suicidal ideation
The nurse practitioner should assess for increased suicidal ideation. The FDA's boxed warnings for selective serotonin reuptake inhibitors such as fluoxetine include an increased risk of suicidality in children, adolescents, and young adults at the initiation of treatment and with dosage changes. Antidepressant discontinuation syndrome usually includes symptoms such as insomnia, flu-like symptoms, nausea, sensory disturbances, imbalance, and hyperarousal. Because fluoxetine 60 mg daily is the recommended daily dosing for the treatment of OCD in an adolescent and 2 months is an appropriate trial length, the maximum therapeutic dose had been reached. Weaning off fluoxetine is the safest approach before initiating any other pharmacological intervention.

173. C) Wernicke encephalopathy
Wernicke encephalopathy is a degenerative brain disorder attributed to thiamine deficiency and is often found in patients with alcohol use syndrome. Its signs include ataxia, confusion, and blurred vision resulting from nystagmus. Detoxification is the safe withdrawal of the substance to which the patient is addicted. Delirium tremens is an acute syndrome of symptoms such as tremors and hallucinations that are brought about when suddenly withdrawing from addictive substances. Korsakoff's amnestic syndrome involves cardiovascular and neurological systems with difficulty focusing and retrieving memories.

174. A) Yoga and guided imagery

Therapies that address spirit-mind-body health include yoga, guided imagery, and acupuncture. Sertraline (Zoloft) is a prescribed selective serotonin reuptake inhibitor; it is not considered alternative therapy that integrates spirit, mind, and body, so it would not be included. Exercise and qigong are therapies for substance abuse, and omega-3 fatty acids and music therapy are used for depression.

175. A) Zero step of evidence-based practice

Evidence-based practice is divided into a series of steps. Cultivating a spirit of inquiry is the zero step. It is challenging prevalent practice and asking questions related to current practice. After generating this spirit, the first step is to ask the questions in a well-defined format. The second step includes collecting the relevant evidence. The third step is to critically appraise to evaluate the validity, reliability, and applicability of the evidence.

Practice Exam 2

1. According to Freud, the age at which a child learns independence and control is:

    A. Birth to 18 months
    B. 18 months to 3 years
    C. 3 to 6 years
    D. 6 to 12 years

2. The psychiatric-mental health nurse practitioner expects that a patient with bulimia nervosa who is experiencing muscle weakness, fatigue, and cardiac dysrhythmias will have a potassium value of:

    A. 3.0 mEq/L
    B. 3.5 mEq/L
    C. 5.1 mEq/L
    D. 5.0 mEq/L

3. After completing the assessment and evaluation of a patient, the psychiatric-mental health nurse practitioner formulates a nursing diagnosis with prioritization of each goal. The standard of practice implied here is standard:

    A. 1
    B. 2
    C. 3
    D. 4

4. A patient who is a binge drinker has been recently diagnosed with Stage I of liver cirrhosis. The patient reports tremors, insomnia, and nausea whenever they stop drinking alcohol. The nurse practitioner will prescribe:

    A. Ramelteon
    B. Tasimelteon
    C. Acamprosate
    D. Agomelatine

5. A patient visits a clinic and reports alteration in sleep patterns and a lack of interest in everyday activities. During physical assessment, the psychiatric-mental health nurse practitioner observes bruises on the patient's skin. The nurse practitioner should assess for an increase in:

    A. C-reactive protein
    B. Urine cortisol level
    C. Acetylcholine
    D. Interleukin-6

6. Resilience assists patients with moving forward in light of situations and setbacks. Resilience can be described as:

   A. Strength and the ability to adapt without making any changes
   B. Acknowledgment and learning from situations to move forward
   C. Frequent reflection on failures as a way to become stronger
   D. Recognition of the use of maladaptive coping mechanisms to heal

7. A patient has been in treatment for 4 months for alcohol use. The psychiatric-mental health nurse practitioner has prescribed medication. The patient is now compliant with taking medication and keeping appointments. The patient recently began going to daily Alcoholics Anonymous meetings. The patient has identified triggers and people, places, and things that are a risk to sobriety. According to the transtheoretical stages of change, the phase of change demonstrated by the patient is:

   A. Precontemplative
   B. Maintenance
   C. Preparation
   D. Action

8. A patient reports insomnia lasting 2 months due to work stress. The psychiatric-mental health nurse practitioner will prescribe a drug that blocks:

   A. Dopamine 2 receptors
   B. Activities of orexin receptors
   C. Serotonin 2A receptors
   D. Stimulation of noradrenergic receptors

9. During a follow-up assessment, a patient previously prescribed sertraline (Zoloft) 100 mg per day for obsessive-compulsive disorder tendencies reports taking St. John's wort to help with their anxiety-related depression. Upon this discovery, the psychiatric-mental health nurse practitioner will:

   A. Provide education on the safe use of herbal supplements
   B. Have the patient discontinue sertraline while taking St. John's wort
   C. Explain that St. John's wort has lethal side effects and must be discontinued
   D. Advise against St. John's wort and suggest golden root or lavender instead

10. In a clinical interview, the psychiatric-mental health nurse practitioner helps a depressed patient to think about alternative explanations regarding problems to:

    A. Alter the depressed mood of the patient
    B. Improve the patient's self-concept
    C. Provide the patient an accurate perception of the world
    D. Provide the patient strength and support

11. If a patient is showing early symptoms of, or has a family history of, early-onset Alzheimer's disease, the psychiatric-mental health nurse practitioner may seek genetic testing for:

    A. *BRCA* genes
    B. *APOE* E4*
    C. Karyotyping and fluorescence in situ hybridization (FISH)
    D. Amyloid precursor protein (*APP*), presenilin-1 (*PSEN1*), and presenilin-2 (*PSEN2*)

12. The diagnostic test results that indicate that it is not safe for a patient to start valproate (Depakote) are:

    A. Aminotransferases (ALT and AST): AST: 570 IU/L and ALT: 620 IU/L
    B. Potassium (K): 4 mEq/L and sodium (Na): 140 mEq/L
    C. Platelet count: 300,000 per uL and white blood cell (WBC) count: 7.2 cells/mm^3
    D. Hemoglobin: 18 g/dL and hematocrit 40%

13. In order for a patient to be diagnosed with major depressive disorder, the patient must present with depressed mood and:

    A. Anhedonia
    B. Weight loss
    C. Grandiosity
    D. Paranoia

14. Substantial increases in body weight can be induced by several antipsychotic drugs, most notably olanzapine (Zyprexa) and clozapine (Clozaril). The neurobiological mechanism thought to cause weight gain is:

    A. Glucagon-like peptide 1 (GLP-1) agonists
    B. Agonism at the 5-HT2C serotonin receptor
    C. Antagonism of H1 histamine and 5-HT2C serotonin receptors
    D. Sodium glucose cotransporter 2 (SGLT-2) inhibitors

15. A patient reports fatigue and drowsiness for the last 3 months that is affecting job performance. The psychiatric-mental health nurse practitioner would prescribe:

    A. Armodafinil
    B. Clomipramine
    C. Desipramine
    D. Diazepam

16. A patient comes to the psychiatric-mental health nurse practitioner to talk about issues with excessive gambling and no-strings-attached relationships. The patient also reveals cheating on their spouse. After hearing the situation, the nurse practitioner should:

    A. Ask the patient to give up gambling
    B. Ask the patient to tell their spouse about the infidelity
    C. Ask the patient to describe the problems and how they affect the patient
    D. Sympathize with the patient about troubled relationships

17. A patient with anger management issues visits a psychiatric-mental health nurse practitioner. Following the proper technique of asking guided questions of the patient, the nurse practitioner will:

    A. Ask focused questions before open-ended questions
    B. Ask for an elaborated response rather than just yes or no
    C. Avoid providing multiple choices for a single question
    D. Avoid repeating patient's response once the patient finishes answering

18. A 6-year-old boy visits the clinic with his parent, who reports that the child is fascinated with lights and often repeats what others say. On examination, the psychiatric-mental health nurse practitioner recognizes the patient's inability to maintain eye contact or engage in conversation. To determine a diagnosis, the next step the nurse practitioner will take is to:

    A. Refer the patient to a neurologist
    B. Assess the patient for abuse
    C. Schedule the patient for cognitive testing
    D. Refer the patient for genetic testing

19. A 65-year-old patient is being treated by the psychiatric-mental health nurse practitioner. The patient is irritated all the time and destroys things at home. The patient has not responded well to the first line of treatment. The nurse practitioner decides to initiate the second line of treatment with a different class of drug. The clinical decision of the nurse practitioner is based on:

    A. Assessment of internal evidence
    B. Patient's preferences or desires
    C. Use of research evidence
    D. Healthcare resources evaluation

20. The action that demonstrates a psychiatric-mental health nurse practitioner's role in patient advocacy is:

    A. Emphasizing to the patient how important it is to follow provider recommendations
    B. Assisting the patient in choosing an aftercare plan that reflects the vegetarian diet the patient prefers
    C. Expressing support for family members' choices for patient treatment to improve family dynamics
    D. Respecting the patient's decision not to take prescribed medications and protecting the patient's accumulation of medications

21. In order to meet the diagnostic criteria for bipolar II, the patient must have hypomanic symptoms and present with:

    A. At least one episode severe enough to cause hospitalization or psychosis
    B. At least one episode of mania
    C. Predominate (more than half the time) mood swings for at least 2 years
    D. At least one major depressive episode

22. A patient reports impulsive behavior, frequent distractions, and restlessness lasting for 6 months. The psychiatric-mental health nurse practitioner observes the patient's tendency to answer questions before the nurse practitioner has completed them. The patient is also observed to be fidgeting and absent-minded. After careful observation and evaluating test results, the nurse practitioner prescribes:

A. Armodafinil (Nuvigil)

B. Flurazepam (Dalmane)

C. Clozapine (Clozaril)

D. Atomoxetine (Strattera)

23. The nurse practitioner provides BASIC guidance on parenting that encourages parent–child attachment and a child's self-confidence, academic readiness, and social and emotional development when the child has:

A. Attention deficit/hyperactivity disorder (ADHD)

B. Major depression disorder (MDD)

C. Generalized anxiety disorder (GAD)

D. Obsessive-compulsive disorder (OCD)

24. Nurse practitioners are required to administer prescribed medications, but patients, at the same time, can refuse them. In these situations, the psychiatric-mental health nurse practitioner decides between:

A. Confidentiality versus duty to warn

B. Justice versus nonmaleficence

C. Nonmaleficence versus fidelity

D. Autonomy versus beneficence

25. A patient with schizophrenia is pregnant. The patient's family urges the patient to terminate the pregnancy. The psychiatric–mental nurse practitioner respects the decision of the patient to carry the pregnancy to term. The nurse practitioner is maintaining the principle of:

A. Confidentiality

B. Autonomy

C. Veracity

D. Justice

26. A patient with a clinical history of diplopia is recently diagnosed with Parkinson's disease. After a few weeks, the patient reports delusions and hallucinations. The psychiatric-mental health nurse practitioner will avoid prescribing:

A. Diphenhydramine

B. Pimavanserin

C. Rivastigmine

D. Benztropine

27. A patient is asked to monitor heart rate, respiratory rate, and blood pressure whenever the patient has episodes of major depression. This type of monitoring is an example of:

    A. Aversion therapy
    B. Interpersonal therapy
    C. Modeling therapy
    D. Biofeedback therapy

28. Antidepressants resolve the depressive episodes associated with deficiency of transmission of monoamine neurotransmitters by:

    A. Stimulating the effects of gamma-aminobutyric acid (GABA)
    B. Stimulating the reuptake of norepinephrine
    C. Stimulating the reuptake of dopamine
    D. Blocking the reuptake of serotonin

29. While assessing a 17-year-old patient, the psychiatric-mental health nurse practitioner observes loss of muscle mass along with edema of the face and extremities. Upon further evaluation, the nurse practitioner finds Russell's sign, parotid swelling, and indications of dental caries. The nurse practitioner will evaluate for the diagnosis of:

    A. Bulimia nervosa
    B. Anorexia nervosa
    C. Depression
    D. General anxiety disorder

30. A patient reports restlessness, lack of concentration, and frequent palpitations that last for a short duration. The patient has a clinical history of substance use disorder. The psychiatric-mental health nurse practitioner would prescribe:

    A. Diazepam (Valium)
    B. Lorazepam (Ativan)
    C. Buspirone (BuSpar)
    D. Alprazolam (Xanax)

31. The psychiatric-mental health nurse practitioner is formulating the treatment plan for a patient with bipolar disorder. The patient's genetic testing results indicate that the patient is homozygous for the A allele of the rs1061235 A > T polymorphism. This patient does not carry the HLA-B*1502 allele or a closely related *15 allele. The medication plan:

    A. Can include lamotrigine (Lamictal)
    B. Cannot include lamotrigine (Lamictal)
    C. Cannot include carbamazepine (Tegretol)
    D. Can include methylphenidate (Ritalin)

32. A patient with hypertension visits the psychiatric-mental health nurse practitioner and reports blisters along with reddish and purplish spots accompanied by fever. The clinical history of the patient involves alcohol addiction, excessive sleepiness, and bipolar depression. The nurse practitioner should ask if the patient takes:

    A. Armodafinil
    B. Carbamazepine
    C. Chlordiazepoxide
    D. Clonidine

33. A patient with a clinical history of attention deficit/hyperactivity disorder (ADHD) is diagnosed with Tourette's syndrome. The psychiatric-mental health nurse practitioner will prescribe:

    A. Amphetamine (D)
    B. Clonidine
    C. Methylphenidate (D, L)
    D. Haloperidol

34. A patient reports hallucinations, delusions, and disorganized speech and has been prescribed medications. The symptoms persist even after the psychiatric-mental health nurse practitioner switches to two different medications over time. The nurse practitioner prescribes another drug and informs the patient that this medication will require weekly monitoring for 6 months. The medication prescribed is:

    A. Bupropion (Wellbutrin)
    B. Memantine (Namenda)
    C. Armodafinil (Nuvigil)
    D. Clozapine (Clozaril)

35. A 5-year-old patient visits the clinic. The patient's parents report that the patient is restless and impulsive and has difficulty doing multiple tasks at a time. After evaluation, the psychiatric-mental health nurse practitioner suggests:

    A. Cognitive behavioral therapy
    B. Atomoxetine
    C. Honey and white rice in the diet
    D. Donepezil

36. An aspect of the consultation room of a psychiatric-mental health nurse practitioner that will provide therapeutic value to the patient is:

    A. A photograph of the nurse practitioner's family
    B. Comfortable furniture and ambient temperature
    C. Chairs placed directly across each other
    D. Soft instrumental music

37. When evaluating an adolescent patient for anxiety, it is important to also assess for:

   A. Agoraphobia
   B. Comorbidities
   C. Socioemotional deficiencies
   D. Separation anxiety

38. The psychiatric-mental health nurse practitioner plans to start carbamazepine (Tegretol) for a 25-year-old female patient with bipolar disorder. Pretreatment evaluation typically includes:

   A. Serum thyroid-stimulating hormone (TSH), blood urea nitrogen (BUN), serum creatinine, and urinalysis
   B. Fasting lipid profile and hemoglobin A1c
   C. Complete blood count (CBC), liver function tests, human chorionic gonadotropin (HCG level), and ECG
   D. No blood levels

39. A child is now able to sort objects according to characteristics such as shapes, types, color, or size, and whether objects are broken and can be fixed. The child can put things in order based on characteristics or criteria. The child can choose between options but is unable to use deductive reasoning, logic, or draw conclusions. According to Piaget, this cognitive ability indicates the child is in the stage called:

   A. Formal operational
   B. Concrete operational
   C. Preoperational
   D. Sensorimotor

40. A psychiatric-mental health nurse practitioner provides a discourse to influence identified plans and addresses other providers to use overlapping skills in order to enhance services. The advanced intervention referred to is:

   A. Milieu therapy
   B. Psychotherapy
   C. Consultation
   D. Prescriptive authority

41. During the physical examination of a newborn, the psychiatric-mental health nurse practitioner observes the infant puckering their lips when the nurse practitioner softly strokes the corner of the infant's mouth. Understanding developmental milestones, the nurse practitioner:

   A. Suspects delayed development
   B. Believes the infant is premature
   C. Continues with the assessment
   D. Orders a neurological consult

42. Neurocognitive disorders with rapid, insidious onset presenting with ataxia, memory loss, and behavior changes are seen in:

A. Down syndrome
B. Huntington's disease
C. Creutzfeldt–Jakob disease
D. Alzheimer's disease

43. According to Erikson's psychosocial stages, one pathological outcome seen in identity versus role confusion conflict is:

A. Midlife crisis
B. Despair
C. Schizoid personality
D. Delinquency

44. A patient's family member reports the patient having sudden-onset auditory hallucinations, tremors, and global disorientation that has been "off and on" for the past 24 hours. The nurse practitioner will evaluate for:

A. Frontal lobe trauma
B. Insomnia
C. Alzheimer's disease
D. Delirium

45. The patient has been diagnosed with Huntington's disease. The psychiatric-mental health nurse practitioner understands the etiology of this disease is:

A. Depletion of inhibitory neurotransmitter gamma-aminobutyric acid (GABA)
B. Low β-amyloid 42 and high tau and phosphorylated tau in cerebrospinal fluid
C. Poor reabsorption of cerebral spinal fluid with ventricle enlargement
D. Rapid eye movement (REM) sleep

46. The dopamine and serotonin level of the patient is lower than normal. The psychiatric–mental health nurse practitioner can assess the patient for:

A. Mania
B. Depression
C. Anxiety
D. Narcolepsy

47. When developing an intensive family intervention module for parents of a child who has begun displaying signs of depression and conflict with parents and who is overweight, the psychiatric-mental health nurse practitioner will build an interdisciplinary team that includes a social worker and a:

A. Family counselor
B. Registered nurse
C. Member of the clergy
D. Dietician/nutritionist

48. The patient is taking St. John's wort (Hypericum perforatum) and warfarin (Coumadin). The psychiatric-mental health nurse practitioner advises the patient to:

   A. Discontinue St. John's wort and monitor the patient's international normalized ratio (INR)
   B. Continue St. John's wort and monitor the patient's INR
   C. Continue St. John's wort and increase warfarin
   D. Discontinue St. John's wort and monitor for signs of bleeding

49. A patient reports being angry and resentful and losing their temper quite often. The psychiatric-mental health nurse practitioner observes the patient blaming others for their own temperament during psychotherapy. To reduce the aggressive symptoms, the patient is prescribed:

   A. Divalproex sodium (Depakote)
   B. Atomoxetine (Strattera)
   C. Paroxetine (Paxil)
   D. Lamotrigine (Lamictal)

50. A psychiatric-mental health nurse practitioner prescribes a drug to a patient with Alzheimer's disease. The drug, which works by inhibiting acetylcholinesterase, is:

   A. Donepezil (Aricept)
   B. Chlorpromazine (Thorazine)
   C. Carbamazepine (Tegretol)
   D. Clomipramine (Anafranil)

51. Neurons that regulate extrapyramidal movement and cognitive functions, especially motivation and reward associations, are due to:

   A. Volume loss of basolateral amygdala (BLA) gray matter
   B. Degeneration of dopaminergic neurons in substantia nigra pars compacta
   C. Dopaminergic neurons in the substantia nigra pars compacta and ventral tegmental area
   D. Hyperactive basolateral amygdala (BLA)

52. A 23-year-old patient is being treated for mania and has been prescribed valproic acid (Depakote). The patient reports loss of appetite, extreme fatigue, and nausea. The urine is dark, and the patient now is jaundiced. There are no other complaints or previous contributing history. Lab results are normal except for moderately elevated liver function tests. Based on the patient history, a possible diagnosis is:

   A. Choledocholithiasis
   B. Drug-induced liver injury
   C. Primary biliary cirrhosis
   D. Hereditary hemochromatosis

53. A patient reports anxiousness, restlessness, and loss of interest in everyday activities for 6 months. On the evaluation of blood reports, the patient's cortisol levels are found to be very high. The psychiatric-mental health nurse practitioner will recommend:

    A. Memantine (Namenda)
    B. Eszopiclone (Lunesta)
    C. Galantamine (Razadyne)
    D. Duloxetine (Cymbalta)

54. At a follow-up visit with a patient diagnosed with schizophrenia who is taking risperidone (Risperdal), it is discovered that the patient has gained 11.5 pounds (5.2 kilograms). To address the weight gain based on evidence, the psychiatric-mental health nurse practitioner will:

    A. Refer the patient to a nutritionist and exercise therapist with instructions to monitor weight on a weekly basis
    B. Provide instruction on proper nutrition, reduce the amount of risperidone taken daily, and provide a tracker for recording daily weight
    C. Add a combination herbal supplement for weight reduction and refer the patient to a personal trainer for daily exercise
    D. Educate the patient on the Dietary Approaches to Stop Hypertension (DASH) diet, include instruction on appropriate exercise, and set up monthly monitoring sessions

55. The psychiatric-mental health nurse practitioner is working on the hospice unit and assessing a patient. Upon examination, the nurse practitioner notes absence of motor responses, corneal reflexes, absent pupillary response to light, and no gag reflex. To confirm the assessment findings, the nurse will order a(n):

    A. ECG
    B. EEG
    C. Complete metabolic panel
    D. MRI of the brain

56. A patient treated with antipsychotics develops neuroleptic malignant syndrome (NMS) with muscle rigidity. The psychiatric-mental health nurse practitioner would expect abnormal laboratory values of:

    A. Elevated prolactin
    B. Elevated creatinine phosphokinase
    C. Low white blood cell count
    D. Low hemoglobin level/hematocrit

57. Essential factors that influence the therapeutic alliance and cannot be learned through training are:

    A. Strict adherence to treatment manual
    B. Circadian physiology
    C. Social rhythms
    D. Emotional style of the therapist

58. The psychiatric-mental health nurse practitioner is assisting patients who have been displaced due to devastation from a hurricane. The first step the nurse practitioner will take is to:

A. Employ a mobile crisis team
B. Refer patients to a board-and-care program
C. Set up a temporary multiservice center
D. Establish a partial hospitalization program

59. A 14-year-old patient comes into the office accompanied by parents with a chief complaint of recent changes in mood. Upon evaluation, the psychiatric–mental health nurse practitioner finds that the patient had a recent concussion while playing soccer. The nurse practitioner best demonstrates clinical decision making by:

A. Further evaluating the patient's mood changes in relation to their being a teenager
B. Employing evidence-based clinical practice guidelines about concussions to drive treatment
C. Referring the patient to a sports medicine specialist
D. Listening to the patient's parents to determine diagnosis and treatment

60. A 68-year-old patient presents to the office of a psychiatric-mental health nurse practitioner for treatment. The nurse practitioner demonstrates their role in patient advocacy by:

A. Ensuring that the patient has a trusted family member to discuss the treatment plan
B. Discussing with the patient's family member without the patient's consent
C. Disregarding information regarding a healthcare power of attorney
D. Prescribing medications without giving time for the patient to ask questions

61. An example of a selective serotonin reuptake inhibitor (SSRI) used to treat depression or anxiety is:

A. Aripiprazole (Abilify)
B. Alprazolam (Xanax)
C. Escitalopram (Lexapro)
D. Clonazepam (Klonopin)

62. The medical nurse practitioner at a nursing home has asked that a psychiatric-mental health nurse practitioner see a patient. The patient is 80-years-old with severe depression and is taking medications for cardiac arrhythmia and breast cancer. After an assessment, the psychiatric-mental health nurse practitioner decides to put the patient on escitalopram (Lexapro) because:

A. Escitalopram is the only FDA-approved medication for older adults
B. Escitalopram does not affect hepatic metabolizing enzymes and is less likely to cause drug interactions
C. Escitalopram is a strong CYP450 2D6 inhibitor of tamoxifen and limits drug interactions
D. Escitalopram has been associated with fewer falls in older adult patients

63. When working with a 9-year-old diagnosed with social anxiety disorder on building a FEAR plan, the second component the nurse practitioner will address is:

    A. Autonomy in decision making
    B. Expecting bad things to happen
    C. Identifying physical symptoms of arousal of anxiety
    D. Self-monitoring of expectations

64. Partnering as a method of skilled interviewing involves:

    A. Identification and acknowledgment of the patient's emotions
    B. Briefing of the patient's story at the interview's end
    C. Expression of commitment to the continued relationship
    D. Making the patient aware before moving to the next topic

65. A patient with hearing loss in one ear visits a psychiatric-mental health nurse practitioner after reporting symptoms of depression. During the clinical interview, the nurse practitioner will:

    A. Face the patient in good lighting
    B. Speak at a higher volume than usual
    C. Look down at papers while interviewing
    D. Explain the instructions verbally before closing

66. In an effort to build a trusting relationship with an adolescent patient who is concerned about confidentiality, the psychiatric-mental health nurse practitioner must practice:

    A. Justice
    B. Fidelity
    C. Veracity
    D. Paternalism

67. A patient visits the psychiatric-mental health nurse practitioner reporting severe restlessness and anxiety. The nurse practitioner observes that the patient is continuously scrubbing their hands and the table with sanitizing wipes. When asked about the behavior, the patient reports a fear of contamination and germs that makes them wash their hands repeatedly and change their clothes six to seven times a day. After a thorough examination and assessments, the nurse practitioner prescribes:

    A. Fluvoxamine (Luvox)
    B. Benztropine (Cogentin)
    C. Valproate (Depakote)
    D. Zopiclone (Imovane)

68. A patient loves to gamble and spends most of their time in a casino. The patient realizes the negative effects of gambling and the impact it has on their life. The patient comes to the psychiatric-mental health nurse practitioner and asks about ways to quit. The first response of the nurse practitioner should be to:

    A. Focus on patient's behaviors and attitude
    B. Be attentive in their behavior toward the patient
    C. Express empathy toward the patient
    D. Encourage the patient in independent problem solving

69. A patient visits the psychiatric-mental health nurse practitioner and reports feeling unmotivated to do even simple tasks. The patient is unable to differentiate left from right and relates experiencing near misses involving accidents. The lobes of the cerebral cortex that have faced disruptions are the:

    A. Frontal and temporal
    B. Temporal and occipital
    C. Frontal and parietal
    D. Parietal and occipital

70. A 67-year-old patient visits the clinic with their spouse, who reports that the patient feels lonely and sad most of the time and does not eat well. Upon further assessment, it is revealed that the couple's daughter passed away 3 months ago. The screening tool the psychiatric-mental health nurse practitioner will use to make an accurate diagnosis is the:

    A. Geriatric Depression Scale (GDS)
    B. Beck Depression Inventory (BDI)
    C. Strengths and Difficulties Questionaire (SDQ)
    D. Hospital Anxiety and Depression Scale (HADS)

71. An example of a positive behavior by a patient in recovery from an addiction would be:

    A. Spending time with old friends who are active substance users
    B. Revisiting places that the patient frequented when actively using
    C. Giving a lecture about the experience of recovery
    D. Calling in sick to a job when not physically ill

72. As complementary and alternative medicine, a nutrition plan for treating children with autism is:

    A. Dietary Approaches to Stop Hypertension (DASH)
    B. Gluten-free/casein-free (GFCF)
    C. Mediterranean diet plan
    D. Ketogenic diet plan

73. An adult patient is brought to the psychiatric-mental health nurse practitioner by their parents. The patient tells the nurse practitioner about having magical powers to make dead people alive by touching them. The nurse practitioner diagnoses:

    A. Erotomaniac delusion
    B. Nihilistic delusion
    C. Grandiose delusion
    D. Persecutory delusion

74. A patient diagnosed with delirium is admitted to the hospital. The psychiatric-mental health nurse practitioner prescribes a combination of:

    A. Ketamine and lorazepam
    B. Haloperidol with lorazepam
    C. Lithium and haloperidol
    D. Amitriptyline and haloperidol

75. A 72-year-old patient presents with early dementia with Lewy bodies. The patient is showing signs of depression. The assessment tool the nurse practitioner will use is the:

    A. Saint Louis University Mental Status Examination (SLUMS)
    B. Cornell Scale for Depression (CSDD)
    C. Rating Anxiety in Dementia (RAID)
    D. Hamilton Rating Scale for Depression (HAM-D)

76. The psychiatric-mental health nurse practitioner is interviewing a patient with suicidal ideation. To know if the patient is suffering from hopelessness, the nurse practitioner should ask if the patient:

    A. Faces issues regarding problem solving
    B. Has become addicted to drugs or alcohol
    C. Feels like a burden on others
    D. Has developed a feeling of isolation

77. A risk factor for obsessive-compulsive personality disorder is:

    A. Being of female sex
    B. Having a first-degree relative with obsessive-compulsive personality disorder
    C. Having a first-degree relative with schizophrenia
    D. Lacking discipline in the family

78. While the nurse practitioner is working the FEAR plan with a 12-year-old patient with social anxiety disorder, the patient successfully engages with a stranger during the initial exposure phase. After assessing the patient's anxiety level and implementing coping strategies, the nurse practitioner determines that the patient is ready for the next move on the hierarchy of anxiety-provoking situations. The next step that would be appropriate for this stage of exposure is:

    A. Accompanying the patient into an elevator full of people
    B. Encouraging the parents to take the patient on a short shopping trip
    C. Having the child initiate a conversation with children on the playground
    D. Including the patient in a sports activity at the local community center

79. When monitoring an infant with suspected fetal alcohol syndrome (FAS), the measurement that is critical in assessing appropriate development is:

    A. Body length
    B. Body mass
    C. Awareness
    D. Head circumference

80. The FDA warning of potential life-threatening drug reactions as a possible side effect of lamotrigine (Lamictal) includes:

    A. Hemophagocytic lymphohistiocytosis and Stevens-Johnson syndrome
    B. Drug reaction with eosinophilia and systemic symptoms
    C. Persistent pulmonary hypertension of the newborn
    D. Dangerous abnormalities in the electrical activity of the heart

81. A medical emergency associated with the use of monoamine oxidase inhibitors (MAOIs) is:

    A. Neuroleptic malignant syndrome
    B. Stevens–Johnson syndrome
    C. Hypertensive crisis
    D. Priapism

82. A patient reports feeling "foggy" and extremely tired and has gained approximately 15 pounds over the course of the past 3 months. When assessing for depressive disorder, the psychiatric-mental health nurse practitioner will rule out:

    A. Hypo-hyperthyroidism
    B. Hypertension
    C. Cardiomyopathy
    D. Blood dyscrasias

83. When working with a 13-year-old on building a FEAR plan, the first component the nurse practitioner will address is:

    A. Expecting bad things to happen
    B. Identifying helpful attitudes and actions
    C. Identifying physical symptoms of arousal of anxiety
    D. Self-rating and self-reward

84. A patient presenting to the emergency department with chest pain and prolonged QRS waves on ECG has a reported history of taking "something for depression." The patient denies using any other medications. With no history of substance use, the psychiatric-mental health nurse practitioner suspects that the antidepressant the patient uses is:

    A. Escitalopram (Lexapro)
    B. Vilazodone (Viibryd)
    C. Trazodone (Desyrel)
    D. Imipramine (Tofranil)

85. A 14-year-old patient presents to the emergency department after attempting suicide. The parents report that the child has been easily frustrated lately and has had issues with impulse control. During the initial interview, the patient reports feeling extremely sad since their favorite actor committed suicide and experiencing sudden urges to harm themselves. The psychiatric-mental health nurse practitioner will determine treatment based on the scientific finding in this age group known as:

    A. Immature prefrontal cortex
    B. Damaged hippocampus
    C. Disconnect in cingulate cortex
    D. Underdeveloped amygdala

86. The court appoints a court-trained volunteer guardian for patients who are:

   A. In restraint or secluded from others
   B. Incompetent in making treatment-related decisions
   C. Going through electroconvulsive therapies
   D. Afraid that their right to confidentiality is being violated

87. In order to diagnose attention deficit/hyperactivity disorder (ADHD), symptoms must include hyperactivity and impulsivity that is:

   A. Inconsistent with the developmental stage
   B. Consistent with the developmental stage
   C. Able to be self-controlled
   D. Resulting in physical harm to self or others

88. The psychiatric-mental health nurse practitioner realizes that a patient poses a danger to self and others. The nurse practitioner will:

   A. Inform the patient's family and staff members
   B. Protect the confidentiality of the patient
   C. Ask the patient to try to stay calm
   D. Discontinue the treatment of the patient

89. The doctrine that guides the psychiatric-mental health nurse practitioner's legal responsibility to educate the patient about the risks and benefits of treatment to allow the patient to make informed decisions about accepting care is:

   A. Confidentiality
   B. Signature form
   C. Health Insurance Portability and Accountability Act of 1996 (HIPAA)
   D. Informed consent

90. A mental status exam for a patient diagnosed with early dementia will include:

   A. Intact orientation
   B. Impaired short-term memory
   C. Hallucinations
   D. Incoherent speech

91. A 30-year-old patient visits a psychiatric-mental health nurse practitioner to report that they are becoming very short tempered with other people and have a tendency to break things. The patient reports an adverse childhood. Past history includes the patient experiencing sexual abuse at the hands of their father after the father's binge drinking episodes. The nurse practitioner understands the patient is at increased risk for:

   A. Conduct disorder
   B. Obsessive–compulsive personality disorder
   C. Oppositional defiant disorder
   D. Intermittent explosive disorder

92. A psychiatric-mental health nurse practitioner believes that the cause of a patient's clinical depression is conflicts with their spouse. The nurse practitioner advises the patient to work on communication with the spouse to improve their relationship. This approach is part of the therapy known as:

    A. Aversion
    B. Behavioral
    C. Interpersonal
    D. Psychoanalytic

93. In Erikson's psychosocial stages, the conflict where the pathological outcome may be schizoid personality is:

    A. Industry versus inferiority
    B. Identity versus role confusion
    C. Intimacy versus isolation
    D. Generativity versus stagnation

94. Another name for assisted inpatient psychiatric treatment is:

    A. Conditional release
    B. Emergency commitment
    C. Involuntary commitment
    D. Unconditional release

95. An adolescent patient visits the psychiatric-mental health nurse practitioner's clinic. The patient is experiencing severe depression, and the mental state of the patient is adversely affecting the family. The patient acknowledges the parents' struggle to give the patient a better life. The nurse practitioner advises family therapy and starts a session by suggesting that the patient:

    A. Join family dinners even if just to sit at the dinner table
    B. Stop engaging in family activities when they are sad
    C. Skip antidepressant medication when they start feeling better
    D. Refrain from sharing their feelings with the family

96. The psychiatric-mental health nurse practitioner teaches good sleep hygiene practices that include:

    A. Exercising before bed
    B. Taking naps during the day
    C. Drinking alcohol before bed
    D. Keeping the bedroom cool

97. Behavior therapy focuses on:

    A. Learning through interacting with the environment
    B. Dealing with problems in a positive manner
    C. Developing a stronger and healthier sense of self
    D. Achieving congruence through the self-concept

98. The 6-year-old patient's chief complaint is inattention. Attention deficit disorder is suspected. The factors the nurse practitioner needs to consider when making differential diagnoses include absence of oppositional or defiant behavior, defiance, factors that may be related to medication, a general medical condition, symptoms of hyperactivity/impulsivity, and the:

A. Length of time the symptom is reported, impact on function in more than one setting, and age of onset
B. Presence of episodic irritability, aggression, and grandiosity in the patient
C. Fact that the patient cannot soothe when angry, rages for hours, and is internally distracted
D. Patient's chronic irritable mood, with frequent explosive outbursts in more than one setting

99. A patient comes to the psychiatric-mental health nurse practitioner's office for the first time and wants advice about family problems. The patient states that the problems are affecting work life and suddenly begins crying. The nurse practitioner should:

A. Ask the patient to stop crying and place a box of tissues near the patient
B. Let the patient cry for some time and then discuss the issues after the patient settles
C. Ask the patient to go outside to cry for some time and then return
D. Let the patient cry and comfort the patient with a hug after some time

100. The medication associated with a reduction in suicide and suicidal attempts for patients diagnosed with bipolar disorder and major depression is:

A. Lamotrigine (Lamictal)
B. Lithium (Eskalith)
C. Carbamazepine (Tegretol)
D. Valproate (Depakote)

101. The most toxic drug used in the treatment of acute mania in bipolar disorder is:

A. Lurasidone (Latuda)
B. Cariprazine (Vraylar)
C. Lithium (Lithobid)
D. Lamotrigine (Lamictal)

102. Without the presence of external life stressors or precipitants, changes in the autonomic nervous system giving rise to sleeplessness, restlessness, despondency, irritability, and a loss of appetite are known as:

A. Atypical features
B. Major depressive disorder
C. Hypomania
D. Psychotic features

103. A failure of professional judgment when a direct provider–patient relationship exists that results in injury, loss, or damage is:

    A. Dereliction of duty
    B. Duty of care
    C. Malpractice
    D. Abandonment

104. After determining that a patient is stable for discharge, the psychiatric-mental health nurse practitioner meets with the patient. The nurse practitioner provides psychoeducation to the patient, who is bilingual, regarding discharge medications and provides current academic research on clinical results for medications. Initially, the patient demonstrates interest in receiving the information. As the nurse practitioner continues to review the clinical data, the patient does not appear to be paying attention. The patient begins to avoid eye contact, does not have any questions, and does not review the discharge instructions or the literature. The most likely reason for the changes in the patient's behavior is that the:

    A. Materials are not written in the patient's language
    B. Patient is unable to read
    C. Materials are not written at a third- to fifth-grade level
    D. Patient is responding to internal stimuli

105. A 70-year-old patient being treated for Parkinson's disease reports reduced appetite, lack of interest in food and drink, fatigue, and dizziness. Upon assessment, purpura is noticed on the lower extremities. The nurse practitioner will first conduct an additional assessment for:

    A. Constipation
    B. Jaundice
    C. Medication
    D. Dementia

106. When developing a treatment plan for a patient with generalized anxiety disorder, the intervention the psychiatric-mental health nurse practitioner includes as a complementary treatment is:

    A. Systematic desensitization/exposure therapy
    B. Electroconvulsive therapy
    C. Transcranial magnetic stimulation
    D. Meditation

107. The family member of a patient with schizophrenia reports the patient has started to show signs of depression and has become apathetic and unmotivated. The psychiatric-mental health nurse practitioner will assess how the patient's medication is affecting the system called:

    A. Mesolimbic
    B. Mesocortical
    C. Nigrostriatal
    D. Tuberoinfundibular

108. While the psychiatric-mental health nurse practitioner is evaluating an older adult patient from a differing culture, the patient's family offers a cultural explanation describing memory loss and confusion. To further assess this patient, the nurse practitioner determines that the most appropriate test is the:

    A. Mini-Cog
    B. Mini Mental Status Exam (MMSE)
    C. Four-object recall
    D. Months backward test

109. The medication to be given to reverse hypotension and respiratory depression in a patient who has overdosed on an opioid is:

    A. Buprenorphine
    B. Methadone
    C. Naproxen
    D. Naloxone

110. A phenomenon in psychotherapy in which a patient directs painful or angry feelings toward the psychiatric-mental health nurse practitioner is:

    A. Positive transference
    B. Positive countertransference
    C. Negative transference
    D. Boundary violations

111. The behavior that is responsible when a patient accepts an intervention and then resists the tasks given by the psychiatric-mental health nurse practitioner is:

    A. Negative countertransference
    B. Negative transference
    C. Positive transference
    D. Positive countertransference

112. To diagnose attention deficit/hyperactivity disorder (ADHD), symptoms of hyperactivity and impulsivity must:

    A. Include a pattern of angry/irritable mood and argumentative behavior
    B. Be accompanied by symptoms of hostility and defiance
    C. Negatively impact functioning and cause distress for the patient
    D. Not cause functional difficulty or impairment in functioning

113. A patient with anger management issues visits the psychiatric-mental health nurse practitioner. During the interview, it is revealed that the patient uses an herb given by a traditional healer of their culture. The patient believes the herb is calming during times of anger and aggression. The nurse practitioner knows that this herb can cause cognitive impairment. The nurse practitioner will:

    A. Encourage the patient to continue using the herb while trying to manage the harmful effects by prescribing an additional medication
    B. Tell the patient to stop taking the herb and not begin conventional treatments until the patient does so
    C. Educate the patient that the herb is harmful and then leave decisions around usage of the herb completely up to the patient
    D. Negotiate with the patient to reduce the quantity and pattern of herb usage in a way that will bring the patient less harm

114. A medical emergency associated with the use of antipsychotics is:

    A. Serotonin syndrome
    B. Neuroleptic malignant syndrome
    C. Stevens–Johnson syndrome
    D. Hypertensive crisis

115. A patient reports sleep disturbances that the psychiatric-mental health nurse practitioner has determined to be sleep fragmentation. After assessing medications and comorbidities, the nurse practitioner will order an EEG to evaluate for:

    A. Loss of awareness during transition between stage 1 (N1) and stage 2 (N2) sleep
    B. Amount of time between wakefulness and rapid eye movement (REM) stage of sleep
    C. Neurophysiologic changes noting transition through non-rapid eye movement (NREM) and REM sleep
    D. Molecular changes in brain chemistry during stage 3 (N3) delta sleep

116. A comprehensive health history should be done for:

    A. New patients
    B. Patients seeking treatment for chronic illness
    C. Patients seeking treatment for particular conditions
    D. Patients visiting frequently for routine check-ups

117. The psychiatric-mental health nurse practitioner protects the confidential information provided by a patient. In doing so, the nurse practitioner is following the ethical principle of:

    A. Beneficence
    B. Nonmaleficence
    C. Justice
    D. Veracity

118. A patient visits the psychiatric-mental health nurse practitioner, who notices that the patient rushes into the room. Suddenly, the patient begins sipping from the nurse practitioner's coffee cup. During the clinical interview, the patient laughs constantly and points to a coat rack, asking if it is a bear. The nurse practitioner prescribes a classical microdialysis test to assess an alteration in the level of the neurotransmitter:

     A. Serotonin
     B. Hypocretin
     C. Norepinephrine
     D. Acetylcholine

119. The 6-year-old child of a patient who recently completed suicide is withdrawing from friends and family and has refused to come out of their bedroom or eat meals. The psychiatric-mental health nurse practitioner schedules the child for psychoeducational therapy to begin focusing on:

     A. Stress reduction
     B. Normalization
     C. Social skills
     D. Grief processes

120. To diagnose attention deficit/hyperactivity disorder (ADHD), consistent symptoms of inattention must be present in at least two of three domains. The domains are academic, social, and:

     A. Physical
     B. Occupational
     C. Behavioral
     D. Cognitive

121. The psychiatric-mental health nurse practitioner is treating a patient with substance use disorder. There is a family history of substance use disorders. The genotype that has been linked to opioid dependence is:

     A. G allele genotype in the A118G SNP of *OPRM1*
     B. Opioid receptor mu 1 (*OPRM1*) genotype
     C. Human leukocyte antigen *HLA-B*57:01 allele.
     D. Amyloid precursor protein (*APP*), presenilin-1 (*PSEN1*), and presenilin-2 (*PSEN2*).

122. According to Peplau, the phase that includes a patient-nurse meeting in which the purpose of the therapy is decided is the phase called:

     A. Preorientation
     B. Orientation
     C. Working
     D. Termination

123. Humanistic psychotherapy differs from other psychotherapies because it focuses on:

    A. Objective experiences of the patient
    B. Overall needs of a human being
    C. Past experiences more than the present
    D. Only one diagnosed issue objectively

124. In the clinic, the psychiatric-mental health nurse practitioner is often asked about how a new antipsychotic drug compares with an older antipsychotic drug in treating patients with bipolar disorder. As per the PICOT format of the question, patient forms the:

    A. P element
    B. I element
    C. C element
    D. O element

125. A 10-year-old boy visits the psychiatric-mental health nurse practitioner with his parents. The parents report that the patient has been very quiet and does not let the parents know when he is sad or angry. They have witnessed issues of social anxiety increasing day by day and have noticed that the patient does not have any friends. The parents say that the patient's uncle suffers from schizophrenia. While assessing the patient by asking him some questions, the nurse practitioner notes that the patient being a boy is a risk factor for the disorder the patient may have. The nurse practitioner is assessing the patient for the personality disorder known as:

    A. Paranoid
    B. Histrionic
    C. Narcissistic
    D. Avoidant

126. The psychiatric-mental health nurse practitioner is practicing within ethical standards of practice and protecting patient rights when:

    A. Disclosing the medical diagnosis to the patient's adult child
    B. Checking a hospitalized friend's medical records for test results
    C. Sending a deceased patient's medical records to an attorney upon request
    D. Participating in interprofessional meetings about treatment

127. An example of how the psychiatric-mental health nurse practitioner can act as an advocate is:

    A. Continuing education
    B. Preceptorship
    C. Participating in the American Psychiatric Nurses Association
    D. Publishing research

128. A psychiatric-mental health nurse practitioner is performing a clinical interview with a patient with depression. To know whether the patient is experiencing impaired coping, the nurse practitioner should ask if the:

    A. Patient feels rejected and not good enough
    B. Patient feels angry at a greater power
    C. Patient's sexual pattern has changed
    D. Patient's problem-solving skills have deteriorated

129. The differential diagnosis for a pediatric patient with a history of group A streptococcal (GAS) infection with sudden anxiety attacks, temper tantrums, new-onset hyperactivity with obsessive-compulsive behaviors, and occasional tics includes:

    A. Neuropsychiatric lupus
    B. Anxiety disorder due to another medical condition
    C. Pediatric acute-onset neuropsychiatric syndrome
    D. Obsessive–compulsive disorder

130. To reduce risk-taking behaviors in adolescent patients experiencing peer pressure, a first-line approach to mental health promotion by the psychiatric-mental health nurse practitioner will include:

    A. Peer level education programs
    B. Coaching on assertiveness
    C. Setting positive examples
    D. Community youth activities

131. A psychiatric–mental health nurse practitioner learns from a blood test report that a patient's cortisol level is lower than normal. The nurse practitioner will assess the patient for:

    A. Schizophrenia
    B. Posttraumatic stress disorder
    C. Anorexia nervosa
    D. Major depressive disorder

132. A patient with chronic anxiety issues visits the psychiatric-mental health nurse practitioner. The patient has panic attacks. She experienced sexual abuse during childhood and sometimes recalls the incidents during the sessions; however, the patient denies that the recollection of sexual abuse bothers her. The patient reports being unable to perform daily tasks like showering or grocery shopping due to low energy levels. The patient has gained 20 pounds and sleeps for a major part of the day. Her son has recently moved to another city for college. The nurse practitioner's first priority should be reducing the:

    A. Potential for panic attacks
    B. Depression-related symptoms
    C. Trauma of the childhood abuse
    D. Impact of the son leaving home

133. The most common underlying contributing factor that the psychiatric-mental health nurse practitioner evaluates for in a patient being monitored after a suicide attempt is:

    A. Chronic history of deliberate self-harm
    B. Presence of a psychiatric disorder
    C. Loss of a family member
    D. Physical illness

134. Based on the standards of practice, the psychiatric-mental health nurse practitioner:

    A. Identifies outcomes only by their own expectations
    B. Verifies issues only with individual patients
    C. Engages alone in patients' culturally sensitive data collection
    D. Prioritizes data collection based on patient condition

135. A 16-year-old patient experiencing posttraumatic stress disorder (PTSD) visits a psychiatric-mental health nurse practitioner. The patient's symptoms appeared 2 years ago after the patient witnessed the death of their best friend in a car crash. The patient has difficulty concentrating in school, remains isolated and disconnected from friends and family, and continues to have visualizations of the incident, making it difficult for the patient to sleep. The intervention that the nurse practitioner would recommend is to:

    A. Electrically stimulate the brain
    B. Provide a role model
    C. Provide worksheets and assignments
    D. Ask the patient to regularly check vitals

136. An example of a violation of the mental health patient's bill of rights is:

    A. Providing the patient with a written treatment plan for the next 10 days with no review or reassessment needed
    B. Completing a treatment plan without the patient's input for a patient who has been committed by court order
    C. Restraining a patient brought to the emergency department who is threatening to harm the staff
    D. Allowing the patient to review treatment plans and other documents in the medical record

137. Ziprasidone (Geodon) can cause ECG changes, including:

    A. QT interval prolongation
    B. Prominent U waves, premature ventricular contractions, T wave and ST-segment changes, and ventricular arrhythmias
    C. Lengthening of the PR, QRS, and QT intervals
    D. Depression of the sinus node

138. A new psychiatric-mental health nurse practitioner joins a hosital. The healthcare management team provides an orientation to explain ways of creating a healthy work environment. The orienting nurse practitioner can explain the importance of:

    A. Prioritizing work over life outside of work
    B. Using interpersonal development opportunities
    C. Recognizing management for achievements
    D. Qualifying as chief nursing officer

139. The best research work or study to use as evidence contains:

    A. Research that has been peer-reviewed
    B. Opinions of experts
    C. Qualitative research
    D. Randomized control trials

140. A patient with vascular dementia has begun demonstrating panic attacks and expressing increased worry about family members. The assessment tool the psychiatric-mental health nurse practitioner will use is:

    A. Saint Louis University Mental Status Examination (SLUMS)
    B. Cornell Scale for Depression (CSDD)
    C. Rating Anxiety in Dementia (RAID)
    D. Hamilton Rating Scale for Depression (HAM-D)

141. The overall goal of youth treatment programs such as the "Coping Cat" is to:

    A. Eliminate all stressors causing anxiety
    B. Recognize signs of internal stress
    C. Recognize stressors and implement coping strategies
    D. Develop alliances with youth and parents to manage stress

142. An patient with Alzheimer's disease has been prescribed donepezil (Aricept). The patient feels sick and has diarrhea and nausea. The appropriate action of the nurse practitioner will be to:

    A. Reduce the dose of the same drug
    B. Replace the drug with a new drug
    C. Augment the drug with a similar drug
    D. Prescribe rivastigmine along with the drug

143. When monitoring pediatric patients for bullying, it is important to recognize that girls are more likely than boys to use:

    A. Physical aggression
    B. Relational aggression
    C. Verbal abuse
    D. Cyberbullying

144. Echoing is a skilled interviewing technique that involves:

    A. Asking questions eliciting "yes" or "no" responses

    B. Repeating the last words of the patient

    C. Offering multiple choices for answering

    D. Asking leading questions

145. To attain good mental health, achieve healthy outcomes, and respond to stress, children develop a coping mechanism known as:

    A. Resilience

    B. Normalization

    C. Invincibility fables

    D. Protective factors

146. A 65-year-old patient comes into the office for an initial visit with the psychiatric-mental health nurse practitioner. Upon assessment, the nurse practitioner diagnoses the patient with generalized anxiety disorder and recommends medication treatment. To adhere to medical decision-making guidelines, prior to prescribing the patient medications, the nurse practitioner should:

    A. Telling the patient not to worry and that everything is going to be all right

    B. Review all pertinent data regarding the patient's history

    C. Prescribe the medication if the patient's spouse agrees

    D. Provide the patient with a list of possible treatments and have the patient decide which to initiate

147. To promote mental health in children, it is important that there is:

    A. Secure attachment through emotional bonds

    B. Progress in developmental stages

    C. Identification of protective factors for disorders

    D. Support of invincibility in adolescents

148. A patient visits the psychiatric-mental health nurse practitioner with symptoms of schizophrenia. The nurse practitioner prescribes two first-generation antipsychotics; one is the antagonist of the D2 receptor for dopamine, and the other is the antagonist of the H1 receptor for histamine. The nurse practitioner will assess for:

    A. Urinary retention, constipation, and dizziness

    B. Weight gain, hyptension, and priapism

    C. Sedation, acute dystonia, and akathisia

    D. Dry mouth, blurred vision, and ejaculatory dysfunction

149. A psychiatric-mental health nurse practitioner has a deeply religious belief system and believes everyone needs the support of a church for their survival. The nurse practitioner is working with an agnostic patient. In the therapeutic relationship with the patient, the nurse understands the differences in the beliefs and values held between them. The nurse continues to serve the patient well, and this behavior of the nurse is a result of:

  A. Self-awareness,
  B. Values
  C. Beliefs
  D. Supervision

150. The psychiatric-mental health nurse practitioner is reviewing autopsy results for a 70-year-old patient with Alzheimer's disease. The report notes that the brain has diffuse atrophy with flattened cortical sulci, enlarged ventricles, and neurofibrillary tangles. The microscopic examination of the brain most likely also shows:

  A. Senile plaques
  B. Argentophyllic globes
  C. Parenchymal lesions
  D. Arteriosclerotic plaques

151. A patient reports hopelessness, suicidal thoughts, and extreme lethargy. The psychiatric-mental health nurse practitioner would prescribe:

  A. Serotonin and norepinephrine reuptake inhibitor
  B. Benzodiazepine
  C. Dopamine receptor antagonist
  D. Anticholinergic

152. Vilazodone (Viibryd) belongs to a class of drugs known as:

  A. Serotonin partial agonist and reuptake inhibitors
  B. Tricyclic antidepressants
  C. Serotonin-norepinephrine reuptake inhibitors
  D. Serotonin antagonists and reuptake inhibitors

153. During the first session with a patient to address treatment, the psychiatric–mental health nurse practitioner discusses with the patient the risks and benefits of various alternatives of psychotropic medications, the treatment plan goals, and the alterations in the treatment plan. The nurse practitioner is nurturing the therapeutic alliance through:

  A. Setting limits or boundaries
  B. Shared decision making
  C. Self-identification as the expert
  D. Creating a safety plan

154. According to the cultural beliefs and values of Western culture, the family members of a patient will think that the patient:

A. Should have information and make decisions related to care

B. Should stay in bed and be cared for by family members

C. Suffers from disease due to lack of harmony between the patient's body and the environment

D. Can be healed only if traditional healers are appointed and traditional remedies are used

155. The psychiatric-mental health nurse practitioner is evaluating an older adult patient being treated with a selective serotonin reuptake inhibitor (SSRI) for major depressive disorder who reports headache, nausea, vomiting, lethargy, and disorientation. While reviewing the patient's laboratory results, the nurse practitioner expects to see:

A. Sodium level of 148 mEq/L

B. Sodium level of 132 mEq/L

C. Potassium level of 3.2 mmol/L

D. Potassium level of 5.5 mmol/L

156. A patient presents with depression that has been treated for >5 years with several antidepressants. The patient states that although the medication seems to work for a month or two, it quickly stops and the patient becomes even more depressed than before. Upon assessment, the psychiatric–mental health nurse practitioner notes symptoms of sad mood, crying, insomnia, irritability, and lack of motivation and energy. The patient was started on bupropion (Wellbutrin) most recently, but symptoms returned after 1 month. The patient then stopped taking medications altogether. The depression symptoms appear to be cyclic for the patient. The nurse practitioner decides the best course of treatment is to:

A. Start a different, newer antidepressant and send the patient for therapy

B. Start a mood stabilizer and have the patient monitor their mood

C. Send the patient for therapy and start an antipsychotic medication

D. Send the patient for an ECG and start a new antidepressant

157. A patient presents to the emergency department with a disheveled appearance, reporting weight loss, slowed thinking, and an overall feeling of apathy. Upon assessment, the psychiatric-mental health nurse practitioner observes affective flattening alogia, as well as red eyes and slowed reaction time. The nurse practitioner further evaluates for differential diagnosis between schizophrenia and:

A. Substance use disorder

B. Hyperthyroidism

C. General anxiety disorder

D. Temporal lobe epilepsy

158. A personal characteristic not required by the nurse practitioner for establishing a therapeutic relationship with a patient is:

    A. Genuineness
    B. Empathy
    C. Positive regard
    D. Sympathy

159. A patient with a long history of bipolar disorder with psychosis is currently taking risperidone (Risperdal) 4 mg daily and lamotrigine (Lamictal) 50 mg daily. The patient reports high irritability and has gained 50 pounds over the last year. Laboratory results reveal a fasting triglyceride level of 203 mg/dL. The psychiatric-mental health nurse practitioner's treatment plan is to:

    A. Stop the lamotrigine and redraw labs in a week
    B. Increase the risperidone to 8 mg daily and schedule a follow-up visit for a week later
    C. Taper the risperidone over 2 or 3 months and redraw labs in 3 months
    D. Admit the patient for testing and start new medications

160. A 68-year-old patient reports new-onset olfactory hallucinations with anxiety and confusion. The nurse practitioner's differential diagnoses include general medical conditions, substance intoxication, substance withdrawal, delirium, previous psychiatric history, and:

    A. History of visual impairment or cataracts
    B. Schizoaffective disorder
    C. Intellectual or cognitive impairment
    D. Temporal lobe epilepsy

161. According to the American Nurses Association (ANA), the definition of cultural knowledge is:

    A. The integration of expertise and skills into practice when a nurse practitioner is assessing, communicating, and providing care for members of their own social or ethnic group
    B. An expected and measurable level of nursing performance that integrates knowledge, skills, abilities, and judgment based on established scientific knowledge and expectations for nursing practice
    C. The integrated enactment of knowledge, skills, values, and attitudes that define working together across professions
    D. The concepts and language of an ethnic or social group used to describe their health-related values, beliefs, and traditional practices, as well as the etiologies of their conditions, preferred treatments, and any contraindications for treatments or pharmacological interventions

162. Psychiatric patients may require hospitalization for observation against their will. The criterion for involuntary hospitalization is that:

   A. The patient is a risk to themselves and others
   B. The patient is a risk to themselves
   C. The patient is a risk to others
   D. Determination has been made by judicial hearing

163. A patient's request to refuse treatment can be denied when:

   A. The patient is brought into the emergency department by a family member
   B. As an inpatient, the patient has a history of making irrational decisions
   C. The patient's commitment has been court ordered
   D. The patient is participating in a research trial for medication

164. The patient is a 20-year-old sexual assault survivor with a high Adverse Childhood Experiences (ACE) score. The best type of psychotherapy for this patient is:

   A. Cognitive behavioral
   B. Trauma informed
   C. Psychodynamic
   D. Dialectical behavior

165. A patient with problems in their marriage visits the psychiatric-mental health nurse practitioner. The patient tells the nurse that they have had conflicts in their marriage before, but they used to figure out the solutions themselves. However, this time, the spouse of the patient has started bringing their best friend into every fight to direct any communication toward the patient. The patient explains that they feel uncomfortable due to the spouse's friend's interventions. This situation is an example of:

   A. Triangulation
   B. Modeling
   C. Cross-generational coalition
   D. Covert coalition

166. The psychiatric-mental health nurse practitioner is assessing a 6-year-old patient who is cognitively impaired, makes poor eye contact, and does not interact socially with peers. The patient was born with spina bifida that required surgery. The patient's mother reports taking medications for a seizure disorder and depression while pregnant. The medication the nurse practitioner suspects the patient's mother was taking during pregnancy was:

   A. Folate
   B. Paroxetine
   C. Lamotrigine
   D. Valproate

167. A patient visits the clinic and reports frequent coughing with mild breathing difficulty. During the clinical interview, the patient reports being addicted to cigarette smoking and feeling agitated, nauseous, and restless whenever trying to give up smoking. After evaluation, the psychiatric-mental health nurse practitioner recommends:

    A. Naltrexone
    B. Clonidine
    C. Nalmefene
    D. Varenicline

168. An example of a paradoxical reaction is when a patient:

    A. Sleeps for 10 hours after the administration of zolpidem (Ambien)
    B. Wakes from an unconscious state after the administration of zolpidem (Ambien)
    C. Experiences sedation after the administration of lorazepam (Ativan)
    D. Experiences drowsiness after the administration of disulfiram (Antabuse)

169. The psychiatric-mental health nurse practitioner is conducting a follow-up assessment on a patient recently discharged after inpatient treatment for bipolar disorder. The patient's Global Assessment of Functioning (GAF) score at admission was 36. During today's visit, the nurse practitioner will determine the most updated functional status of the patient by using the tool called the:

    A. Beck Depression Inventory (BDI)
    B. Hamilton Anxiety Rating Scale
    C. World Health Organization Disability Assessment Schedule (WHODAS)
    D. Conners Rating Scale

170. The psychiatric-mental health nurse practitioner is evaluating a 13-year-old patient. The parent states, "He has tantrums like a 6-year-old. When he is not having tantrums, he is just angry at the world. He's lost most of his friends. He has been like this for the past 2 years, and it is just getting worse." In order to rule out mood disorders with overlapping clinical symptoms, the nurse practitioner asks:

    A. "Have your child's mood problems been episodic?"
    B. "Has your child ever shown physical aggression toward animals?"
    C. "Has there been any suspected abuse of your child?"
    D. "Are there any difficulties with distraction or hyperactivity?"

171. The psychiatric-mental health nurse practitioner is treating a patient who comes to the office with multiple bruises. The patient admits to being abused often by their spouse. The patient is depressed and would benefit from medication, but refuses because the spouse does not believe in medication. The statement that supports the nurse practitioner's duty to respect the patient's autonomy is:

    A. "The medication is good for you. You can hide it from your spouse."
    B. "I understand and respect your decision. Please contact the office when you are ready to follow medical recommendations."
    C. "Why don't you bring your spouse to the office to discuss what is going on at home?"
    D. "I understand. Let's make another appointment next week. I would like to check in with you."

172. To differentiate between bulimia and binge eating disorder, the psychiatric-mental health nurse practitioner will ask the patient:

    A. "Do you eat to the point of feeling too full and then feel as if you may vomit?"
    B. "Do you feel bad about yourself or have feelings of guilt after eating?"
    C. "After eating, have you ever attempted to get rid of the food by vomiting or taking laxatives?"
    D. "Have you ever felt as if your eating was out of control, or that eating controlled your life?"

173. The statement that indicates that a patient is in the maintenance phase of change is:

    A. "I don't need help. I am not perfect, but my drinking is not a problem."
    B. "I would like to get help. I know I need to stop drinking. I am trying to figure it out."
    C. "I have been sober for 4 months. Every day is a battle, but I am going to meetings."
    D. "I am better, sober for 9 months. I am afraid I could relapse; I need help."

174. A patient presents with hyperverbal speech, sexual indiscretions, flight of ideas, and decreased need for sleep. The patient also reports extended periods of low mood, anhedonia, weight loss, lack of concentration, and feelings of excessive guilt. In order to rule out the first differential diagnosis associated with these symptoms, the psychiatric-mental health nurse practitioner must ask the patient:

    A. "Do your friends ever tell you that you are talking too fast?"
    B. "Have you had periods where you are snapping at people?"
    C. "How long have you had these symptoms?"
    D. "Are you easily distracted?"

175. After a patient reports feeling anxious and experiencing nausea at the first medication follow-up visit, the psychiatric-mental health nurse practitioner assesses the patient's medications. The nurse practitioner will say:

    A. "Have there been improvements in your emotional state since your last visit?"
    B. "Please supply a list of side effects from all of the medications you take."
    C. "What herbal and vitamin supplements and over-the-counter medications do you take?"
    D. "Over-the-counter medications are not regulated. They may be dangerous, and you should not take them."

Practice Exam 2 Answers

1. B) 18 months to 3 years

According to Freud, the age at which a child learns independence and control is 18 months to 3 years and is the anal stage. Birth to 18 months is the oral stage; 3 to 6 years is the phallic stage and 6 to 12 years is the genital stage.

2. A) 3.0 mEq/L

A patient with bulimia nervosa will often present with hypokalemia due to vomiting, abuse of laxatives, and/or use of diuretics. Signs of hypokalemia include muscle weakness, fatigue, and cardiac dysrhythmias. A value of 3.0 mEq/L would be considered mild hypokalemia and may be corrected with dietary supplementation of potassium-containing foods or oral potassium supplements. Normal potassium levels are 3.5 to 5.1 mEq/L. Potassium levels of 3.5 mEq/L, 5.1 mEq/L, and 5.0 mEq/L are within the normal range. Patients in the normal range would not exhibit muscle weakness, fatigue, or cardiac dysrhythmias due to hypokalemia.

3. D) 4

Standard 4 deals with the planning and prioritization of expected outcomes and goals. Standard 1 deals with the collection of healthcare data required for diagnosis. Standard 2 is related to analyzing the assessment data for diagnosis. The identification of expected outcomes and goals falls under Standard 3.

4. C) Acamprosate

The symptoms of the patient are a result of alcohol withdrawal. To combat this, acamprosate can be prescribed; it functions as "artificial alcohol" by reducing glutamate activity. Ramelteon and tasimelteon are beneficial in treating insomnia. Prescribing these medications will only promote sleep without treating other symptoms and their causes. One of the atypical antidepressants is agomelatine. It is not beneficial in treating alcohol withdrawal symptoms and, in contrast, has insomnia and liver toxicity as its adverse effects.

5. C) Acetylcholine

Symptoms of depression may be due to alterations in different neurotransmitters, including an increase in acetylcholine. Increased acetylcholine can also cause increased risk of bruising or bleeding in patients. The patient is more likely to have an increased amount of C-reactive protein and interleukin-6 in the plasma during stressful times rather than during depression. Cortisol level is also higher during stress because it is released in response to it.

6. B) Acknowledgment and learning from situations to move forward

Resilience is a person's ability to adapt and process through setbacks in life without dwelling on things that did not go as planned. It allows for a person to acknowledge and learn from situations and to move forward in life. It includes strength but it encourages the person to move forward with openness toward change. While it is good to reflect on lessons as a form of healing, focusing on failures and not working through them does not help develop resilience. Recognizing maladaptive coping mechanisms is part of cognitive behavioral therapy and is not a description of resilience.

7. D) Action

During the action phase, the patient is actively engaging in therapeutic behavior for a period of less than 6 months. In the precontemplation stage, the patient has no intention to change. During the maintenance stage, the patient has engaged in behaviors to prevent relapse for more than 6 months. When in the preparation stage, the patient is ready for change and shows evidence of readiness for action.

8. B) Activities of orexin receptors

The nurse practitioner will prescribe an orexin receptor antagonist like suvorexant. These drugs bind to orexin receptors (orexin 1 and orexin 2), blocking them from wakefulness promotion and inducing sleep. Drugs that block dopamine 2 receptors fall under conventional antipsychotics. They help in lowering psychosis positive symptoms and are preferable for treating psychotic disorders, not insomnia. Drugs that restrict serotonin 2A receptors are used for treating cognitive and affective symptoms. Stimulation of noradrenergic receptors is responsible for nightmares. Blocking stimulation of these receptors helps in reducing nightmares during sleep. The reason for the patient's insomnia is not nightmares; therefore, such drugs are not preferable.

9. D) Advise against St. John's wort and suggest golden root or lavender instead

St. John's wort, when taken with selective serotonin reuptake inhibitors (SSRIs), can increase the risk of serotonin syndrome. Therefore, the nurse practitioner will advise against the use of St. John's wort and suggest other supplements such as golden root or lavender if the patient feels strongly that herbal supplements are important in their treatment. Simply providing education on the safe use of herbal supplements would not offer the patient the accurate and important information they need when taking a supplement that would interact with prescribed medication. The patient would not be instructed to stop the prescribed medication without further assessment. While St. John's wort does have interactions with other prescribed medications, the nurse practitioner stating that the supplement is lethal is not an accurate explanation and does not provide the patient with information that addresses the concern of anxiety.

10. A) Alter the depressed mood of the patient

Helping the patient to consider problems in a different way will help the patient to gain a hopeful attitude about the future and will improve the patient's mood. Exercise can aid in improving self-concept. Identification of cognitive distortions is necessary for providing the patient proper conception regarding the world and the self. Religious or spiritual support can give the patient strength.

11. D) Amyloid precursor protein (*APP*), presenilin-1 (*PSEN1*), and presenilin-2 (*PSEN2*)

Mutations in the *APP* gene on chromosome 21, the *PSEN1* gene on chromosome 14, and the *PSEN2* gene on chromosome 1 have been identified, and they account for approximately 50% of all cases of early-onset familial Alzheimer's disease. *BRCA1* and *BRCA2* (breast cancer genes 1 and 2) are the most well-known genes linked to breast cancer. Karyotyping and FISH are studies that detect fetal chromosome abnormalities. The *APOE* E4* gene is associated with late-onset Alzheimer's disease.

12. A) Aminotransferases (ALT and AST): AST: 570 IU/L and ALT: 620 IU/L

Valproate is contraindicated in patients with hepatic impairment. High ALT and AST are indicators of liver disease. The levels reported are abnormally high. The normal AST range is 8 to 42 IU/L, and the normal ALT range is 3 to 30 IU/L. The other laboratory results are all within normal range.

13. A) Anhedonia

A patient with major depressive disorder must have five the following symptoms: depressed mood, lack of interest or pleasure (anhedonia), weight loss or weight gain, increased or decreased activity, feelings of hopelessness/worthlessness or guilt, fatigue/loss of energy, insomnia or hypersomnia, diminished ability to think or concentrate, and/or recurring thoughts of death or suicide. At least one of those symptoms must be depressed mood or lack of interest or pleasure (anhedonia). Weight change may be weight gain, not necessarily weight loss. Grandiosity is associated with bipolar disorder. Paranoia is associated with thought disorders.

14. C) Antagonism of H1 histamine and 5-HT2C serotonin receptors

Antagonism at certain receptors, particularly 5-HT2C and histamine H1 receptors, is implicated in weight gain with atypical antipsychotics. H1 receptor antagonism interferes with satiety signals from the gut. 5-HT2C receptor antagonism increases food intake. Diabetes drugs in the GLP-1 agonists class include dulaglutide (Trulicity), exenatide extended release (Bydureon), exenatide (Byetta), semaglutide (Ozempic), semaglutide (Rybelsus), liraglutide (Victoza), and lixisenatide (Adlyxin). Agonism at the 5-HT2C serotonin receptor is thought to reduce both energy intake and body weight. Lorcaserin is an example of a selective 5-HT2C receptor agonist. SGLT-2 inhibitors are associated with weight loss and improved blood sugar control. These include canagliflozin (Invokana), dapagliflozin (Farxiga), and empagliflozin (Jardiance).

15. A) Armodafinil

The nurse practitioner would prescribe armodafinil, a wakefulness-promoting drug. It functions by boosting hypothalamic wakefulness center activity. Clomipramine, desipramine, and diazepam are sleep-inducing drugs beneficial in treating insomnia and therefore are not recommended for excessive drowsiness. The two tricyclic antidepressants, clomipramine and desipramine, function by blocking the norepinephrine and serotonin transporters. Diazepam, a benzodiazepine, functions by increasing gamma-aminobutyric acid inhibitory actions.

16. C) Ask the patient to describe the problems and how they affect the patient
The practitioner should try to inquire more about the issues that the patient is facing concerning gambling and disloyalty. The goals of psychotherapy are usually decided mutually. Unless the patient asks the practitioner for help with quitting gambling, the practitioner should not immediately provide suggestions like ceasing gambling altogether. The practitioner should refrain from bringing the patient's spouse into the session because the therapy is focused on the patient. Unless the therapy is related to improving the couple's relationship, the spouse should not be informed about anything being discussed in the session by the practitioner. Whether the patient tells the spouse about infidelity has to be decided by the patient only. The practitioner can empathize with the patient instead of sympathizing. Sympathizing is feeling pity for the patient; however, empathizing will ensure that the patient feels safe to express their problems.

17. B) Ask for an elaborated response rather than just yes or no
When conducting a patient interview, the nurse practitioner should ask guided questions that require more elaborated responses and refrain from asking questions having yes or no as answers. The nurse practitioner should first ask open-ended questions and then ask focused questions. The nurse practitioner can offer the patient multiple choices to reduce bias. During an interview, the nurse practitioner should repeat the patient's wording. This behavior reflects careful listening and encourages a patient to express their feelings without hesitation.

18. B) Assess the patient for abuse
The first action of the nurse practitioner would be to assess for physical or emotional abuse that could cause the patient to be nonverbal or not engage in interaction. Once abuse has been ruled out, the nurse practitioner can then schedule cognitive testing and refer the patient for genetic testing or neurology if needed.

19. A) Assessment of internal evidence
There are four components in the clinical decision-making model: internal evidence, patient preferences, research evidence, and healthcare resources. The drug class is changed after observing the internal evidence and clinical state of the patient. The first line of treatment has not worked, so the nurse practitioner changes the drug based on the patient outcome. The patient is not asked before changing the line of drugs. The second line of treatment is not initiated because the nurse practitioner refers to any research evidence or expert panels. The decision is made based on the condition of the patient. Since the provided treatment did not work, it is changed. The nurse practitioner changes the drug without considering other factors such as the availability of new drugs or the insurance coverage of the patient.

20. B) Assisting the patient in choosing an aftercare plan that reflects the vegetarian diet the patient prefers
Advocacy is generally described as defending the rights and property of others. In nursing, it has been defined as being a patient representative, defending the patient's rights and universal rights, protecting the interests of the patient, contributing to patient decision making, and supporting the patient's decisions. Adherence to the provider's treatment plan is important, but compliance is different from choice. Supporting family wishes is appropriate only when it is aligned with the patient's choices. Respecting a patient's decision not to take medication is appropriate, but allowing the patient to hoard medications that could be used for a suicide attempt is not in the patient's best interest.

21. D) At least one major depressive episode

In order for a patient to meet the diagnostic criteria of bipolar II they must meet criteria for a hypomanic episode, which includes having at least three of the following symptoms: flight of ideas, rapid speech, distractibility, insomnia, risk taking behaviors, inflated self-esteem, and distractibility. The symptoms must have lasted for at least 4 consecutive days and no >6 days. The patient must also meet criteria for a major depressive episode, which can only be met if at least one of the five symptoms of major depression is either depressed mood or anhedonia lasting for at least 2 consecutive weeks. Episodes generally do not require hospitalization; if the patient is psychotic then they meet mania criteria for bipolar I. Mood swings lasting at least half the time in a 2-year period is a symptom of cyclothymic disorder.

22. D) Atomoxetine (Strattera)

The patient shows symptoms of attention deficit/hyperactivity disorder. Atomoxetine (Strattera) is an FDA-approved non-stimulant drug that is a preferred choice for the treatment of attention deficit/hyperactive patients. Armodafinil (Nuvigil) is commonly used for the treatment of excessive sleepiness associated with narcolepsy. Flurazepam (Dalmane) is a benzodiazepine that has inhibitory actions on sleep centers, which results in sedation; it is prescribed to treat insomnia. Clozapine (Clozaril) is an antipsychotic drug that is commonly prescribed for treatment-resistant schizophrenia and not for attention deficit/hyperactivity disorder.

23. A) Attention deficit/hyperactivity disorder (ADHD)

The Incredible Years BASIC program provides parents and children support through psychoeducational programs geared toward behavior and emotional disorders such as ADHD. A diagnosis of MDD calls for treatment involving family and individual therapy. Identifying cognitive distortions and using cognitive behavioral techniques are associated with better outcomes. GAD calls for teaching relaxation techniques. OCD involves techniques such as systematic desensitization.

24. D) Autonomy versus beneficence

Patient autonomy can go against medical directives, despite clearly defined needs. Patients have a right to refuse all medical care and to make choices for themselves regarding their own healthcare. The principle of beneficence is the obligation to act for the benefit of the patient and prevent harm. Although it may not be in the patient's best interest to refuse treatment, when competent, it is their right to do so. Nonmaleficence is the obligation not to harm the patient. The ethical principle of fidelity is the obligation to prevent harm and the obligation to fulfill commitments to one's duties.

25. B) Autonomy

Autonomy refers to the right that informed patients have to make their own clinical decisions. The nurse practitioner is maintaining autonomy by letting the patient decide about continuing the pregnancy. Confidentiality refers to maintaining and protecting a patient's information and refraining from disclosing it to others, including family members, without the patient's consent. Veracity is a principle that requires truth-telling and conducting honest interactions with the patient. Veracity would be demonstrated when the nurse practitioner provides patient teaching regarding the risks to fetal development associated with medications. Justice refers to the distribution of resources and care equally among patients with no room for any sort of discrimination.

26. D) Benztropine

Benztropine is an antiparkinson agent, highly recommended for treating Parkinson's disease. However, it involves diplopia as its side effect. Therefore, the nurse practitioner should avoid prescribing this drug as it can worsen the condition. Diphenhydramine is an anticholinergic agent prescribed for Parkinson's disease. It has only minor side effects like dry mouth, dizziness, nausea, and constipation and therefore can be recommended. Pimavanserin is approved for treating hallucinations as well as delusions as a result of Parkinson's disease due to its atypical antipsychotic property. Because the patient is experiencing hallucinations and delusions, it can be prescribed. Rivastigmine acts as a cholinesterase inhibitor and is recommended for treating cognitive impairment due to Parkinson's disease.

27. D) Biofeedback therapy

The patient measuring vital signs is a part of biofeedback therapy. In this therapy, interventions help to gain a better understanding of the physiology of the patient, based on which further pharmacological and psychological interventions can be made. Aversion therapy is used where the patient needs to quit a habit like smoking or significant alcohol use. Interpersonal therapy focuses on improving social and personal life by resolving interpersonal conflicts. Modeling therapy focuses on changing the patient's behavior by providing a model to the patient that the patient can then imitate the model to change concerning behavior.

28. D) Blocking the reuptake of serotonin

Selective serotonin reuptake inhibitors block the reuptake of serotonin by blocking the 5-HT2 receptors. Blocking the reuptake of these neurotransmitters makes them available at the synapse in a larger quantity, which helps in alleviating depression. Stimulating the effects of GABA inhibits neuronal activity and is used to treat seizure disorders. Reuptake of norepinephrine and dopamine would not help because their presence at the synapse is needed to alleviate depression.

29. A) Bulimia nervosa

The patient is exhibiting signs of bulimia nervosa, which include Russell's sign, or calluses on the hand indicative of self-induced vomiting. Anorexia nervosa does not present with Russell's sign because purging is not seen in these patients. While loss of muscle mass may be due to decreased appetite in general anxiety disorder and depression, these disorders will not manifest with Russell's sign, parotid swelling, or edema.

30. C) Buspirone (BuSpar)

Buspirone (BuSpar) is commonly prescribed for the long-term treatment of anxiety disorder characterized by restlessness, lack of concentration, and frequent palpitations. It is a safe medication to prescribe to patients with a history of substance use disorder as it does not cause dependence. Diazepam (Valium), lorazepam (Ativan), and alprazolam (Xanax) are benzodiazepines and are not recommended for long-term usage, especially in patients with substance use disorder, because they may cause dependence.

31. A) Can include lamotrigine (Lamictal)

The patient can start lamotrigine or carbamazepine for the treatment of bipolar disorder. This patient is homozygous for the A allele of the rs1061235 A T polymorphism, indicating the absence of the HLA-A*3101 allele. This patient does not carry the HLA-B*1502 allele or a closely related *15 allele. This genotype suggests a lower risk of serious hypersensitivity reactions, including Stevens–Johnson syndrome, toxic epidermal necrolysis, maculopapular eruptions, and drug reaction with eosinophilia and systemic symptoms when taking certain mood stabilizers. Methylphenidate is not indicated for bipolar disorders. If treating attention deficit disorder, the patient should be homozygous for the G allele of the −1291G C polymorphism in the adrenergic alpha-2A receptor gene. This genotype suggests a normal response to certain attention deficit/hyperactivity disorder medications.

32. B) Carbamazepine

Stevens–Johnson syndrome is a life-threatening side effect of carbamazepine, which is recommended for bipolar disorder. Headache, insomnia, and anxiety are adverse effects of armodafinil, which is prescribed for wakefulness promotion. Hepatic dysfunction, renal dysfunction, and blood dyscrasias are rare but life-threatening side effects of chlordiazepoxide, which is prescribed for alcohol withdrawal symptoms. Dry mouth, dizziness, major depression, and sedation are side effects of clonidine, which is prescribed for hypertension.

33. B) Clonidine

Clonidine is an antihypertensive agent and acts as a nonstimulant for ADHD. It acts centrally on the alpha 2 receptors found in the prefrontal cortex. It is also used to treat Tourette's syndrome. Therefore, the nurse practitioner would recommend clonidine to the patient. Amphetamine (D) and methylphenidate (D, L) are recommended to patients with ADHD as they improve the symptoms by increasing dopamine and norepinephrine activities. However, these drugs should be avoided if the patient is also diagnosed with Tourette's syndrome because they may worsen that condition. Haloperidol is beneficial in treating Tourette's syndrome by blocking the activities of dopamine 2 receptors in the nigrostriatal pathway. However, this mode of action is not beneficial in treating ADHD; instead, it can be used for schizophrenia.

34. D) Clozapine (Clozaril)

Clozapine is a second-generation antipsychotic that is prescribed for the treatment of schizophrenia when at least two medications have failed to have any prominent results. The patient shows symptoms of schizophrenia, and since two previous medications have already been changed, clozapine should be prescribed. It suppresses bone marrow, making the patient susceptible to infections, so the patient's absolute neutrophil count should be monitored. Bupropion is an antidepressant that is commonly prescribed for smoking cessation and does not require monitoring of absolute neutrophil count. Memantine is used for the treatment of Alzheimer's disease. Armodafinil (Nuvigil) is commonly used for the treatment of excessive sleepiness associated with narcolepsy.

35. A) Cognitive behavioral therapy
The patient shows symptoms of attention deficit/hyperactivity disorder (ADHD). Cognitive behavioral therapy is highly recommended as it helps in management of everyday tasks and management of time, and it improves productivity. Atomoxetine is a drug prescribed for ADHD, but it should be given only to patients older than 6 years. Patients with ADHD should strictly avoid honey and white rice in the diet as these may worsen ADHD symptoms. Donepezil is also recommended for ADHD but should not be given to patients younger than 8 years.

36. B) Comfortable furniture and ambient temperature
Comfortable furniture and comfortable room temperature help to put the patient at ease and assist them in developing trust. A photograph of the nurse practitioner's family offers no therapeutic value. Chairs must be placed at an angle of 45°, and the room must be quiet with no music or other distractions.

37. B) Comorbidities
Many adolescents with anxiety disorders have other conditions such as attention deficit/hyperactivity disorder) and health-related issues. Often the combination of disorders can lead to generalized anxiety disorder, separation anxiety disorder, and social anxiety disorder. Therefore, assessing for separation anxiety would not be an initial assessment to determine comorbidities. Agoraphobia and socioemotional deficiencies are often the result of anxiety, but are not disorders that should be assessed for at this stage.

38. C) Complete blood count (CBC), liver function tests, human chorionic gonadotropin (HCG level), and ECG
Carbamazepine may produce changes in the levels of white blood cells, platelets, and red blood cells. ECG is done to rule out problems with cardiac conduction (QTc and QRS prolongation). A pretreatment urine pregnancy test is obtained in women of childbearing years because various congenital abnormalities can occur. Lithium pretreatment includes TSH, BUN, serum creatinine, and a urinalysis. Fasting lipid profile and hemoglobin A1c are measured with the use of antipsychotics. Ordering no blood levels is beneath the standard of care for patients starting carbamazepine.

39. B) Concrete operational
The child is in the concrete operational stage at around age 7 to 11 years. It is the third stage of intellectual development. This stage brings an increasing orientation to the reality-based world and more organized, coherent mental structures that allow for internal, rather than action-oriented, problem solving. Children in this age group are unable to use deductive reasoning. Thinking is concrete and lacks moral reasoning abilities. The formal operational stage is present from 11 through adolescence. During this stage, there is a shift to higher-level abstract thinking and hypothetical deductive reasoning. They are able to reason and change their thinking. The preoperational stage (from 18 months to 7 years) is marked by object permanence and imitation. Thinking is egocentric. They view the world from their point of view. They ask "why" questions. They cannot reason, use logic, or combine ideas. They have trouble assessing between quantity and appearance. In the sensorimotor stage (birth to 18 months), the child actively constructs information about the world via physical explorations and actions. They lack object permanence.

40. C) Consultation
Consultation is a practice that the nurse practitioner provides by giving a discourse to influence identified plans and addressing other providers to enhance services. Milieu therapy refers to the philosophy of providing a secure environment. Psychotherapy includes the principles of therapeutic communications. Prescriptive authority is the authority to prescribe treatments under the law.

41. C) Continues with the assessment
The nurse is assessing the rooting reflex, which when elicited should cause the infant to pucker their lips and turn their head to the stimulated side and suck. This is a normal finding, and the nurse practitioner should continue with the examination. This reflex should be observed in both full-term and preterm infants. If the infant had not responded, then the nurse practitioner would order a neurology consult, suspecting the infant has a developmental or central nervous system disease.

42. C) Creutzfeldt–Jakob disease
Prion disorder (Creutzfeldt–Jakob disease) is represented by a single gene mutation on the prion protein gene and manifests as progression of impaired motor function resulting in ataxia or monoclonus, memory loss, and behavior changes. Progression of the disease has a rapid, insidious onset that can be fatal. Alzheimer's disease is a form of progressive dementia seen commonly in older adults with impairments in several memory tasks. Mutations on the amyloid precursor protein gene are highly indicated in Alzheimer's, leading to the amyloid plaques that are the hallmark of this disease. Down syndrome is caused by an extra copy of chromosome 21. Huntington's disease is caused by a defective gene on chromosome 4.

43. D) Delinquency
According to Erikson's psychosocial stages, the pathological outcome seen in identity versus role confusion conflict is delinquency. Midlife crisis is seen as a pathological outcome of the generativity versus stagnation conflict; despair is seen in the ego integrity versus despair conflict; and schizoid personality is seen in the intimacy versus isolation conflict.

44. D) Delirium
The patient is exhibiting signs of delirium, which occurs rapidly and fluctuates over a 24-hour period with auditory or visual hallucinations, or both, and tremors, global disorientation, and decreased cognition and consciousness. Frontal lobe trauma would manifest as an inability to regulate critical thinking and emotions, which often leads to risky behaviors. Insomnia would not present with tremors or hallucinations. Alzheimer's disease is a form of dementia that does not have a rapid onset of symptoms.

45. A) Depletion of inhibitory neurotransmitter gamma-aminobutyric acid (GABA)
Evidence supports the hypothesis that disrupted GABAergic circuits underlie Huntington's disease pathogenesis. Low β-amyloid 42 and high tau and phosphorylated tau is found in Alzheimer's disease. Poor reabsorption of cerebrospinal fluid with ventricle enlargement is indicative of normal pressure hydrocephalus. A distinctive clinical feature of Lewy body disease is that REM sleep behavior disorder is a frequent concomitant and often precedes cognitive symptoms.

46. B) Depression

Levels of dopamine and serotonin remain low in cases of depression. In a patient with mania, the levels of gamma-aminobutyric acid decrease, while dopamine increases. Anxiety is characterized by increased levels of norepinephrine and low levels of gamma-aminobutyric acid. Hypocretin levels remain increased in the case of narcolepsy.

47. D) Dietician/nutritionist

When working with a child who is displaying signs of depression and conflict and who is overweight, it is important to build an interdisciplinary team that includes the psychiatric-mental nurse practitioner, a social worker, a recreational therapist, and a dietician/nutritionist who has experience in working with parents on delivering interventions. A family counselor would be included when there are issues with the parents themselves, such as separation or divorce. A registered nurse would be included if there are comorbid disorders that need to be monitored. A member of the clergy would be included at the parents' request and at not the discretion of the nurse practitioner when building the team.

48. A) Discontinue St. John's wort and monitor the patient's international normalized ratio (INR)

Discontinuing the St. John's wort is necessary because St. John's wort can activate the cytochrome P-450 3A4 detoxification system in the liver, which reduces the therapeutic effect of warfarin. Warfarin interacts with St John's wort, leading to a reduction in the anticoagulant effect of warfarin. Therefore, the INR may increase upon discontinuation and needs to be monitored. Patients are prescribed warfarin to decrease the clotting tendency of their blood to prevent life-threatening blood clots. The blood test used to measure clotting time is referred to as protime (PT) and reported as the INR. The dose of warfarin may need to be adjusted according to clotting time. The INR is always monitored when taking warfarin. Continuing St. John's wort is contraindicated due to the risk of affecting the patient's INR level. Increasing coumadin to adjust to continuing St. John's wort is risky and not practical. Discontinuing St. John's wort is advisable; however, monitoring for signs of bleeding is not done in lieu of clinically indicated blood tests, specifically the INR.

49. A) Divalproex sodium (Depakote)

The patient shows symptoms of the oppositional defiant disorder. Divalproex sodium (Depakote) is an anti-seizure medication that is commonly prescribed to treat aggression in patients diagnosed with oppositional defiant disorder. Atomoxetine (Strattera) is a nonstimulant used to treat attention deficit/hyperactivity disorder and should not be prescribed as the symptoms of the patient correlate with the diagnostic criteria of oppositional defiant disorder. Paroxetine (Paxil) is a selective serotonin reuptake inhibitor that is commonly prescribed to treat depression. Lamotrigine (Lamictal) is used to treat bipolar disorder. The patient does not show symptoms of bipolar disorder with manic or depressive episodes.

50. A) Donepezil (Aricept)

Donepezil (Aricept) is an acetylcholinesterase inhibitor that is prescribed for the treatment of Alzheimer's disease. It works by inhibiting acetylcholinesterase, which increases the availability of acetylcholine, thereby compensating for degenerating cholinergic neurons involved in memory processes. Chlorpromazine (Thorazine) is a conventional antipsychotic that is prescribed for schizophrenia. It works by blocking dopamine 2 receptors, thereby reducing positive symptoms of psychosis. Carbamazepine (Tegretol) is prescribed for the treatment of seizures. It works by blocking voltage-sensitive sodium channels. Clomipramine (Anafranil) is a tricyclic antidepressant that works by blocking serotonin and norepinephrine reuptake.

51. C) Dopaminergic neurons in the substantia nigra pars compacta and ventral tegmental area

Midbrain dopaminergic (DA) neurons in the substantia nigra pars compacta and ventral tegmental area regulate extrapyramidal movement. DA neurons in the ventral tegmental area and retrorubral field regulate cognitive functions, including emotion, motivation, reward, and addictive behaviors. Studies have identified volume loss in BLA gray matter in patients with mood disorders. Functional changes have suggested the BLA to be hyperactive in a range of mood disorders. Selective degeneration of DA neurons in substantia nigra pars compacta is a key neuropathological feature in Parkinson's disease.

52. B) Drug-induced liver injury

The patient's symptoms are acute, not chronic. Medications such as Depakote are common causes of acute liver injury. Choledocholithiasis, a stone in the bile duct, presents acutely with jaundice, fever, and loss of appetite. It is associated with severe abdominal pain. The acute presentation is not consistent with primary biliary cirrhosis, a chronic liver disease usually occurring in the 40- to 50-year-old age group. Hemochromatosis is a chronic hepatocellular disease. Excessive iron accumulates in the liver and other organs. The onset of symptoms in female patients is usually after menopause. The acute onset of symptoms, the relatively young age, and the sex of the patient are not consistent with hemochromatosis.

53. D) Duloxetine (Cymbalta)

The patient's symptoms correlate to major depressive disorder. The nurse practitioner should prescribe duloxetine (Cymbalta), which works by inhibiting the reuptake of serotonin and norepinephrine and is commonly used as a first-line treatment for major depressive disorder. Memantine (Namenda) is an N-methyl-D aspartate receptor antagonist that is used for the symptomatic treatment of Alzheimer's disease. It is involved in improving the memory processes and is not helpful to treat major depressive disorder. Eszopiclone (Lunesta) is a non-benzodiazepine hypnotic that is prescribed to patients diagnosed with insomnia. Galantamine (Razadyne) is a cholinesterase inhibitor that is prescribed for the treatment of Alzheimer's disease. It works by inhibiting cholinesterase, which increases acetylcholine availability. It has no significant role in treating major depressive disorder.

54. D) Educate the patient on the DASH diet, include instruction on appropriate exercise, and set up monthly monitoring sessions

Research supports the DASH diet, or a similar nutritional program, and activity for weight reduction for patients with serious mental illness. Weight management monitoring should be scheduled at least once monthly. It is not necessary to refer a patient to a nutritionist or exercise therapist at this point in therapy. Reducing the prescribed medication is not the most appropriate option because the dosage will alter the therapeutic effect. Adding combination herbal supplements is not an appropriate intervention because many herbs have serious interactive effects with prescribed medications.

55. B) EEG

The assessment findings are associated with brain death. An EEG is used to confirm brain death. The absence of brain waves confirms brain death. A comprehensive metabolic panel assesses liver and kidney function, an ECG will assess cardiac rhythm, and MRI of the brain will not detect brain waves.

56. B) Elevated creatinine phosphokinase

A patient with NMS would present with elevated creatinine phosphokinase, liver enzymes, plasma myoglobin, and myoglobinuria, which may be associated with renal failure. NMS is a complication that occurs during the course of antipsychotic treatment and is considered a medical emergency. Symptoms include muscle rigidity, dystonia, akinesia, agitation, hyperthermia, diaphoresis, tachycardia, and hypertension. Hyperprolactinemia is. associated with the use of atypical antipsychotics; the most common agent is Risperdal. Symptoms of hyperprolactinemia do not include muscle rigidity or NMS. Low white blood cell count is associated with the use of antipsychotics, most significantly clozapine (Clozaril). A low hemoglobin/hematocrit count indicating anemia is associated with the use of carbamazepine (Tegretol). Muscle rigidity is not reported.

57. D) Emotional style of the therapist

Therapeutic skills and variable treatment modalities can be learned; however, therapists bring lifelong personal variables such as their individual personality and emotional style to the process. Dispositions are preexisting. Therapy results and the strength of the therapeutic alliance are affected by these factors. Strict adherence to the treatment manual is not the goal; techniques are delivered with an integrated blend of technical content and the personality of the therapist. Circadian physiology and social rhythms are a series of neurohormonal events, such as timing of cortisol and melatonin secretions, sleep-wake cycles, and the relationship of these patterns to mood. Disruption in these cycles affects the patient's mood and function. They are not associated with the strength of the therapeutic alliance.

58. A) Employ a mobile crisis team

The first step in an emergency such as a disaster is to employ a mobile crisis psychiatric service team to assess patients and provide emergency medications. Once the team has provided initial emergency evaluation, patients can be referred to housing services such as board-and-care homes and partial hospitalization programs. Setting up a multiservice center would be a step to take for maintenance once patients have been stabilized.

59. B) Employing evidence-based clinical practice guidelines about concussions to drive treatment

Employing evidence-based clinical practice guidelines to guide screening and diagnostic activities as available and appropriate is a competency of the assessment done by the nurse practitioner. Assuming that the patient's mood changes are related to being a teenager and immediately referring the patient to a sports medicine specialist do not demonstrate an understanding of the nurse practitioner's role in decision making due to elimination of the patient's history of a recent concussion. While listening to the patient's parents may be important, it should not be a major component in clinical decision making when additional history is omitted.

60. A) Ensuring that the patient has a trusted family member to discuss the treatment plan

The nurse practitioner has a duty to advocate for patients, which includes actions such as having trusted family members to ensure understanding of the treatment plan. Failure to obtain patient consent and disregarding information for the patient's healthcare power of attorney demonstrate lack of advocacy for the patient. Education is a significant component of advocacy to ensure the patient is able to make informed decisions about treatment.

61. C) Escitalopram (Lexapro)

Escitalopram is an example of an SSRI medication used to treat depression and anxiety. Additional SSRI medications are citalopram (Celexa), fluoxetine (Prozac), paroxetine (Paxil), and sertraline (Zoloft). Aripiprazole is an antipsychotic. Alprazolam and clonazepam are benzodiazepines used to treat anxiety.

62. B) Escitalopram does not affect hepatic metabolizing enzymes and is less likely to cause drug interactions

Escitalopram is an antidepressant that does not affect the metabolizing enzymes in the liver. It is less likely to cause a drug interaction with cardiac medications. Escitalopram is not the only FDA-approved medication for older adults. It is not a CYP450 2d6 inhibitor of tamoxifen, and it is associated with increased falls in older adult patients.

63. B) Expecting bad things to happen

The FEAR plan includes a four-step method to address the psychoeducational needs of children with anxiety disorders. The first half is building the plan, which includes addressing feeling frightened (F), expecting bad things to happen (E), attitudes and actions that might help (A), and results and rewards (R). The first component to be addressed is feeling frightened, which identifies the physical symptoms of arousal in anxiety feelings. From this, the patient is taught relaxation techniques to overcome the physical reactions of anxiety. Expecting bad things to happen is the second component in the plan and addresses how to manage maladaptive expectations through cognitive restructuring. During this phase, the patient will engage in modeling and role-playing to identify challenges that can be restructured to realistic perceptions. Attitudes and actions involve problem solving and building confidence to make appropriate decisions. The results and reward area focuses on self-monitoring and how to achieve realistic expectations.

64. C) Expression of commitment to the continued relationship

Partnering is an expression of commitment to the existing or ongoing relationship between the patient and the practitioner. It is one of the vital components of the skilled interviewing process and assures the patient that support from the practitioner will always be there. This helps strengthen mutual trust. Effective reassurance is achieved by recognizing and accepting the emotions of a patient. This helps in building up a connection and makes the patient understand at the interview's end the ways to deal with situations or concerns. Briefing the patient's story at the end of an interview is called summarization. It is another important method of skilled interviewing that makes the patient feel that their concerns and emotions were addressed and listened to carefully. It also helps to address if there is anything more for the nurse practitioner to know. Making patients aware before moving on to different topics is known as transitioning.

65. A) Face the patient in good lighting

During a clinical interview with a patient with hearing loss, the nurse practitioner should face the patient in good lighting. This helps the patient in lip reading. The rate of speaking of the nurse practitioner should be slow. Also, the nurse practitioner should avoid looking down while speaking. Speaking at a high volume and not looking directly at the patient make lip reading difficult for the patient. The nurse practitioner should provide written instructions in addition to explaining the instructions verbally before closing the clinical interview.

66. B) Fidelity

Fidelity is a commitment to obligation and duty that is executed as keeping promises. Maintaining fidelity is of utmost importance when building a trusting patient-provider relationship. Patients are more likely to discuss deeper issues with the provider when they feel they can trust that person. Justice is the duty to treat everyone fairly and is important in distributing equal access to resources. Veracity is the duty, or obligation, to tell the truth. While this is an important ethical characteristic, it often conflicts with mental health recovery and therefore is not the characteristic needed to establish a trusting relationship. Paternalism is based on using professional knowledge and education to make decisions for the good of the patient.

67. A) Fluvoxamine (Luvox)

The patient shows symptoms of an obsessive-compulsive disorder. The nurse practitioner would prescribe fluvoxamine, which is used for the treatment of obsessive-compulsive disorder. Benztropine is commonly prescribed for parkinsonism. Valproate is used to treat mania associated with bipolar disorder. Zopiclone is commonly prescribed for the treatment of insomnia.

68. A) Focus on patient's behaviors and attitude

The first step is to recognize the patient's behaviors and identify the reasons behind the patient's responses. This also helps in the construction of other ways to view the patient's thinking and behavior, which is necessary before taking the process further. Attending is a type of listening that entails a level of presence with the patient in order to build a positive connection. Once the nurse practitioner knows the reasons behind the patient's behaviors, they should empathize with the patient. Empathy occurs when the nurse practitioner tries to comprehend the world from the patient's point of view. Once enough progress has been made, the nurse practitioner must encourage the patient toward independent problem solving, which is important to minimize the dependency of the patient.

69. C) Frontal and parietal

The right and left orientation of a person is controlled by the parietal lobe of the cerebral cortex, and the frontal lobe helps people to stay motivated to work. Hence, the patient is facing disruptions in the frontal lobe and the parietal lobe. The temporal lobe aids people to express emotions. It also helps in language comprehension and storing sound into memory. The occipital lobe helps in interpreting a visual image. It also keeps visual memories in storage and helps in language formation as well.

70. A) Geriatric Depression Scale (GDS)

The GDS is used for older adult patients. The GDS Long Form is a 30-item questionnaire to which participants are asked to respond by answering yes or no in reference to how they felt over the past week. A Short Form GDS consisting of 15 questions was developed in 1986. Questions from the Long Form GDS that had the highest correlation with depressive symptoms in validation studies were selected for the short version. Scores of 0 to 4 are considered normal, depending on age, education, and complaints; scores of 5 to 8 indicate mild depression; scores of 9 to 11 indicate moderate depression; and scores of 12 to 15 indicate severe depression. The BDI is commonly used to assess patients for depression but would not be the most appropriate tool for older adults. The SDQ is a self-evaluation tool for children with conduct and/or emotional problems. HADS is used to assess depression related to inpatient care.

71. C) Giving a lecture about the experience of recovery
Giving a lecture regarding an experience is a healthy way to reflect and grow from a situation and positively apply life lessons. In addition, it can help others who are struggling find hope and learn from the speaker's experience and use it in their life situations. While spending time with friends is a healthy part of recovery, a past circle of friends may have contributed to addiction. An essential part of recovery is for patients to place distance between themselves and people or places that potentially may lead to relapse. Calling in sick when not physically ill is dishonest and suggestive of manipulation, which is against the tenets of recovery behavior that promote honesty and responsibility.

72. B) Gluten-free/casein-free (GFCF)
A GFCF diet plan avoids foods that contain gluten (found in many breads and cereals) and casein (found in milk products). Gluten-free diets are the first-line treatment for celiac disease and are used in cases of nonceliac gluten sensitivity and wheat allergy. Casein-free diets exclude the use of casein, which is a protein found in dairy products. Following both of these diets creates a gluten-free and casein-free dietary protocol, which has been used for several years as a nontraditional treatment approach for patients with autism. The DASH diet is designed to help treat or prevent high blood pressure (hypertension). The Mediterranean diet and the ketogenic diet are nutrition plans for general wellness and are not used for autism.

73. C) Grandiose delusion
When a patient believes that they possess exceptional abilities that are false or unbelievable, those beliefs are regarded as diagnostic features of grandiose delusion. Erotomanic delusion deals with a false belief of the patient that a person loves the patient romantically. Nihilistic delusion is a reasonless belief that some major catastrophe is about to take place. In persecutory delusion, a patient thinks that other people are trying to harass or harm the patient.

74. B) Haloperidol with lorazepam
Haloperidol in combination with lorazepam is beneficial in treating delirium. Haloperidol works by blocking the activity of dopamine 2 receptors, whereas lorazepam works by increasing gamma-aminobutyric acid inhibitory effects. Ketamine is beneficial in treating pain and inducing anesthesia. It acts as N-methyl-D-aspartate receptor antagonist and is generally not recommended to be used with lorazepam as they are incompatible. Lithium is beneficial in treating bipolar and manic depression. It acts as a mood stabilizer and therefore is not recommended for delirium. If given with haloperidol, it increases the risk of the encephalopathic syndrome. Amitriptyline is a tricyclic antidepressant as well as a noradrenaline and serotonin reuptake inhibitor. It helps in treating fibromyalgia, depression, and insomnia but is not beneficial in the case of delirium. Amitriptyline and haloperidol together may increase the tricyclic antidepressant blood concentration.

75. D) Hamilton Rating Scale for Depression (HAM-D)
The HAM-D uses a scale of 0 to 4 with questions that require a yes or no answer and is an easy tool for older adults to self-administer and understand. This is a tool that is used to assess depression in patients with dementia when they are cognizant and capable of answering questions. When a patient with dementia begins to demonstrate signs of anxiety or additional deterioration in mood stability, the RAID scale is a tool used to assess worry, apprehension, phobias, and panic attacks. The SLUMS is a tool used to assess for schizophrenia. The CSDD is a tool for assessing depression using information from the patient and outside informants and is used in patients with limited ability to express themselves.

76. D) Has developed a feeling of isolation
Feeling of isolation is related to hopelessness. The problem of impaired coping brings issues in problem solving and can cause a person to develop addiction issues with drugs or alcohol. Considering oneself to be a burden on others is a sign of having chronic low-esteem.

77. B) Having a first-degree relative with obsessive-compulsive personality disorder
A risk factor for obsessive-compulsive disorder is having a first-degree relative with the same disorder. In general, male patients suffer more from obsessive-compulsive personality disorder than female patients. Having a first-degree relative with schizophrenia is not a risk factor for obsessive-compulsive personality disorder. Having a family background with harsh discipline, not lack of discipline, is a risk factor for obsessive-compulsive personality disorder.

78. C) Having the child initiate a conversation with children on the playground
The next appropriate step for the patient is to initiate a conversation with a small group of children on the playground. This is a safe environment that involves activities the child would enjoy, and therefore it will be a less threatening situation. Accompanying the patient on a full elevator would not be appropriate and would induce great anxiety in the patient, thus risking the progress of the therapy. Encouraging the parents to take the patient on a short shopping trip would be appropriate after the patient initiates contact with more than one person, such as a group of children. Likewise, including the patient in a large group activity such as those at a community center would overstimulate the patient.

79. D) Head circumference
Infants with FAS typically have a smaller head circumference, indicating an underdeveloped brain. Body length, body mass, and awareness are not measurements that are critical in assessing appropriate development as these do not reflect the cognition and intellectual development most often at risk in FAS.

80. A) Hemophagocytic lymphohistiocytosis and Stevens–Johnson syndrome
Lamotrigine has an FDA warning label identifying hemophagocytic lymphohistiocytosis and Stevens–Johnson syndrome as potential risk factors. Carbamazepine is known to have a risk for drug reaction with eosinophilia and systemic symptoms. Persistent pulmonary hypertension of the newborn is associated with selective serotonin reuptake inhibitor antidepressant use during pregnancy. Dangerous abnormalities in the heart's electrical activity are associated with the FDA dosing and warning recommendations for the antidepressant citalopram hydrobromide (Celexa).

81. C) Hypertensive crisis

Hypertensive crisis occurs with concurrent use of MAOIs and tyramine-containing foods such as smoked fish, cured meats, red wine, beer, aged cheese, or fermented foods like sauerkraut. Symptoms of hypertensive crisis include high blood pressure, stiff neck, headache, sweating, and nausea and vomiting. Stevens–Johnson syndrome is associated with the use of lamotrigine or carbamazepine. Neuroleptic malignant syndrome is associated with the use of antipsychotic drugs. Priapism is associated with the use of trazodone.

82. A) Hypo-hyperthyroidism

Endocrine disorders such as hypo–hyperthyroidism can present as depressive disorders. Hypothyroidism signs and symptoms may include depression, fatigue, and memory problems. Symptoms of hyperthyroidism also include complaints of nervousness, restlessness, and irritability. Hypertension, cardiomyopathy, and blood dyscrasias may be comorbidities of a depressive disorder but are not part of a differential diagnosis.

83. C) Identifying physical symptoms of arousal of anxiety

The FEAR plan is a four-step method to address the psychoeducational needs of children with anxiety disorders. The first half is building the plan, which includes addressing feeling frightened (F), expecting bad things to happen (E), attitudes and actions that might help (A), and results and rewards (R). The first component to be addressed is feeling frightened, in which the patient identifies the physical symptoms of arousal in anxiety feelings. From this, the child is taught relaxation techniques to overcome the physical reactions of anxiety. Expecting bad things to happen is the second component in the plan and addresses how to manage maladaptive expectations through cognitive restructuring. Attitudes and actions involve problem solving and building confidence to make appropriate decisions. The results and reward area focuses on self-monitoring and how to achieve realistic expectations.

84. D) Imipramine (Tofranil)

Tricyclic antidepressants such as imipramine (Tofranil) have a risk for cardiac conduction effects. Although all selective serotonin reuptake inhibitors and serotonin antagonist and reuptake inhibitors, such as escitalopram, vilazodone, and trazodone, can lengthen QT intervals, it is usually in combination with an antipsychotic medication.

85. A) Immature prefrontal cortex

Due to an immature prefrontal cortex, adolescents are prone to impulse control issues as well as poor judgment and frustration. This causes adolescent patients to be at higher risk for high stress levels that, when combined with suicidal ideations, may lead to lethal outcomes. The hippocampus is responsible for memory and learning, and the amygdala influences motivation and the response to fear. The cingulate cortex is involved in emotion and cognition, and a disconnect is not a cause for altered executive functioning of the brain.

86. B) Incompetent in making treatment-related decisions

The court appoints court-trained volunteer guardians to incompetent patients in case the family members of the patients are absent or do not intend to be the guardians. Therefore, the volunteers make treatment-related decisions on the patients' behalf. Patients can be kept in restraint or secluded from others if they are at risk of harming themselves or others. Court-trained volunteer guardians are not associated with restraints or seclusion. Patients going through electroconvulsive therapies or fearing violation of their right to confidentiality are not appointed guardians.

87. A) Inconsistent with the developmental stage
The diagnosis of attention deficit/hyperactivity disorder and impulsivity requires symptoms that are not consistent with the patient's developmental level. Consistency with the developmental stage would involve appropriate behaviors for the age, including slight inability to focus and excessive energy. The ability to self-control is a positive sign and not part of the hyperactivity spectrum. Impulsivity that results in physical harm to self and others falls under many other mental health disorders, but not ADHD.

88. A) Inform the patient's family and staff members
In cases where the patient poses a danger to self and others, the nurse practitioner should inform the patient's family and the hospital staff to warn them. The nurse practitioner can breach the patient's confidentiality when required to protect the patient and others from any impending harm. Asking the patient to be calm does not minimize the risk of harm that the patient poses. The nurse practitioner cannot discontinue treatment with the patient without safely reassigning the patient to another nurse practitioner.

89. D) Informed consent
Informed consent is a doctrine that providers must adhere to, inclusive of risks versus benefits of care offered, allowing the patient to make an informed decision about accepting care. A signature form is not specific to healthcare ethics. Confidentiality is based on the duty to protect a patient's health information. HIPAA involves restriction to access of individuals' private health information.

90. A) Intact orientation
Patients with early dementia are oriented in all spheres. Dementia and delirium are both cognitive disorders; however, dementia has an insidious course, and deficits worsen progressively over the years. Patients with delirium have deficits in short-term memory; patients with early dementia do not exhibit short-term memory problems. Hallucinations or perceptual deficits are usually not present in early dementia, except in Lewy body dementia. Incoherent speech is often present with delirium; patients with early dementia have difficulty with word-finding.

91. D) Intermittent explosive disorder
Being sexually abused and having a family history of substance use disorder are risk factors for intermittent explosive disorder. Adverse childhood experiences result in conduct disorder and oppositional defiant disorder as well, but generally in these disorders, neglect or conflict between parents is the risk factor. The most common risk factor of obsessive-compulsive personality disorder is harsh discipline in the house, which the patient has not experienced.

92. C) Interpersonal
Interpersonal therapy improves the interpersonal relationships and social interactions of the patient. Aversion therapy is used to treat issues such as alcohol disorder, shoplifting, or self-harm. Behavioral therapy changes maladaptive behaviors by targeting problems like gambling, anger issues, or alcohol use disorder. It is also used for disorders like phobias or anxiety. Psychoanalytic therapy believes that the root cause of mental illness is childhood trauma and is not considered a valid approach today.

93. C) Intimacy versus isolation
In Erikson's psychosocial stages, the conflict where the pathological outcome is schizoid personality is intimacy versus isolation. Inertia is the pathological outcome of industry versus inferiority; delinquency is the pathological outcome of identity versus role confusion; and midlife crisis is observed as a pathological outcome in the generativity versus stagnation conflict.

94. C) Involuntary commitment
Involuntary commitment is also known as assisted inpatient psychiatric treatment. Assisted outpatient treatment and conditional release are similar: The patient is released with certain conditions. Emergency commitment occurs when the patient applies for admission with written consent. It is also known as a temporary commitment or emergency admission. Unconditional release is release from the hospital after admission, which signifies the termination of any relationship between the institution and the patient.

95. A) Join family dinners even if just to sit at the dinner table
The patient joining the family at dinnertime will give the family a chance to sit together and share thoughts. If the patient stops engaging in family activities when sad, it may create a distance between the patient and other family members. The discontinuation or alteration of the medication regimen is done only after an evaluation by the nurse practitioner. Feeling better is not a criterion to discontinue the medication. Sharing feelings is a positive approach that helps the patient connect and realize that they are not alone.

96. D) Keeping the bedroom cool
Sleep hygiene practices include keeping the bedroom cool, dark, and quiet; keeping a regular bedtime schedule; exercising during the day; and taking time to wind down before bed. Drinking alcohol before bed, taking naps during the day, and exercising before bed will not promote sleep; they may induce insomnia and should be avoided.

97. A) Learning through interacting with the environment
Behavior therapy is a type of psychotherapy. It is used for bringing a change in the behavior pattern of a patient. Behaviorism is a popular concept that is based on the idea that all behaviors are learned through interaction with the environment. Cognitive behavioral therapy aims to help a person deal with overwhelming problems in a more positive way by breaking them down into smaller parts. Humanistic therapy helps the patient develop a stronger and healthier sense of self by focusing on the individual's strengths and values. Client-centered therapy involves achieving congruence by adjusting the self-concept.

98. A) Length of time the symptom is reported, impact on function in more than one setting, and age of onset

The chief complaint of inattention may be present in multiple diagnoses, such as oppositional defiant disorder, bipolar disorder, mood disorders, and disruptive mood dysregulation disorder. It is often a challenge to differentiate between attention deficit disorder and oppositional defiant disorder, bipolar disorder, mood disorders, and disruptive mood dysregulation disorder. The differential diagnosis would include age of onset, the length of time symptoms are present, and the impact on function in more than one setting. In order for a patient to be diagnosed with attention deficit disorder, the age of onset must be before age 12, with symptoms interfering with function in two or more settings. The presence of episodic irritability, aggression, and grandiosity suggests bipolar disorder. The inability to soothe when angry and raging for hours also suggests bipolar disorder. Chronic irritable mood with frequent explosive outbursts in more than one setting is indicative of disruptive mood dysregulation disorder. Patients with attention deficit disorder present with a more stable mood, are externally distracted, and are able to be soothed. Explosive outbursts are infrequent for both bipolar disorder and disruptive mood dysregulation disorder. Considering the differential diagnosis carefully is imperative because bipolar disorder may be worsened with the use of stimulants and carries a significant mortality risk.

99. B) Let the patient cry for some time and then discuss the issues after the patient settles

The nurse should give the patient time to cry and offer empathy. Crying helps suppressed emotions to surface and enables the nurse practitioner to communicate with the patient. The nurse practitioner should not ask the patient to stop crying because this would suppress the expression of the patient. The practitioner can provide tissues to the patient and wait until the patient feels like speaking again. The practitioner should not ask the patient to go outside to cry because this will not help the office provide a safe space for open communication. Hugging or touching a patient depends on several factors. The practitioner should usually refrain from physical contact with the patient as it can cause ethical issues. Hugging a patient is a personal decision; however, generally, it is not an appropriate response to a crying patient.

100. B) Lithium (Eskalith)

Based on multiple research studies, lithium is recognized as having anti-suicidal effects for patients with mood disorders, particularly major depression and bipolar disorder. Reduced suicide risk is not associated with the benefits of lamotrigine, carbamazepine, or valproate for patients with mood disorders.

101. C) Lithium (Lithobid)

Lithium is approved by the FDA for treating acute mania. It is usually supplemented in the early phases of treatment. Lithium has incredible clinical benefits but is highly toxic. The second-generation antipsychotic drug lurasidone is used for treating bipolar depression and is known to be less toxic. Cariprazine is an FDA-approved drug that does not fall into the most toxic category. Lamotrigine is an antipsychotic drug recommended for treating bipolar depression that has fewer side effects than lithium and is generally safe.

102. B) Major depressive disorder

Symptoms of major depressive disorder include sleeplessness, restlessness, despondency, irritability, and a loss of appetite. Atypical and psychotic features are specifiers used for major depressive disorder, and signs or symptoms of hypomania may include being abnormally upbeat, increased activity or energy, decreased need for sleep, exaggerated sense of self-confidence or well-being, unusual talkativeness, and distractibility.

103. C) Malpractice

Malpractice is defined as a failure of professional judgment that results in injury, loss, or damage. The legal requirement for malpractice must include duty to care for the patient, dereliction of duty, direct causation, and damage. Duty to warn refers to the responsibility of a mental health clinician to inform third parties or authorities if a patient poses a threat to themselves or another identifiable individual. Abandonment is considered a breach of duty and is defined as unilateral termination of the provider-patient relationship without adequate notice for the patient to obtain substitute medical care.

104. C) Materials are not written at a third- to fifth-grade level

Guidelines for Developing Patient Education Materials recommend choosing books, pamphlets, and/or brochures written at a third- to a fifth-grade level. Teaching material that is at a higher academic level does not consider the educational level of the patient. The patient is bilingual. Asking the patient what language they prefer would be clinically appropriate, but there is no suggestion of a language barrier. While literacy deficits can be missed, the patient was initially engaged and appeared to lose interest as the teaching continued. Attention to nonverbal behavior suggests communication problems began when the subject matter was reviewed. As the patient was assessed in order to be able to be discharged, it is less likely there is an active perceptual problem.

105. C) Medication

Medications such as amantadine, used to treat Parkinson's disease, have side effects that include anorexia, fatigue, and dizziness. Purpura is often a more serious side effect found in amantadine use; therefore, the nurse practitioner would first assess medications for side effects and contraindications. Constipation is due to decreased bowel movement. Jaundice has an increase in bilirubin due to hepatitis, gallstones, or tumors. Dementia is deterioration of cognitive functions and would not be a first assessment for anorexia, fatigue, or purpura.

106. D) Meditation

Meditation is a popular complementary and alternative treatment. Meditation is defined as the intentional self-regulation of attention from moment to moment. This technique calls for an intentional and self-regulated focusing of attention to relax and calm the mind and body. Systematic desensitization/exposure is a form of psychotherapy used for patients with phobias, not generalized anxiety. Electroconvulsive therapy and transcranial magnetic stimulation are medical treatments for treatment-resistant and severe depression.

107. A) Mesolimbic

The mesolimbic pathway connects the ventral tegmental area to the nucleus accumbens and is associated with reward, motivation, and emotion. Mesocortical pathways are linked to cognitive function, executive function, and negative symptoms of schizophrenia. Nigrostriatal pathways are responsible for purposeful movement. The tuberoinfundibular pathway is responsible for the regulation of prolactin.

108. A) Mini-Cog
Compared to the MMSE, the Mini-Cog test for dementia avoids cultural bias and insensitivity. Three-word recall is part of the Mini-Cog test; there is no test involving recall of four objects. The months backward test may be used to test for cognitive impairment but is not the preferred test to avoid cultural bias.

109. D) Naloxone
Naloxone is an opioid antagonist that is given to reverse the effects of opioid intoxication such as hypotension and depressed respirations. Buprenorphine is an antagonist used for heroin and morphine, naproxen is an anti-inflammatory drug, and methadone maintenance is a treatment for opioid addiction.

110. C) Negative transference
Negative transference may result in the patient directing painful or angry feelings toward the nurse practitioner. The nurse practitioner may need to explore negative transference that threatens the nurse–patient relationship. If, however, a patient is motivated to work with the nurse practitioner, completes assignments between sessions, and shares feelings openly, it may be that the patient is experiencing positive transference. Countertransference occurs when the nurse practitioner unconsciously displaces feelings related to significant figures in the nurse practitioner's past onto the patient. Boundary violations are characterized by a reversal of roles wherein the needs of the nurse practitioner are being met rather than the needs of the patient.

111. B) Negative transference
The patient may have feelings for the nurse practitioner, possibly because the patient sees a significant other (e.g., a parent) in the nurse practitioner. The behavior of the patient can then be affected by their feelings or thoughts toward that significant other. This is called transference. When the patient has hostile or negative feelings associated with the significant other, the patient can transfer those negative feelings to the nurse practitioner as well. This is known as negative transference. Here, the patient resists the tasks given because of negative feelings. Negative countertransference occurs when the nurse practitioner has prejudices or negative feelings for the patient because the patient resembles someone the nurse practitioner dislikes. Positive transference occurs when the patient has affectionate or positive feelings toward the nurse practitioner. The patient may become too responsive or might overexpress in the session because of this. Positive countertransference occurs when the nurse practitioner is extra-protective toward a patient because the patient resembles someone the nurse practitioner likes or loves. The nurse practitioner will then show abnormally high concern toward the patient.

112. C) Negatively impact functioning and cause distress for the patient
ADHD symptoms must negatively impact function and cause distress for the patient. A pattern of angry/irritable mood and argumentative behavior plus hostility and defiance is part of the criteria for oppositional defiant disorder.

113. D) Negotiate with the patient to reduce the quantity and pattern of herb usage in a way that will bring the patient less harm

One way the nurse practitioner helps a patient who is highly reluctant to stop using a harmful substance is negotiation. The nurse practitioner can try to negotiate with the patient about repatterning the usage of the herb so that they can come to a mutual understanding. The nurse practitioner will not encourage the patient to continue using the herb in the same manner. The nurse practitioner will not tell the patient to stop taking the herb, but instead will educate the patient about the harm caused by the herb and repattern and restructure the usage if the patient does not want to completely give up the herb. The nurse practitioner will educate the patient regarding the harmful effects of the herb but will not then leave the decision entirely in the patient's hands; instead, the nurse practitioner will negotiate with the patient.

114. B) Neuroleptic malignant syndrome

Neuroleptic malignant syndrome is a medical emergency associated with the use of antipsychotic drugs. The symptoms include hyperthermia, muscle rigidity, autonomic instability, catatonic stupor, parkinsonian symptoms, and elevated creatine phosphokinase. Serotonin syndrome is associated with the use of antidepressants, namely serotonin reuptake inhibitors or monoamine oxidase inhibitors (MAOIs) in combination with each other or with other serotonin-increasing drugs. Stevens–Johnson syndrome is associated with the use of lamotrigine or carbamazepine. Hypertensive crisis is associated with use of MAOIs concurrently with tyramine-containing foods.

115. C) Neurophysiologic changes noting transition through NREM and REM sleep

EEG recording, known as a hypnogram, measures the distinct physiological states of sleep: NREM and REM. The transition through each stage is measured for sleep continuity and to record any disruptions between the two stages. NREM is divided into three stages (N1, N2, N3), characterized by the progression of sleep from wakefulness to deep sleep known as REM. REM sleep involves an absence of skeletal muscle tone and rapid eye movement and is the deepest sleep stage. Loss of awareness is normal between N1 and N2 stages. The amount of time between wakefulness and REM sleep, and molecular changes in brain chemistry, are not what an EEG specifically records.

116. A) New patients

A comprehensive health history is done in the cases of new patients. By understanding a patient's comprehensive health history, the psychiatric-mental health nurse practitioner will be able to select particular elements and provide recommendations for quick recovery and for the overall well-being of the patient. Self-management of the patient, life quality, and response to provided treatment should be the main focus for patients seeking treatment for chronic illness or in cases of ongoing treatment. Problem-oriented history or focused history should be done for patients seeking treatment for specific conditions. The interview in such cases should be limited to determining the particular health condition. A nurse practitioner should discuss sexual behavior and smoking or drug use with patients visiting frequently for routine check-ups.

117. B) Nonmaleficence

The ethical principle of nonmaleficence instructs the nurse practitioner to do no harm to the patient, and not breaking the patient's confidentiality is part of this. The ethical principle of beneficence deals with aiding the patient to get well by promoting the patient's health. The ethical principle of justice teaches the nurse practitioner to divide resources and care among all the patients equally. Veracity is the ethical principle that tells the nurse practitioner to communicate truthfully with the patients.

118. C) Norepinephrine

Rushing, hallucinations, and exhibiting boundary impairment by regarding other's things as one's own are all symptoms of schizophrenia. Collectively grouping the symptoms, the nurse practitioner can prescribe a classical microdialysis test to check if the patient's norepinephrine level has increased, as the increased level of this neurotransmitter results in schizophrenia. Serotonin alteration is not related to schizophrenia but may lead to depression. Hypocretin decreases narcolepsy. Acetylcholine increases in depression and decreases in Parkinson's disease, Alzheimer's disease, and Huntington's disease.

119. B) Normalization

Many therapeutic modalities help to promote mental health in children who have experienced trauma. Psychoeducational programs are designed to teach basic coping skills for stress by focusing on normalization. Teaching normal behaviors to a 6-year-old patient is instrumental during this developmental stage to reduce risks for issues with anger, behavior, or socioemotional status. Stress reduction, social skills, and grief processes are important in a developing child; however, this child's focus should be on what is normal and what is not due to the fact that suicide has played a large part in the psychological and emotional aspects of the patient's life.

120. B) Occupational

ADHD is characterized by consistent symptoms of inattention in at least two of three domains, identified as academic, social, or occupational. Physical, behavioral, and cognitive are not domains.

121. B) Opioid receptor mu 1 (*OPRM1*) genotype

The *OPRM1* has clear involvement in mediating the analgesic and rewarding effects of endogenous and exogenous opioids and has been tightly linked to the development of addiction disorders due to its involvement in the brain reward pathway. The *OPRM1* gene encodes for the mu opioid receptor, and sequence variants within its coding region are the most frequently studied candidates in association with opioid dependence. Patients positive for *HLA-B*57:01* are associated with higher adverse reaction risk (hypersensitivity reactions) for HIV patients treated with abacavir (Ziagen). *APP, PSEN1*, and *PSEN2* mutations cause autosomal dominant forms of early-onset Alzheimer's disease (AD-EOAD).

122. B) Orientation

The orientation phase can last for a few meetings or extend over a longer period of time. During the orientation phase, the patient may begin to express thoughts and feelings, identify problems, and discuss realistic goals. The preorientation phase begins with preparing the assignment of the patient's condition, learning about prescribed medications, and understanding laboratory results. The termination phase is the final, integral phase of the nurse–patient relationship. A strong working relationship allows the patient to safely express concerns. During this phase, the nurse works on providing and evaluating solutions for the patient. Before this phase, the major purpose of the therapy has already been discussed in the orientation phase.

123. B) Overall needs of a human being

Humanistic psychotherapy differs from psychoanalytical and behavioral therapy because it focuses on the overall needs of the patient. The focus is on the subjective experiences of the patient. It is more focused on the present than the past, unlike psychoanalytical therapy, in which the root cause of mental illness is mostly supposed to be an unresolved past conflict. Humanistic therapy does not focus on one issue only because it takes care of the overall experiences of the patient.

124. A) P element

The PICOT format is used for asking clinical questions. P here is population or person. The patient represents the P element. I is the issue or intervention made. The intervention can be prescribing new drugs. C stands for comparison. The efficacy of the two drugs is to be compared at this stage. O refers to the outcome of the intervention made, and T refers to the time needed to achieve the outcome.

125. A) Paranoid

In paranoid personality disorder, patients become quiet and do not have friends because they become suspicious of other people. The risk factor for this disorder is having a relative with schizophrenia. This disorder occurs more often in male patients than in female patients. Those with histrionic personality disorder remain emotionally expressive from their childhood; this nature works as a predisposing factor for the occurrence of the disease. Those with narcissistic personality disorder generally have a relative with the same disorder, not with schizophrenia. Male sex is not a risk factor for avoidant personality disorder; it has an equal chance of occurring in male and female patients.

126. D) Participating in interprofessional meetings about treatment

The psychiatric-mental health nurse practitioner role includes participation on interprofessional teams, and adherence to ethical standards of practice includes addressing risks, benefits, and outcomes for each patient. In compliance with ethical standards regarding patient confidentiality, providers may not speak with family members without patient consent. It is a breach of confidentiality to review records that are not for the nurse practitioner's patient. Only direct caregivers may access patient information without patient consent. In order to maintain adherence to ethical practice standards, all information shared between providers must be exchanged per the patient's consent. Medical records cannot be released unless under subpoena, even after patient death.

127. C) Participating in the American Psychiatric Nurses Association

Participating in the American Psychiatric Nurses Association is an example of promoting mental health as an advocate. Roles of the nurse practitioner include avenues of scholarly activities such as publishing, lecturing, journal clubs, preceptorship, and continuing education. These examples are ways to continue competency through scholarly activity.

128. D) Patient's problem-solving skills have deteriorated

Deterioration of problem-solving skills is associated with impaired coping. Social isolation causes feelings of being rejected and not being good enough. Spiritual distress makes one angry toward a greater power, and impaired sexual functioning can change sexual patterns. To determine the condition of impaired coping in a patient, the nurse practitioner should question the problem-solving skills of the patient.

129. C) Pediatric acute-onset neuropsychiatric syndrome

PANDAS is a subset of pediatric acute-onset neuropsychiatric syndrome (PANS), which is thought to be triggered by pharyngitis with GAS infection. Anxiety disorder due to another medical condition and obsessive-compulsive disorder diagnosis may be considered due to some of the symptoms, but not all are present, and neither is linked with GAS. Systemic lupus erythematosus is a chronic, multisystem autoimmune disease with some overlapping psychiatric symptoms, but a history of GAS infection is not associated with this condition.

130. A) Peer level education programs

First-line approaches for mental health promotion in adolescent patients include intervening through education directed at the peer group and peer level. This can include alternative recreational activities and peer counseling. Coaching on assertiveness is a second-line approach, and setting positive examples and community youth activities are third-line interventions.

131. B) Posttraumatic stress disorder

Posttraumatic stress disorder is caused by traumatic past experiences. In this disorder, the cortisol level of the blood is reduced. In disorders like schizophrenia, anorexia nervosa, and major depressive disorder, an increase in cortisol levels is observed.

132. A) Potential for panic attacks

The first goal should be to focus on eliminating the panic attacks. The nurse practitioner can help the patient understand the early signs of panic attack and the causes of stress. The patient's symptoms of oversleeping, weight gain, and low energy can be resolved over a period of time with the help of pharmacological interventions; however, panic attacks are the primary concern during the initial phase of therapy. Tapping into unresolved childhood conflicts can be done at later stages, especially given that the patient does not seem to be ready to discuss the issue in detail with the nurse practitioner at this point. The patient is going through an "empty nest" transition phase and will require the support of her spouse. This is a working-phase patient goal where the focus should be on emotional intimacy between the patient and her spouse.

133. B) Presence of a psychiatric disorder

Suicide and suicidal ideation, as well as anxiety and depression, are prominent in patients with mental health disorders. History of deliberate self-harm is defined as willful self-injurious acts without intent to die. The loss of a family member and physical illness are considered risk factors, but neither are among the most significant risk factors.

134. D) Prioritizes data collection based on patient condition

The nurse practitioner should prioritize the collection of data on the basis of the patient's condition or needs. The nurse practitioner should not identify outcomes only by their own expectations but should also involve other healthcare professionals and the patient. Any issues or diagnoses should be verified not only with the patient but also with the patient's family and interprofessional colleagues. For the collection of culturally sensitive data, the nurse practitioner should engage other healthcare professionals along with the patient. These acts are necessary to achieve better and desired outcomes.

135. C) Provide worksheets and assignments

Cognitive behavioral therapy is designed to allow the patient to challenge their negative thoughts and substitute them with positive, rational thoughts. Worksheets and assignments are the common interventions used in this therapy because they allow the patient to write their negative thoughts and substitute them with positive thoughts. Electrical stimulation of the brain is used to treat psychiatric and neurological disorders. Modeling involves providing a role model to allow the patient to learn a particular behavior through imitation. Biofeedback is employed to control the body's physiological response to stress and anxiety by making certain changes in the body, such as by eliminating pain or relaxing the muscles.

136. A) Providing the patient with a written treatment plan for the next 10 days with no review or reassessment needed

All treatment plans, regardless of time limitations, are to have a review and reassessment periodically so that appropriate revisions can be made to treatment and patient goals. Completing a treatment plan without the patient's input is appropriate in cases where the patient has been committed by court order. Patient restraining is appropriate if the patient is in an emergency situation and there is possibility of self-harm or harm to others. Patients have the right to access their medical records.

137. A) QT interval prolongation

Ziprasidone (Geodon) prolongs QT interval more than other antipsychotics. Thioridazine (Mellaril) is known for prominent U waves, premature ventricular contractions, T wave and ST-segment changes, and ventricular arrhythmias. Tricyclic antidepressants are linked with the lengthening of the PR, quasirandom signal (QRS), and QT intervals. Lithium (Eskalith) therapy can impair sinoatrial node function.

138. D) Qualifying as chief nursing officer

The orienting nurse practitioner must demonstrate the pathway to excellence program, which should involve the role of a chief nursing officer (CNO). The CNO is a qualified healthcare professional who is involved at all levels of the healthcare system and also plays a major role in clinical decision making. The orienting nurse practitioner should also encourage nurse practitioners to prioritize a balanced lifestyle because a lack of work-life balance can result in fatigue and other health issues due to stress. The orienting nurse practitioner should promote professional development. The orienting nurse practitioner should encourage the recognition of nurse practitioners for achievements, not recognition of management alone.

139. D) Randomized control trials

Randomized control trials (RCTs) are considered the best evidence, or Level 1 evidence, in evidence-based practice. The systemic review of relevant RCTs (more than one) is performed. When the results of these multiple RCTs are the same, the knowledge can be applied or used as evidence. RCT studies usually provide clear-cut results and apply to other cases as well. Level 2 pieces of evidence are usually obtained from at least one RCT and do not apply to a larger group of patients. This is why RCT studies are preferred as evidence over Level 2 pieces of evidence. Peer-reviewed articles can be used to gain insight into the issues of a patient; however, they are considered a lower level of evidence. Opinions are not used as evidence because they are not based on research methods or conducted trials. Qualitative research can be useful as literary assistance to understand patients and associated impacts on them due to a mental illness, but for treating a patient, evidence is required to apply knowledge from different sources in evidence-based practice.

140. C) Rating Anxiety in Dementia (RAID)
When a patient with dementia begins to demonstrate signs of anxiety or additional deterioration in mood stability, the RAID scale is a tool used to assess worry, apprehension, phobias, and panic attacks. The SLUMS is a tool used to assess for schizophrenia. The (HAM-D and the CSDD are tools for assessing depression.

141. C) Recognize stressors and implement coping strategies
The overall goal for intervention and treatment programs such as the "Coping Cat" is to recognize the stressors and signs of anxious arousal and to develop and implement strategies for coping with distress and anxiety, not to eliminate all anxiety or stressors. The program's goal is not to simply recognize signs of internal stress or to develop alliances with parents, as these are only small components of the plan that will help the child to better develop coping skills.

142. A) Reduce the dose of the same drug
Donepezil is a selective acetylcholinesterase inhibitor. It is given to enhance cognitive function. Nausea, diarrhea, and vomiting are common side effects of acetylcholinesterase inhibitors. To help with the side effects, the dose can be reduced. Replacing it with a new drug is not an appropriate option because other approved drugs for Alzheimer's disease (acetylcholinesterase inhibitors) have similar side effects. The drug can augment with antidepressants or atypical antipsychotics for depression or behavioral disturbances, not for reduction of nausea and diarrhea. Rivastigmine is also an acetylcholinesterase inhibitor; two such drugs are not prescribed together as they can cause acetylcholine toxicity.

143. B) Relational aggression
Girls are more likely to engage in relational aggression with their group of peers to disrupt relationships by spreading rumors, excluding, and/or manipulating others. Boys tend to be more physically aggressive, often abusing weaker or smaller children. Verbal abuse is a tactic used by both boys and girls equally, as is cyberbullying.

144. B) Repeating the last words of the patient
The psychiatric-mental health nurse practitioner should repeat the last words of the patient because it makes the patient comfortable and encourages them to express their feelings. This method is called echoing. Questions resulting in a "yes" or "no" response from the patient should be strictly avoided; instead, questions encouraging a graded response are more encouraged, and this is a skilled interviewing technique. Offering multiple choices for answering is also a process of guided questioning and is therefore encouraged because it helps in limiting bias. It also encourages patients in explaining their symptoms. Leading questions should be strictly avoided; instead, neutral questions should be asked while interviewing. Leading questions discourage the patient from expressing their symptoms, resulting in very short responses.

145. A) Resilience
Resilience is a characteristic developed by children and adolescents at risk for psychopathology to attain good mental health and achieve healthy outcomes while also maintaining hope and responding to life stressors. Normalization is a form of psychoeducational therapy that teaches families and children normal behaviors and the expected responses. Invincibility fables are thought patterns that adolescents develop in which they feel they are immune to anything bad happening to them. Protective factors are characteristics that reduce the probability of a child developing mental illness.

146. B) Review all pertinent data regarding the patient's history
To adhere to medical decision-making guidelines, the nurse practitioner must review all pertinent data prior to prescribing medication. Telling the patient not to worry invalidates any concerns the patient may have. Medical decision making may include family members upon the patient's consent, but family consent is not a necessary factor for pursuing treatment. Providing treatment alternatives is appropriate; however, the nurse practitioner's role is to make the recommendation and prescribe according to the evaluation and perceived benefit of different options.

147. A) Secure attachment through emotional bonds
To promote mental health in children, it is important that there is a secure attachment established through emotional bonding between parents and children at an early age. Secure attachment allows a child to develop positive social relationships and an easily adaptable temperament, which reduces the risk for mental illness. Progress through developmental stages is important for growth, but not key to promoting mental health in children. Identification of risk factors for psychopathology is key and is tied to building protective factors, but protective factors themselves are not a method of promotion of mental health. Invincibility fable is common in adolescents and results in risky behaviors due to the feeling of being immune to danger. This behavior should not be supported and must be monitored when promoting mental health.

148. C) Sedation, acute dystonia, and akathisia

The antagonist of the D2 receptor of dopamine can cause extrapyramidal symptoms like acute dystonia and akathisia. The side effects caused by the antagonists of H1 receptors include sedation. The antagonists of muscarinic cholinergic receptors for acetylcholine can bring side effects of urinary retention and constipation, while dizziness is caused by the antagonists of α1 receptors for norepinephrine. Weight gain and hypotension are side effects of the antagonists of 5-HT2 receptors for serotonin; priapism can be caused by α2 receptors for norepinephrine. Dry mouth and blurred vision are the side effects of the antagonists of muscarinic cholinergic receptors for acetylcholine, and ejaculatory dysfunction can be caused by the antagonists of α1 receptor of acetylcholine and 5-HT2 receptor of serotonin.

149. A) Self-awareness

The nurse practitioner understands that values and beliefs guide behavior, but self-awareness helps them to accept the uniqueness and differences among different beliefs. Self-awareness is self-knowledge, knowledge about one's own actions. Values are abstract standards and represent an ideal, either positive or negative. A belief is a concept that is held as true by a person. It is not the rational concept of believing in something to be true. Supervision is an important factor in building ethically and legally sound therapeutic relationships. Supervision involves a third person supervising or looking over the behavior of the nurse practitioner. In this case, the relationship is between the nurse practitioner and the patient only.

150. A) Senile plaques

Alzheimer's disease is characterized by diffuse atrophy of the brain with flattened cortical sulci, enlarged cerebral ventricles, neurofibrillary tangles, and senile plaques, also known as amyloid plaques. The presence of senile plaques strongly indicates Alzheimer's disease. Argentophyllic globes are seen in patients with Pick's disease. Vascular dementia is characterized by arteriosclerotic plaques, multiple parenchymal lesions that spread over the brain. They affect primarily small- and medium-sized cerebral vessels and many small infarctions of the white matter, with the exception of the cortical regions.

151. A) Serotonin and norepinephrine reuptake inhibitor

The patient's symptoms suggest the patient has major depressive disorder. This can be treated with the help of a serotonin and norepinephrine reuptake inhibitor, which functions by restricting the norepinephrine and dopamine reuptake pumps. Benzodiazepines are commonly prescribed for anxiety. They reduce anxiousness and insomnia by increasing gamma-aminobutyric acid activities. They have little effect on the symptoms of depression. A dopamine receptor antagonist is beneficial in treating schizophrenia, nausea, and bipolar disorder. It lowers psychotic symptoms by restricting dopamine 2 receptors. The patient does not show any symptoms of psychosis; therefore, this drug should not be prescribed. Anticholinergic drugs are used for treating Parkinson's disease and function by restricting acetylcholine neurotransmitters. Their mode of action shows no improvement of symptoms of depression.

152. A) Serotonin partial agonist and reuptake inhibitors

Vilazodone belongs to the group of serotonin partial agonist and reuptake inhibitors. It stimulates the 5-HT1A receptor as a partial agonist and inhibits serotonin reuptake. Desipramine (Norpramin) is a tricyclic antidepressant that acts by blocking the reuptake of both serotonin and norepinephrine. Venlafaxine (Effexor) is a serotonin-norepinephrine reuptake inhibitor that works by increasing the serotonin and norepinephrine in the synaptic region by blocking neuronal reuptake. Nefazodone is a serotonin antagonist and reuptake inhibitor that acts by inhibiting the reuptake of serotonin and blocking the 5-HT2A receptors. It also weakly blocks the reuptake of norepinephrine.

153. B) Shared decision making

Shared decision making forms the basis of any therapeutic alliance. Soliciting the patient's perspective through shared discussion around decision making begins the therapeutic alliance. Setting limits or boundaries is a factor in the relationship, but the initial session priority is forming the therapeutic alliance. Self-identification as the expert is a paternalistic approach that diminishes the patient's power to be capable of self-determination. Creating a safety plan may be appropriate in cases where suicidal risks exists, but without the presence of a therapeutic alliance, the patient may not feel safe enough to disclose.

154. A) Should have information and make decisions related to care

Regarding a patient with a disease, in Western culture, family members typically allow the patient to know about the disease and ask the patient to make their own decisions. The patient will be asked to be self-independent and do their own work as much as possible. The family members consider things like toxins and mutant cells as causes of the disease, not lack of harmony with the environment. For the treatment of the patient, they will prefer medical technology and provider-prescribed medications rather than traditional healers and remedies.

155. B) Sodium level of 132 mEq/L

Hyponatremia is caused when sodium levels fall below 135 mEq/L and includes symptoms of headache, nausea, vomiting, lethargy, and disorientation. If left untreated, it can cause seizures, coma, and death. Hyponatremia is common in older adults being treated for depression who are taking SSRIs. The syndrome of inappropriate secretion of antidiuretic hormone is a well-known adverse effect of SSRIs. Risk factors for the development of hyponatremia with SSRIs include older age, female sex, concomitant use of diuretics, low body weight, and lower baseline serum sodium concentration. A sodium level of 148 mEq/L indicates hypernatremia. Although the symptoms of hypernatremia are similar to those of hyponatremia, hypernatremia is not associated with the use of antidepressants or SSRIs. Antidepressants or SSRIs are not associated with increased or decreased potassium levels.

156. B) Start a mood stabilizer and have the patient monitor their mood

The patient appears to have cyclic depressed mood. A mood stabilizer is the better option to control symptoms, especially after multiple attempts at antidepressants. Starting another antidepressant will most likely cause the same issues. Although therapy is important, an antipsychotic will not target the symptoms of depression. There is no indication for an ECG.

157. A) Substance use disorder

The patient is experiencing signs that are indicative of schizophrenia as well as substance use disorder; therefore, the nurse practitioner will further evaluate for additional cues that the patient is dependent on a substance or that schizophrenia treatment needs to be addressed. Weight loss can be seen in patients with hyperthyroidism and general anxiety disorders, but these disorders are not typically associated with alogia, red eyes, slowed reaction time, and slowed thinking. Patients with temporal lobe epilepsy will often have memory loss and slowed thinking, but not weight loss, alogia, and red eyes.

158. D) Sympathy

Rogers and Truax identified three personal characteristics of the practitioner that help promote change and growth in patients—factors still valued today as vital components for establishing a therapeutic relationship. They are (1) genuineness, (2) empathy, and (3) positive regard. Sympathy is similar to empathy, but there is a slight difference. A simple way to distinguish them is that in empathy, the nurse practitioner understands the feelings of others, and in sympathy, the nurse practitioner feels pity or sorrow for others.

159. C) Taper the risperidone over 2 or 3 months and redraw labs in 3 months

The patient's fasting triglycerides are very high, and because this is coupled with weight gain, the risperidone should be tapered down first. If need be, the lamotrigine can also be tapered down at a later date. Labs will need to be redrawn in 3 months, and the patient's weight will need to be monitored. The patient does not meet criteria for inpatient care at this time.

160. D) Temporal lobe epilepsy

Hallucinations can occur with any of the five senses; however, olfactory hallucinations are rare and are the hallmark of organic brain disease, specifically temporal lobe epilepsy. Auditory hallucinations are most common. Tactile, olfactory, and gustatory hallucinations are unusual and suggest the presence of a medical or neurological disorder. Differentiating from medical conditions is a broad-based review; however, the presence of olfactory hallucinations should lead to a neurological workup. Certain medical symptoms and conditions are linked to types of hallucinations. It is important to investigate when the hallucination occurs, as well as how often and whether it is disturbing the patient. Patients that are visually impaired due to cataracts are prone to visual hallucinations. Patients with substance misuse history experiencing related tactile hallucinations (e.g., bugs crawling under the skin) suggests cocaine use. Hallucinations in combination with cognitive impairment can be related to a dementia diagnosis. The presence of hallucinations is indicative of types of schizophrenia; however, the new-onset olfactory hallucinations with no previous history strongly suggest a neurological cause.

161. D) The concepts and language of an ethnic or social group used to describe their health-related values, beliefs, and traditional practices, as well as the etiologies of their conditions, preferred treatments, and any contraindications for treatments or pharmacological interventions

According to the ANA, cultural knowledge refers to the concepts and language of an ethnic or social group used to describe their health-related values, beliefs, and traditional practices, as well as the etiologies of their conditions, preferred treatments, and any contraindications for treatments or pharmacological interventions. Cultural skills is defined by the integration of expertise and skills into practice when assessing, communicating, and providing care for members of any social or ethnic group, not only the group(s) the nurse practitioner belongs to. Competency is defined as an expected and measurable level of nursing performance that integrates knowledge, skills, abilities, and judgment, based on established scientific knowledge and expectations for nursing practice. Interprofessional is defined as integrated enactment of knowledge, skills, values, and attitudes that define working together across the professions.

162. B) The patient is a risk to themselves

The criterion for involuntary hospitalization is that the patient presents a risk of direct harm to themselves through direct injury. Other criteria include if there is a direct physical threat to others or if the patient is unable to care for themselves. The definition of what constitutes harm or direct danger varies by state; however, all states allow for short-term confinement with the requirement of psychiatric evaluation by specific licensed mental health professionals. All states have a variable maximum length of time for evaluation before the need for a judicial hearing.

163. C) The patient's commitment has been court ordered

According to the Patient's Bill of Rights, each patient has the right to refuse care unless they are in a dangerous situation or in such situations as a court-ordered commitment. The patient's being brought to the emergency department does not automatically mean the situation is dangerous, so the patient's rights would still be followed. Likewise, a patient's making irrational decisions does not mean they are not competent or cannot make decisions regarding refusal of care. Participating in experimental treatments or research trials is not reason to deny a patient the right to refuse care.

164. B) Trauma informed

An ACE score refers to the results of the Adverse Childhood Experiences scale. Patients with a high ACE score have had traumatic experiences or exposure. Adverse childhood experiences can have an impact on future violence victimization and perpetration; they can also result in lifelong health consequences. Traumatic experiences in childhood and the teenage years may put patients at risk for violence, chronic health problems, mental illness, and substance abuse in adulthood. Trauma-informed therapy recognizes the impact of trauma and recognizes the signs and symptoms of trauma in patients, families, staff, and others involved with the system. The therapy is performed by responding with an integrative approach, and the therapist is especially aware of the risk of re-traumatization. Cognitive behavioral therapy combines the theory and techniques behind both cognitive and behavioral therapies. This approach examines the relationship among a person's negative thoughts, fears, behaviors, and physical responses to various experiences. It is an option for this patient; however, it is not the best one based on past history of trauma and current sexual assault history. Psychodynamic therapists are trained in psychoanalysis to help patients explore how their early-life experiences may have led to the consequent emotions and beliefs that govern their lives. Once the patient understands how they have come to feel, think, and behave in ways that are causing them distress, they are then empowered to change those patterns in a way that will help them reach their goals. This may be an approach for the patient in the future, but it is not the best approach now. Dialectical behavior therapy involves both individual psychotherapy and group skills training. It is associated with borderline personality disorders and suicidal behavior. It is not the first therapeutic approach indicated for this patient.

165. A) Triangulation

Bringing in a third person to resolve conflict is triangulation. Triangulation can be with a child, parent, sibling, or close friend. Modeling occurs when a person imitates the behavior of another in order to alter their own behavior. A cross-generational coalition occurs when one person makes a coalition with another person from a different generation. The parent–child coalition is an example of such a coalition. A covert coalition occurs when the coalition is not so apparent. The coalition here is visible and direct; it is not covert.

166. D) Valproate

Valproate is associated with neural tube defects, such as spina bifida. Furthermore, valproate is associated with cognitive decline in school-age children, and it may increase the risk of autism spectrum disorder. Folate, given in supplements as folic acid, is used to protect the neural development of a fetus, and all pregnant patients should be instructed to take folic acid. Although paroxetine is a teratogen, it does not cause neural tube defects, but is associated with cardiac malformations. Lamotrigine is associated with cleft palate.

167. D) Varenicline

The patient's symptoms are due to nicotine withdrawal. The patient is addicted to nicotine and should be prescribed varenicline. It acts as a partial agonist and functions by blocking alpha-4-beta-2 nicotinic acetylcholine receptors. Naltrexone, clonidine, and nalmefene help in treating alcohol and opioid withdrawal symptoms, but are not useful for nicotine withdrawal symptoms. Naltrexone acts as a mu-opioid receptor antagonist, whereas nalmefene acts as a mu and delta-opioid receptor antagonist. The antihypertensive property of clonidine helps in reducing alcohol and opioid dependency.

168. B) Wakes from an unconscious state after the administration of zolpidem (Ambien)

A genetically abnormal sensitivity to a drug can cause a paradoxical reaction; that is, one that is the opposite of what is expected. Zolpidem is a drug for treating insomnia. It belongs to the short-acting non-benzodiazepine class of drugs and increases the activity of gamma-aminobutyric acid (GABA) by binding to GABA receptors at the same location as benzodiazepines. Paradoxically, zolpidem has been reported to restore neurologic deficits, including consciousness levels, in patients with chronic consciousness disorder. It is expected that patients would sleep after receiving zolpidem, be sedated after lorazepam, and be drowsy after receiving disulfiram until acclimated to the medication.

169. C) World Health Organization Disability Assessment Schedule

The GAF was Axis V in the DSM-IV and measured psychological, social, and occupational functioning. It is no longer part of the DSM-5. The WHODAS measures cognition, mobility, self-care, getting along with others, life activities, and community activities; all are items used to document a patient's functional status. The BDI measures depression only, the Hamilton Anxiety Rating Scale measures only the degree of anxiety, and the Conners Rating Scale is used for attention deficit/hyperactivity disorder diagnosis.

170. A) "Have your child's mood problems been episodic?"

The nurse practitioner is evaluating the patient for disruptive mood dysregulation disorder (DMDD). The clinical presentation is distinctive and involves chronic, nonepisodic, and persistent irritability and temper tantrums disproportionate with the trigger. The symptoms of DMDD must be differentiated from bipolar disorder because some of the features of DMDD are similar to those of bipolar disorder. Determining whether or not the symptom presentation is episodic will help rule out other pathology. Aggression toward animals can be an indicator of abuse; asking about this and about suspected abuse is directed toward investigating trauma-related causes for the patient's behavior. Asking about difficulties with distraction or hyperactivity seeks to rule out the presence of attention deficit disorder, which is not a mood disorder.

171. D) "I understand. Let's make another appointment next week. I would like to check in with you."

Communicating understanding and allowing the patient to choose the course of treatment they feel is best supports the patient's right of autonomy. Telling the patient to hide the drug from their spouse is a paternalistic response and diminishes the patient's opinion with disregard for safety. Respecting a patient's decision communicates understanding, but it does not support the decision, and telling the patient to contact the office when the patient is ready is dismissive and paternalistic. Telling the patient to bring an abusive spouse to the office is an inappropriate intervention because it empowers the spouse and may add to the patient's risk of harm from domestic violence.

172. C) "After eating, have you ever attempted to get rid of the food by vomiting or taking laxatives?"
To differentiate between a diagnosis of bulimia and binge eating disorder, it is important to determine if the patient engages in actions that facilitate ridding the body of the food, either by using laxatives or by vomiting. Purging is the differentiation factor between these two eating disorders. Asking the patient if they eat to the point of feeling full, have feelings of guilt after eating, or have feelings of being out of control with eating habits are all cursory interview questions to determine if there is an eating disorder and do not address the differentiating factor of purging.

173. D) "I am better, sober for 9 months. I am afraid I could relapse; I need help."
The statement "I am better, sober for 9 months. I am afraid I could relapse; I need help," indicates that the patient is in the maintenance stage. The patient has made significant changes for >6 months but recognizes help is needed to prevent relapse. The patient may find it difficult to maintain the changes. There is a recognition of improvement. Denying a problem or refusing help indicates that the patient is in the precontemplation change. The contemplation stage is indicated when the patient acknowledges that there is a problem and/or expresses the desire to change; the patient is trying to understand the problem but has not committed to change. The action phase reflects that the patient has been engaged in changing the behavior pattern for <6 months, has maintained sobriety, and admits to the struggle.

174. C) "How long have you had these symptoms?"
The patient is experiencing symptoms of bipolar, and in order to differentiate between bipolar I or bipolar II, it is essential to determine if the symptoms are mania (bipolar I) or hypomania (bipolar II). This is determined by the timing of the symptoms. If it is less than 1 week, then it is hypomania, or bipolar II. If it is greater than 1 week it is mania, or bipolar I. Bipolar I and II may be further differentiated by psychotic symptoms or such a severe presentation of the mania that hospitalization is required. If that is the case, it does not matter how the long the symptoms last; it is automatically considered a manic episode, or bipolar I.

175. C) "What herbal and vitamin supplements and over-the-counter medications do you take?"
When patients use complementary and alternative treatments such as herbal supplements, unpleasant effects may result from interaction with prescribed medications. Therefore, the patient must be reminded to disclose all medications to avoid drug interactions. However, the patient may wish to take herbal supplements or other over-the-counter products, and the nurse practitioner should respect the patient's choices while still explaining the potential unpleasant effects. The patient is not responsible to know and report all side effects of all medications; it is the responsibility of the practitioner to educate the patient on this information. Improvements in emotional status should be discussed, but for this patient, medications are the primary focus at this time.

Printed in the United States
by Baker & Taylor Publisher Services